# The Complete Guide to Medical Writing

# The Complete Guide to Medical Writing

Edited by

Mark C Stuart

BPharm PGDipCDDS DipBotMed MRPharmS

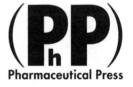

London · Chicago

Published by the Pharmaceutical Press
An imprint of RPS Publishing
1 Lambeth High Street, London SE1 7JN, UK
100 South Atkinson Road, Suite 200, Grayslake, IL 60030-7820, USA

(PhP) is a trade mark of RPS Publishing
RPS Publishing is the publishing organisation of the
Royal Pharmaceutical Society of Great Britain

First published in 2007

Typeset by J&L Composition, Filey, North Yorkshire
Printed in Great Britain by TJ International, Padstow, Cornwall

ISBN 978 0 85369 667 4

# Contents

# Foreword

I am in the habit of referring to medical writing as a blossoming niche. In fact, that is an understatement. Medical writing is undergoing something equivalent to the Big Bang.

Historically, scientific documentation was prepared by only those individuals who had done the research. They designed the experiments, thought about how to analyse the data and wrote up the findings themselves. Over time, specialists such as statisticians were added to the pool of authors. The writing, however, was not seen as something one needed to be specialised in, and continued to be written by the clinician or scientist who had something to say.

It has only been in the last 10 years that people have begun to recognise that writing is a skill, and that having writing as a specialized function can improve the effectiveness of communicating. Once this idea took hold, it began to spread like wildfire.

We are now at a point where medical writing is generally acknowledged as a fundamental skill set in the task of scientific communication. As a result, the demand for medical writers has grown enormously over a short period of time. This led to the 'Catch 22' situation of many people with no experience seeking to begin a career as a medical writer but employers seeking to hire only those with years of professional experience.

As Vice President of the European Medical Writers Association (EMWA) I am exposed to the many different facets of writing that belong under the single umbrella of medical writing. The spectrum includes writing an advertisement campaign and branding of pharmaceutical images, as well as writing a clinical study report or scientific manuscripts. I interact with the people in these hugely varying fields of medical writing and see what their concerns are, what hurdles they are faced with and what their end of the industry is about. This gives me a fascinating and integrated perspective into the world of medical writing from the writer's viewpoint.

On the other side, as the Managing Director of my own medical writing company, I am exposed to what the clients are looking for from the writers they hire. What they need are not only writers who can craft well-written text and data presentations, but who also understand the purpose of the document they have been hired to write. Medical writers need to bring a toolbox full of skills to ply their trade, and the clients don't want to have to fill it for them.

This is why I was so pleased when I heard that this book was being written. With ever-increasing numbers of new writers entering the arena, we need to collect and pass on knowledge from experienced writers. Training is one means of doing this, but a resource book that someone can refer to over and over again is irreplaceable.

This book is just that. It is ambitious in its scope, touching on just about anything a medical writer may ever need to write. It covers all angles of scientific and medical documentation, from the regulatory domain to the advertising arena. It covers fundamental principles of good writing techniques and delves into a broad spectrum of documents, providing tips on how to write each different kind of document and explaining their purpose. A book like this has been long awaited in the medical writing community, and I applaud those who finally sat down and brought it together.

Julia Forjanic Klapproth, PhD
Vice President
European Medical Writers Association
January 2007

# Preface

This book has been written to enable medical professionals and students to communicate scientific and medical information effectively.

From the time of entry into undergraduate studies at college or university, medical and life science students undertake medical writing in one form or another. This skill in communicating medical information quickly becomes an integral and evolving part of their professional lives.

As a student you begin to employ medical writing skills to write up laboratory reports, create presentation materials and write your dissertation or thesis. As a graduate healthcare professional you will probably give expert presentations and provide medical information to patients and peers. You are also likely to be involved in communicating written advice at a public level, which may involve the general media and popular press. After establishing yourself as an expert in the medical community, you may even write or edit your own book. Similarly, as an academic, writing presentation materials and examinations becomes a part of your professional life. If you work in the pharmaceutical industry, you may be involved in writing copy for advertisements or in applications for new drug licences.

Presenting and communicating information effectively in any medical document is of paramount importance. The facts must be presented in such a way that they can be understood as intended. Many medical manuscripts are used for the diagnosis and treatment of patients: if they are misinterpreted, the consequence could be harm to the patient. Far too many errors that occur in medical practice are the result of poorly written documents, which in turn can result in miscommunication of information.

Medical and scientific concepts can be complex and challenging to understand, even for the experts, but regardless of your field or level of expertise the standards of good medical writing should still apply. The aim is to present clear and accurate information that can be interpreted, validated and used safely. This book will help you do this. It also covers many ethical and legal principles, such as copyright and patient confidentiality, which are commonplace in medical communications.

This book is also a valuable tool for medical editors who must help authors communicate their information effectively, when their expertise and training in their medical field may not always be matched by their writing skills. In medical writing, the editor is the link between the reader's need to understand and the author's need to be understood.

The examples used throughout have a pharmacy and pharmaceutical slant, which will appeal to people with backgrounds in these fields working in medical communications. Yet the concepts presented also apply to the full spectrum of medical specialties.

This book is designed to be used as a reference that can be accessed whenever you need guidance on effective, written medical communication, rather than to be read from cover to cover. It has been broadly divided into a number of subsections to reflect the specialist nature of some topics and the audience that the type of medical writing is aimed at. In addition, the appendices will provide a quick ready-reference for common terms and values when writing.

The authors of this book are experts from a cross-section of the pharmacy, medical and literary fields, with first-hand experience in the topics they cover. I am sincerely grateful for their dedication and commitment to producing the book, and for the support of Pharmaceutical Press. A special thank you to my family and friends in Australia, the UK and the USA, who have also offered their valuable support.

Mark Stuart
March 2007

# About the editor

## Mark C Stuart
BPharm PGDipCDDS DipBotMed MRPharmS

Mark has experience as a pharmacist in community and hospital phar-
macies in both Australia and the UK. He was formerly an editor for the
*British National Formulary*, Senior Medical Editor for the National
Institute for Health and Clinical Excellence (UK) and Deputy Editor of
*MIMS* Australia. Mark is currently Clinical Editor for *BMJ Clinical
Evidence*, BMJ Publishing Group.

Mark studied pharmacy at Sydney University. He has postgraduate
qualifications in clinical drug dependence (Macquarie University, Sydney)
and botanical medicine.

With a keen interest in drugs in sport, Mark has worked as a pharmacist and with doping control for the Sydney, Athens and Turin Olympic
Games, and for the Manchester and Melbourne Commonwealth Games.
He has contributed chapters to books on sports medicine, reviewed
educational material for pharmacists on the topic, and edits a website
for pharmacists involved in sports medicine (www.sportspharmacy.com).
As a freelance writer Mark has been published in numerous journals and
magazines.

# Contributors

**Jennifer Archer,** MSc, HRD, FCIPD

Jennifer is the Assistant Director, Centre for Pharmacy Postgraduate Education (CPPE). She is involved in activities such as identifying learning needs, project management, developing learning programmes, and managing the delivery and evaluation of learning.

Jennifer has a diverse experience in pharmacy and HRD organisations, particularly in behavioural science and CPD. She has held many different positions in a range of pharmacy organisations and has undertaken consultancy work. Jennifer was awarded the RPSGB Synergy Award in 2001 for her outstanding contribution to pharmacy. She is a regular speaker at national and international events.

**Lilian M Azzopardi,** BPharm (Hons), MPhil, PhD

Lilian is a Senior Lecturer in the Department of Pharmacy, Faculty of Medicine and Surgery, University of Malta. She has been involved in pharmacy practice teaching and research since 1994. Lilian is responsible for coordinating the teaching of pharmacy practice, including planning, organisation and assessment during the undergraduate course and the preregistration period. In 1997 she received an award from the FIP Foundation for Education and Research, and in 1999 the ESCP German Research and Education Foundation grant. She is the author of *Validation Instruments for Community Pharmacy* published by Pharmaceutical Products Press (USA) and the editor of *MCQs in Pharmacy Practice* and *Further MCQs in Pharmacy Practice* published by Pharmaceutical Press (UK).

**Helen Barnett,** BPharm, MSc, LicAc, BAcC

Helen is an Associate Editor with *Drug and Therapeutics Bulletin* and also works part-time as an acupuncturist in North London.

**Angela Bussey,** MRPharmS, DMS

Angela is the Principal Pharmacist for Medicines Information Projects, at London and South East Medicines Information Service, Guy's and St Thomas NHS Foundation Trust. She is involved in several local and national medicines information projects, including development and review of medicines information services and working with partner organisations. She has broad clinical and management experience in hospital and community pharmacy, across the NHS and independent sectors.

Angela was previously Chief Pharmacist at the independent King Edward VII Hospital, Midhurst, Sussex. Her community pharmacy roles range from locum to Regional Professional Services Development Manager for Lloydspharmacy.

## Sue Childs, BSc, MSc, MCLIP

Sue is the editor of the journal *He@lth Information on the Internet* published by the Royal Society of Medicine Press. She also compiled *Info@UK*, a newsletter and website on Information Society topics, for the British Council. Sue is a researcher in the Information, Knowledge and Systems Research Group, School of Computing, Engineering and Information Sciences, University of Northumbria. She researches on information issues, with a particular interest in health information. Her background is in biology and she is a qualified librarian. Sue is a Member of the Chartered Institute of Library and Information Professionals and Research Fellow for University of Northumbria, Newcastle upon Tyne, UK.

## Richard Clark, BSc, DPhil

Richard is Director of Vitruvian Medical Writing Ltd, Oxford. He is a freelance medical writer based in Oxford, where he gained his doctorate (DPhil) in biochemistry from Trinity College, University of Oxford. Richard has written an awful lot, and some of it even has his name on as an author. This includes over 300 reviews and other peer-reviewed publications. He is a member of the European Medical Writers Association (EMWA), edits and occasionally publishes articles on medical writing in their journal *The Write Stuff*. Further details of his services can be found on the EMWA freelance list: *http://www.emwa.org/FreeListing.html.*

## Linda Dodds, BPharm, MSc, MRPharmS

Linda has a joint post as a specialist pharmaceutical adviser working across primary care trusts in the southeast of England and as a teacher practitioner at the Medway School of Pharmacy, where she is programme head for postgraduate education. She has written many articles and a number of peer-reviewed research papers during her career as a hospital and primary care pharmacist. She is also editor and a contributor to a clinical teaching manual for pharmacists entitled *Drugs in Use*, which is now in its third edition. Linda continues to submit articles for publication and is currently writing and editing material for a multidisciplinary distance learning Masters' programme in Medicines Management.

## Robin J Harman, PhD, MRPharmS

Robin is an Independent Pharmaceutical and Regulatory Consultant, based in Farnham, Surrey. He is an experienced author and editor, and has four books published by the Pharmaceutical Press: *Handbook of Pharmacy Health-Care* (with Pamela Mason), *Handbook of Pharmacy Health Education*, *Patient Care in Community Practice*, and *Development and Control of Medicines and Medical Devices*. He carries out a wide range of regulatory work for the pharmaceutical industry and also writes frequently for pharmaceutical and regulatory publications.

## Paula Hayes, BPharm, ClinDip, MRPharmS

Paula works for Programme Design and Support, The Centre for Pharmacy Postgraduate Education (CPPE) at the School of Pharmacy and Pharmaceutical Sciences, University of Manchester, UK. Her role is to develop learning programmes and to deliver learning support to the pharmacy team. Paula's key work is the development of a programme of CPD support for pharmacy technicians. She has also been involved in the organisation, planning and delivery of many learning events to support the implementation of the new pharmacy contractual framework. She is the project head for the online MUR Assessment developed as a result of collaboration between the University of Manchester and CPPE.

Paula is a hospital pharmacist by training, with clinical interests in paediatrics and cystic fibrosis.

### Ike Iheanacho, BSc, MBBS

Ike is the editor of *Drug and Therapeutics Bulletin*. He was formerly the deputy editor, having previously been a hospital doctor.

### Steven Kayne, BSc, PhD, MBA, LLM, MSc (SpMed), DAgVetPharm, FRPharmS, FCPP, FIPharmM, MPSNZ, FNZCP

Steven Kayne was a community pharmacist in Glasgow for 35 years before retiring to take on a consultancy role. He writes and lectures both at undergraduate and postgraduate levels on topics associated with pharmacy practice in the UK and overseas, and has written, edited and contributed to several books. Steven sits on three UK Government Expert Advisory Committees, is a visiting lecturer at the University of Strathclyde, Glasgow, and Joint Director of the Royal Pharmaceutical Society veterinary pharmacy teaching programme. He is also a member of the Scottish Executive of RPSGB and Chair of the College of Pharmacy Practice in Scotland.

### John Kirkman, MA, PhD, FISTC

John was formerly Director of the Communication Studies Unit at the University of Wales Institute of Science and Technology, Cardiff (now Cardiff University), UK. Since 1983 he has worked full-time as a consultant on scientific and technical communication. He has consulted for more than 350 organisations in 23 countries.

John has been a Visiting Lecturer in Technical Communication at the University of Michigan, USA, and at the Massachusetts Institute of Technology, USA, and a Visiting Fellow in Linguistics at Princeton University, USA. He has published more than 70 articles, and has written, edited or contributed to 10 books, including *Effective Writing* (with Christopher Turk, Spon, 1989), *Good Style: writing for science and technology* (2nd edition, Routledge, 2005), and *Full Marks: advice on punctuation for scientific and technical writing* (3rd edition, Ramsbury Books, 1999). The Society for Technical Communication (USA) gave him its Outstanding Article Award in 1974, and an Award for Distinguished Technical Communication (shared with Peter Hunt) in 1987.

The John Kirkman Communication Consultancy specialises in training writers and editors.

### Maria Kouimtzi, BPharm, MRPharmS, PhD

Maria obtained her Bachelor in Pharmacy (with Honours) from the University of Bath. After completing her preregistration training she moved to London, where she obtained a PhD from the School of Pharmacy, University of London. Since 2000 she has worked full-time as an editor and editor in charge of editorial procedures at the

*British National Formulary*, Royal Pharmaceutical Society of Great Britain. She has recently joined the BMJ Publishing Group as a clinical editor of *BMJ Clinical Evidence*.

## Pamela Mason, BSc, PhD, MRPharmS

Pamela is a pharmaceutical writer and consultant based in Grosmont, Monmouthshire, south Wales. She qualified as a pharmacist at Manchester University and completed postgraduate studies, including an MSc and PhD in nutrition, at King's College, London. She is the author of four books and over 300 articles. She has run workshops for pharmacists on writing for publication.

## Melissa McClean, BSc (Hons), MSc, PhD

Melissa graduated from the University of Sydney, Australia, with a BSc (Hons Class I) and an MSc majoring in pharmacology. Following graduation, Melissa worked in the Department of Respiratory Medicine at Royal North Shore Hospital, Sydney, investigating the mechanics of airway smooth muscle. She also has had articles published in scientific journals such as the *European Respiratory Journal* and *Thorax*. Melissa completed her PhD in 2005 and is now a Research Fellow with the Woolcock Institute of Medical Research at the University of Sydney, where she continues to investigate the mysteries of respiratory disease.

## Paul McManus, MRPharmS

Paul is an Associate Editor with *Drug and Therapeutics Bulletin* and works part-time as a prescribing adviser in North Yorkshire.

## Genevieve Meier, BPharm(Hons)

Genevieve is the director of a recently established medical informatics consultancy. She is a South African-born pharmacist who has been fortunate enough to work with several of the major multinationals on some of their most successful blockbuster products and campaigns. Starting her career as a manufacturing pharmacist, she moved swiftly into medicine registration but did not stop there. Genevieve moved into the field of health technology assessments and is currently completing her MSc in Health Economic Evaluation. During the various projects and campaigns the marketing aspect of pharmaceuticals has always been an interest. Genevieve also runs a tutorial programme for A-level students wishing to follow a career in medicine.

## Plain English Campaign

Founded in 1979 by Chrissie Maher, the Plain English Campaign is a self-funded pressure group that fights for public information to be written in plain English. It believes that all public documents should be written so that the intended audience can read, understand and act on them in a single reading. Its commercial services, which include editing and training, allow the Campaign to remain completely independent. Its internationally recognised Crystal Mark appears on over 12 000 public documents, ranging from bills and application forms to leaflets and magazines. The Crystal Mark shows that these documents have reached Plain English Campaign's high standards of clarity.

### Anthony Serracino-Inglott, BPharm, Pharm D

Anthony is the Professor and Head, Department of Pharmacy, Faculty of Medicine and Surgery at the University of Malta. Anthony carried out his undergraduate studies at the University of Malta and continued his studies at the University of Cincinnati, Ohio, where he also underwent a residency programme at the Medical Center Cincinnati General Hospital. He co-founded and was director of the Institute of Health Care at the University of Malta, where training programmes for paramedical professionals are provided. He was chairman of a number of examination boards and has a vast experience in the setting of assessments and in continuing education programmes for healthcare professionals.

### Matthew Shaw, BPharm, MRPharmS

Matthew Shaw is assistant director at the Centre for Pharmacy Postgraduate Education in England. As well as being the line manager for half of their tutor workforce, Matthew shares responsibility for the design, development and maintenance of their wide range of learning materials.

Previously, Matthew worked for the NPA as a community pharmacy co-ordinator. As part of this role, Matthew collaborated with Regional, Health Authority, PCT, LPC and Pharmacy Development Group personnel, as well as individual pharmacists.

Working with local pharmacy teams, Matthew has supported head louse infection management services and HbA1c monitoring through community pharmacies.

### Tania Thomas, BPharm, MSc, MRPharmS

Tania is an expert in regulatory affairs, specialising in the quality assessment of medicinal products and regulatory strategy. She has completed a pharmacy degree at the School of Pharmacy, University of London and a postgraduate degree in International Management at King's College, London. She has a broad interest in pharmacy, including anti-doping testing at sport events.

### Paul J Weller, BSc, MSc, CChem MRSC

Paul is the Development Director for Pharmaceutical Press, the publications department of the Royal Pharmaceutical Society of Great Britain, London, UK. He has over 15 years of book, journal and electronic STM publishing experience. He was originally an analytical chemist by training, having studied chemistry at University College London and analytical chemistry at Birkbeck College, University of London.

### Maurice Zarb-Adami, BPharm (Melit), BPharm (Lond), PhD

Maurice is a Senior Lecturer at the Department of Pharmacy, Faculty of Medicine and Surgery at the University of Malta. Maurice studied at the University of Malta and at Chelsea College of Pharmacy, London University. He carried out his research work on Pharmacoeconomics and has examined students in pharmaceutics for the past 30 years. He is interested in the use of information technology in teaching and in its application in assessment procedures. He has vast experience in the evaluation of health personnel, as he was attached to the Ministry of Health as head of the civil service.

# Section One

Medical writing essentials

# 1

# Style for accurate and readable medical writing

*John Kirkman*

## Reading is language processing

### Efficient exchange of information in code

Writing and reading together constitute an exchange of information in code. Writing is an encoding process. The efficiency of the text produced depends principally on the writer's understanding of the conventions of the code used (English, French, Spanish . . .) and his or her ability to handle those conventions skilfully and appropriately for the given aim, audience, and context. Reading is a decoding process. From the reader's point of view, an efficient text is one that presents information about the subject matter accurately, in appropriate detail, and in forms of the code that are instantly recognisable and easy to comprehend.

---

➤ To develop skill as a writer, it is essential to recognise what happens during the activity of reading, so that you can give readers as much help as possible with decoding your text.

---

Reading is signal processing. The writer's task is to deliver a stream of signals that readers can process — that is, recognise and interpret — rapidly and comfortably. As their eyes and minds move from left to right across the lines of a text written in English, readers must more-or-less simultaneously:

- recognise vocabulary;
- recognise what is implied by the placing of words in structures;
- recognise the logical and rhetorical implications of the punctuation signals provided;
- recognise the relationships between word-groups within sentences, between sentences within paragraphs, and between paragraphs within larger sections of the argument.

Readers will feel that a text seems easy to read if they are able to move unhesitatingly and comfortably along the stream of signals. Any need to stop — and even worse, to look back — at least disturbs decoding and comprehension, and at worst brings it to a complete halt. Accordingly, writers must try to ensure that the vocabulary they use is familiar, that the relations between words are immediately clear, and that meaning-boundaries are marked with appropriate punctuation signals.

## Helping readers keep moving forward: choosing familiar words

➤ As you write, keep in mind constantly the interrupting effect of unfamiliar words.

If the words we meet as we move along the stream of signals are familiar, we progress comfortably, but if we arrive at a word we have never seen before, we have to pause and make a quick decision: shall we continue, hoping the writer will explain the meaning he or she wants the word to carry; shall we look at the surrounding text to see if we can find clues to the intended meaning; shall we leave the text and consult a dictionary; shall we ask someone else if they know what the word is normally used to mean? Whatever decision we make, the damage has been done: our concentration on the argument of the text has been disturbed.

Obviously, the special terms of science are possible causes of disturbance. If readers arrive at a special term they have never seen before, comprehension stops. A basic rule of good scientific writing, therefore, is that we must be confident our audience will understand all the special terms we introduce, or we must explain them as soon as we introduce them. But comprehension can be stopped by unfamiliar general vocabulary, too. I have shown the following statement to many groups of medical people, and can confirm that not only readers using English as a second language, but also many native speakers of English, cannot understand it:

More information can be educed from the proportions of . . .

The word *educe* is not in common use. The word *drawn* would give exactly the same meaning, and is available in the general vocabulary of far more readers. It would be processed without hesitation, and would therefore have been a preferable choice for clear and immediate communication.

Note: all the examples used in this chapter are genuine. If you are tempted to think 'But surely no-one would write like that', someone did.

### Helping readers keep moving forward: putting words in conventional positions

Readers will expect the stream of words you deliver to be arranged in accordance with established conventions — the grammar of English. The grammar of English is the set of conventions about the structures and inflections (changes in word-forms) we use to signal the relations we intend between words. We may learn the conventions formally in classes, or informally by imitating the usage of other people. Irrespective of how we learn, we develop expectations about how the words we meet in the text will be combined, structured, and inflected.

For example, we expect an adjective to relate to the first noun that follows it, so when I arrived at the words *elderly sample* in an article on dentistry, my first interpretation was that the sample was elderly:

> Two years after restoration of lower shortened arches for an elderly sample of patients, there was . . .

Clearly, such an interpretation was nonsense, so I looked for a more likely meaning. Obviously, the writer meant 'a sample of elderly patients', so I substituted that for my first interpretation, and continued along the line of words. The adjustment to the decoding process took far less time than it has taken me to write about it: there was only a minor hesitation in my concentration on the argument of the text, but there was a hesitation; the damage had been done; my smooth progress along the line of text had been interrupted.

One small hesitation usually does not destroy our concentration on the argument of a text, but an accumulation of hesitations develops into a sense that we are having to work harder than necessary to decode that argument.

---

➤ The main reason for asking writers to conform to the normal conventions of English is to try to ensure that their texts are easy to interpret unhesitatingly and reliably, not just to fulfil an obligation to an abstract set of rules.

---

**Helping readers keep moving forward: using punctuation signals**

Even if the words we meet as we move along the lines of text are familiar and arranged in a conventional order, our processing activity needs help from punctuation signals. At first reading, I misunderstood the following statement in an abstract at the start of a journal article:

> The focus is on drugs, which have the potential to partition (dissolve) in a lipid membrane but do not perturb membranes.

That statement tells us that the focus is on drugs, and adds a comment that all drugs have the potential to dissolve in a lipid membrane. In fact, the writer meant to say that the focus is only on drugs that have the potential to dissolve in a lipid membrane, not on all drugs. The *which* clause was intended to define, not to comment. However, I had moved several lines further through the text before I realised that fact. I had to look back to the statement about focus, cancel my first interpretation, and form a new interpretation. Once again, this took far less time than it has taken me to write about it, but it was an interruption to my smooth forward progress through the text. It affected my sense of the readability of the abstract.

Writers should aim to enable readers to decode their texts comfortably and confidently in a single, continuous pass along the lines. Readers may choose to stop to reflect on the acceptability of the argument being presented, but a decision to stop moving forward should arise from difficulty with concepts, or from difficulty in accepting the logic of the argument, not from difficulty with language.

## Creating easily processable text

### Creating sentences

A common cause of difficulty for readers is that writers encode within the conventions of English, but the stream of signals they transmit is difficult to process. To make your texts easy to process, judge carefully the amount and the pattern of information you deliver in a single string or sentence.

Be careful not to pack into single sentences more information than readers can process comfortably at just one reading. I had to read the following sentence twice:

> *From a discussion of the importance of genetic testing to confirm clinical diagnoses in the management of fertility.*

[... In addition, a broad range of other gene mutations and genetic syndromes are associated with male and female infertility.] For counselling of patients (parental genetic factors can be transferred to offspring that probably would not have been conceived by natural means), for optimizing the therapeutic concept as well as to basically understand how genetic factors affect fertility, it is important to include cytogenetic (and/or in the case of molecular genetic) laboratory testing to screen for genetic alterations in both partners before assisted reproduction [9–12]. [65 words]

That sentence does not break the rules of English grammar, and the vocabulary is familiar, but the decoding task is difficult because the writer delivers more than our short-term memories can accept in a single connected string. I would have found the statement easier to process if it had been broken into smaller units, arranged to give me the main assertion at the beginning, followed by the details of the tests and why they are important. Perhaps the following would have been better:

Before assisting reproduction, it is important to test both partners for genetic alterations. Cytogenetic tests are important because parental genetic factors can be transferred to offspring that probably would not have been conceived naturally. Additionally or alternatively, laboratory tests for molecular genetic factors are important. [Results from] tests help in counselling patients, optimizing the therapeutic concept, and gaining basic understanding of how genetic factors affect fertility [9–12]. [64–66 words]

This example illustrates an important point: frequently, a text that is a struggle to read is difficult because the writer tries to deliver an awkward pattern of thought, not because it contains unfamiliar vocabulary or grammatical errors.

➤ The patterns of language used to deliver an awkward pattern of thought inevitably seem awkward to process, but to make the text easier to interpret we need to rearrange the ideas into more manageable patterns, not just to adjust the encoding.

## Building compound and complex structures

In English, we build statements in three main ways: by linking simple clauses into strings, by choosing one main clause and attaching further clauses to it in subordinate relationships, or by combining the previous two methods. The three structures are outlined in Figure 1.1. In all three cases, if we include too much information we overwhelm our readers' short-term memories.

Two factors make sentences overwhelming: their length and their structural complexity. Both of these stem from the information the writer tries to present. If too many items of information are strung together, readers cannot digest comfortably all the information being delivered in the stream. If, in addition, the statement is made in a complex pattern, in many subclauses and in many parentheses, readers' short-term memories have even greater difficulty in coping with the information load.

My short-term memory would have been helped by more thoughtful delivery of the following information:

> *From a discussion of an individual with virological failure to all three antiretroviral drug classes*
> Long-term virological suppression is unlikely to be achievable for the foreseeable future for many patients with three-class failure (as supported by recent findings from the T-20 vs Optimised Regimen Only trials[33,34]), and therefore in such patients the goal of antiretroviral therapy needs to be adapted to preservation and, if possible, increase in the CD4-cell count, with the long-term aim of maintaining low mortality. [64 words]

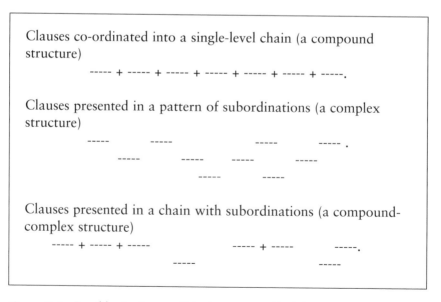

**Figure 1.1**  Possible structures to link clauses in an English sentence.

I would have found the stream of signals easier to process if the writer had paused after the brackets and given me time to digest the first part of the statement before I began to process the rest:

> . . . as supported by findings from the T-20 vs Optimized Regimen Only trials[33,34]). Therefore, in such patients, the goal of antiretroviral therapy needs to be . . .

That adjustment seems minor, but the provision of an extra microsecond of time for digestion of the information makes a great deal of difference to ease of processing.

We cannot blame the English language for complicated statements. A complicated sentence *reflects* a complicated thought — it does not *create* it.

Sometimes, complicated sentences are necessary for the expression of complicated arguments. All too often, however, we have to struggle with complicated sentences just because writers have not considered how easy or difficult it will be for our eyes and minds to process the text. To write readably, we need to develop a reader-friendly attitude — a determination to organise and express information in ways that make minimum demands on readers' language-processing abilities.

## Processability of parenthetical information

Part of the difficulty in processing the long sentences I have just discussed was caused by the delivery of some information in parentheses. Parentheses signal an aside, an explanation, or supplementary information. Readers have to evaluate the parenthetical information quickly, and decide either to discard it or to try to hold it in mind while they continue reading the still-incomplete main statement.

Scientific writers commonly need to add $P$ values to support their statistical statements. As these values are essentially supplementary information, a natural and conventional way to include them in your text is to add them in parentheses, but wherever possible, allow readers' minds to close round a complete phrase structure before you add the supplementary information. The following example has an uncomfortable break in the phrase *significant . . . reduction*:

> Arthroscopic synovectomy led to an overall significant ($P$ between .005 and .05) reduction of the acute inflammatory infiltrates by 82.1%, but to a significant reduction of chronic inflammatory infiltrates by only 62.5%.

The break in *significant . . . reduction* is uncomfortable to process. As the *P* value seems to relate to both sets of measurements, it could have been left more conveniently and comfortably until the end of the statement, as follows:

> Arthroscopic synovectomy led to an overall significant reduction of the acute inflammatory infiltrates by 82.1%, but to a reduction of chronic inflammatory infiltrates by only 62.5% (*P* between .005 and .05).

One parenthetical item is usually manageable: several cause a major disruption to comfortable processing, especially when there are not only parentheses within the main clause but also parentheses within the parentheses:

> However, Lesar *et al.* noted that the rate varied between classes of drugs (most commonly antibiotics (13.5 errors per 1000 orders) cardiovascular (5.0 per 1000) and gastro-intestinal drugs (3.4 per 1000), and specialities (surgical (40.9%), medical (38.8%), paediatric (9.1%), obstetric and gynaecology (6.2%) and emergency (5.0%))).

## Processability of signals that make us look back: respectively

The following statement of results is exceedingly uncomfortable to read, partly because of the array of parentheses, but mainly because of the use of *respectively* at the end:

> After adjustment for covariates, carriers of the *ABCB1* 1236T variant allele had a greater reduction in total cholesterol and low-density lipo-protein cholesterol with simvastatin treatment, as compared with homo-zygotes with the wild-type allele (–29.0% [95% confidence interval (CI), –25.9 to –32.5] versus –24.2% [95% CI, –19.0 to –29.3] [*P* = .042] and –39.6% [95% CI, –35.8 to –44.0] versus –33.8% [95% CI, –27.4 to –40.2] [*P* = .042], respectively).

*Respectively* asks us to relate two or more separated elements, usually variables and numbers, presented before we arrive at *respectively*. The need to look back to check which variable is supposed to be related to which number almost always disturbs our comfortable concentration on the argument of the text, even if the statement is short. Compare the processability of the following two statements:

> Sensitivity, specificity, PPV, and NPV of NMP22 to detect recurrent blad-der carcinoma in the total group of patients was, respectively, 50, 68, 22, and 89%. [25 words]

In the total group of patients, NMP22 detected recurrent bladder carcinoma with 50% sensitivity, 68% specificity, 22% PPV, and 89% NPV. [21 words]

As you write *respectively* at the end of a statement, or *it, this, that, the latter* at the beginning, ask yourself if your reader will be able to remember instantly which previous word(s) you are referring back to.

The time required for checking back as we read a text is insignificant in itself, but the cumulative effect of frequent check-backs on the readers' sense of forward progress is substantial.

## Processability of excessive pre-modification

Within a sentence, a feature of scientific writing that frequently causes difficulty for processing eyes is excessive 'pre-modification' — the piling up of several qualifying words in front of a noun.

The structural conventions of English allow us to add qualifying words either before or after a noun or noun phrase. We can pre-modify the noun *diseases*, and talk about *hypertension-related diseases*, or we can post-modify the noun and talk about *diseases related to hypertension*. Usually, we can handle just one or two pre-modifiers comfortably: for example *daily fluoride consumption*, or *observed pharmacokinetic differences*; but when we read about *sequential radionuclide ejection fraction measurement*, we can be forgiven for wondering whether *sequential* is intended to qualify *radionuclide, radionuclide ejection, radionuclide ejection fraction*, or *measurement*.

Wherever possible, create a left-to-right sequence of words that delivers information to your reader in the order in which it is to be interpreted:

| | |
|---|---|
| *Not:* | sequential radionuclide ejection fraction measurement |
| *Prefer:* | sequential measurement of radionuclide ejection fractions |
| *Not:* | None of the above-mentioned conditions were thought to be trial or dietary related |
| *Prefer:* | None of the above-mentioned conditions were thought to be related to the trial or the diet |

The sequence … *to support legislation for improved car occupant protection* made me smile at the notion of improving car occupants. Of course, the writer intended to talk about *improved car-occupant protection*, using *car-occupant* as a compound adjective qualifying *protection*, but omission of the hyphen led me into a momentary false interpretation. I would have been helped if the idea had been presented to me in the order in which the words were to be interpreted: ... *to support legislation for improved protection of car occupants.*

When we see a preposition such as *for, through, on, by, across, under,* or *of,* we expect it to be followed closely by the noun that is its complement: for example '*for* protection', '*through* the door', or '*on* the table'. We are accustomed to finding one or two adjectives between the preposition and its noun: '*for* lasting protection', '*through* the heavy wooden door', or '*on* the dining-room table'; but more than one or two pre-modifiers are often difficult to process. Especially, if the word immediately following the preposition looks as if it could be the complement, we may be misled:

| | |
|---|---|
| *Not:* | High doses of X could present a risk factor for calcium oxalate urolith formation |
| *Prefer:* | High doses of X could be a risk factor for formation of calcium oxalate uroliths |
| *Or:* | High doses of X could risk formation of calcium oxalate uroliths |

Mental reorganisations such as I have described cause only a momentary flicker in our concentration on the argument of a text. Nevertheless, even a momentary flicker is damaging to our comfort as we process the signals, and if flickers become frequent, we begin to feel that we are having to work harder than is necessary to understand the information the writer is trying to deliver.

## Choosing words: weight, familiarity, and accuracy

As you write, keep clearly in mind the audience for your text. That is easier to say than to do. In life sciences and medicine, the audience may have widely varying backgrounds, and in my experience, editors, academic supervisors, and line managers in business and industry frequently give little or no guidance on the assumptions you should make.

▶ Adopt a 'safety first' policy on choice of words. To make your information available as quickly and comfortably as possible to the widest possible range of readers, use special terms only when they are unavoidable, and surround those special terms with the shortest, most common general words you can find that will express your meaning adequately.

Special terms — jargon — are frequently essential for accurate communication of scientific information, but they have two disadvantages: they are often longer than everyday words, and they *exclude* people from understanding what you are saying. Of course, people with expertise matching your own will understand, but other readers who need your information but are not so familiar with the special terms will not have access to it. So, although your expert readers may be familiar with the jargon of your speciality, it is wise to keep it to a minimum. Use special terms if you must; avoid them if you can.

I am not recommending that you use casual, informal language, which is usually inappropriate because it is imprecise; nor am I suggesting that the information in your text should be distorted or reduced in order to avoid special terms. I am urging you to consider the recognisability of the words you use and the 'weight' of those words: that is, recognise that your readers have to cope not only with an information load, but also with a syllable load in the stream of signals you create.

If you are writing about *hyperprolactinemic* drugs, *parameningeal rhabdomyosarcoma*, or an *endoscopic transsphenoethmoid approach*, your text is inevitably going to be heavy reading, so it is worth taking every opportunity to use short words and the most direct phrasing possible to express what you want to say around those words.

Examine your motive for choosing to write about an *odontogenic developmental programme*. Ask yourself if your text would be easier to read yet just as accurate if you wrote about a 'tooth-development pro-gramme'. Is it really necessary to write *such a complaint is usually pathognomonic of* when (I understand) there would be no loss of meaning in 'such a complaint is usually a sign of', or 'such a complaint usually indicates that'?

From the point of view of accurate and readable communication, is there any added value in writing *a 20G cannula was inserted into a suitable vein on the dorsum of the non-dominant hand* rather than 'a 20G cannula was inserted into a suitable vein on the back of the non-dominant hand'?

I am not querying the use of these special terms because they are inaccurate: my point is that there are always a great many heavyweight words that you cannot avoid in a text for a professional scientific audience, so it is worthwhile removing any that are not essential.

Remove unnecessarily heavyweight general vocabulary, too. Was it really necessary to use the chunky phrase *Methodological heterogenicity* in the statement *Methodological heterogenicity and problems in study design make it difficult to compare results*? I suspect the writer meant no more than 'varied methods', 'varying methods', or 'variation in methods'. All of those alternatives would have saved weight. Write *ends* rather than *terminates*; write *the use of partial-liver grafts* rather than *the utilisation of partial-liver grafts*; write *have higher/more symptoms* rather than *have higher symptomatology*; write *did not explore causes* rather than *did not explore causality*; write *tumour cells that resist killing* rather than *tumour cells that are refractory to killing*.

These are points about tactics, not about grammar. They are points about the processability of your text for the majority of readers, and about how your text will sound, not about accuracy of communication.

Recognise that many readers of your text will be working in English as a foreign language, and as far as possible, choose both special and general vocabulary accessible to those readers. In recent papers, I have met 'Due to the *paucity* of whole organs from paediatric donors' and 'the *putative* transgenerational effect of stilbestrol'. The italicised words are general vocabulary, not technical terms, but they would send many non-native readers (and some native readers) to their dictionaries for help. Judging from the contexts, I believe the intended meanings could have been expressed without loss of accuracy and more inclusively in familiar general words: 'the relatively few whole organs' or 'the scarcity of whole organs', and 'the generally accepted transgenerational effect' or 'the commonly assumed transgenerational effect'.

## Choosing words: borrowings from Latin and other languages

Avoid words and phrases borrowed from Latin and other languages, which present difficulties for readers who are native speakers of English as well as for readers using English as a foreign language.

How would you interpret *the tooth per se is not tender to percussion*? The *New Shorter Oxford English Dictionary* says that *per se* is used to mean 'by or in itself', 'intrinsically', and 'essentially'. Webster's *Ninth New Collegiate Dictionary* (for US usage) adds 'as such'. Dictionaries do not prescribe meanings: they simply record the ways in which words are used. To me, the four interpretations given by those dictionaries are not synonyms. If the writer meant simply 'the tooth itself is not tender to percussion', use of *itself* rather than the borrowed Latin phrase would have been a more reliable encoding.

I must warn you that you cannot rely on everyone sharing your interpretation of *de novo* in scientific texts. I acknowledge that the expression *de novo* is in good dictionaries of English, but it is not an expression that would be taught early in a programme of English as a foreign language, and it is a phrase that most native speakers pick up by hearing other people use it. Consequently, understanding of what it is usually used to mean can vary widely. Consider the following statements:

- ... putty prepared from powder was intramuscularly implanted in athymic rats and *de novo* bone formation quantified (6.7% + 3.5% new bone formation with 49% of ...).
- Dr X presented results from a double-blind study of 157 *de novo* patients.
- PCP may result from *de novo* infection.
- The replacement of subunit X (delta) and Y (MB1) by *de novo* synthesised LMP-2 and LMP-7 in proteasomes of 1FN-γ/treated cells has been described.
- Gestational hypertension was defined as hypertension arising *de novo* in pregnancy without proteinuria.

I have asked many groups of scientists to tell me what meaning they take from *de novo* in those statements. Interpretations have been: 'new', 'primary', 'newly', 'renewed', 'from scratch', 'freshly'. Although all of these cluster round the idea of newness, they are far from identical. The *New Shorter Oxford English Dictionary* explains *de novo* as equivalent to 'de nouveau', 'from new, afresh, starting again from the beginning'. I do not recognise the intended meaning of a *de novo patient* or of *a new cell domain is formed de novo*. At best, *de novo* seems redundant in the last example.

Is *all de jure residents were included* [in a medical study] more likely or less likely to be understood by a majority of your readers than 'rightful residents', 'lawful residents', or 'legitimate residents'? Does *Pain on eating is not a sine qua non* [in a report of symptoms of trouble] mean more than 'Pain on eating is not inevitably present'? If you are tempted to write *Anti-immunisation feeling is almost de rigueur in some circles,* or to describe someone as a *soi-disant expert,* pause to consider whether all your audience will be familiar with French. Do you understand *de rigueur* to mean 'obligatory', or 'customary', or 'fashionable'? These interpretations are not synonyms. Do you understand *soi-disant* to mean a 'so-called' expert or a 'self-styled' expert?

This discussion is not about the use of necessary special terms for which no adequate familiar vocabulary is available. It is about the use of expressions that are likely to puzzle some at least of the typical readers of the journals in which they occurred. I advise 'safety-first writing'. If you mean 'new', write *new*; if you mean 'freshly', write *freshly.* Our objective as writers should be to choose only words that will be instantly and reliably understood by our readers. Often, that is difficult. Deciding whether or not a special term will be comprehended instantly depends on how much we know about the scientific knowledge likely to be held by the audience we are addressing. Similarly, deciding whether or not to use an item of general vocabulary depends on how familiar we are with the range of general vocabulary at the disposal of a typical reader. The onus for making our meaning clear lies on us, the writers: it is not reasonable to ask readers to work out what we probably mean. If in doubt about the instant and reliable recognisability of any word, we should either explain it or find a way of expressing the required meaning in familiar language.

## Choosing words: 'roundabout' phrasing

I have recommended that you keep your text as 'light' as possible by adopting a policy of removing every unnecessary syllable from your text. Similarly, remove every unnecessary word.

---

➤    Unnecessarily long-winded phrasing — roundabout phrasing — is an unfortunate feature of much scientific writing.

---

Compare the following pairs of phrases. Is the first more accurate than the second, or is it simply unnecessarily long-winded?

- Advice on the management of HIV infection is subject to rapid change
  Advice on the management of HIV infection changes rapidly
- The continuous (positive) line on the wick exhibited varying levels of thickness
  The thickness of the continuous (positive) line varied
- Several patients have experienced a reaction . . .
  Several patients have reacted . . .

As these examples show, long-winded phrasing often introduces what language specialists call *nominalisation* — focusing on abstract nouns where it would be possible to write more directly and economically by focusing on a verb. The writer of the final example uses *have experienced a reaction* rather than *have reacted*.

Verbs are the hearts of our statements. They tell readers about the action or state involved. Verbs used to support nominalisations express little meaning in themselves. In the following statement, the writer tells us that the whole spine curvature did some *showing*; wiser writing would have focused on what the whole spine curvature actually did — it *improved*:

*Not:*        The whole spine curvature showed an improvement in 5
              patients
*Prefer:*     The whole spine curvature improved in 5 patients

In the following examples, the verbs tell us about some *exhibiting*, some *carrying out*, some *conducting*, and some *performing*.

- The epithelial cells *exhibit* proliferation
- The development of the index *was carried out* in the pilot study
- We *conducted* comparisons between men and women. . .
- Preparation of chromosomal DNA for ribotyping *was performed* as described by . . .

The following suggested revisions focus on meaningful actions: some *proliferating*, some *developing*, some *comparing*, and some *preparing*:

- The epithelial cells *proliferate*
- The index *was developed* in the pilot study
- We *compared* men and women
- Chromosomal DNA *was prepared* for ribotyping as described by . . .

The common use of roundabout phrasing by scientific writers is a curious phenomenon. They frequently try to excuse uncomfortably compressed writing by saying the number of words they may use is tightly constrained by supervisors and editors, yet they use much redundant wording. I acknowledge that journal editors are usually firm about limiting the length of articles. Their point of view is understandable: many more papers are offered than they can accommodate in their journals, so they try to make space available to as many writers as possible, asking everyone to be brief and to accept limits on the length of articles. However, in trying to compress their information into the smallest number of words and symbols, writers often produce overloaded and puzzling text.

Brevity is a desirable quality in scientific writing, but accuracy and readability should have equal or higher status.

If you have been given a maximum word limit for an article or thesis, my prioritising of accuracy and readability may worry you, but I am confident that, if you use the tactics recommended in this book, you will usually be able to reduce the word-count of your first draft.

We do not need to be told that writers *observed* a phenomenon, *found* a result, *saw* an increase, or *undertook* an examination:

- A reduction in potency in both assays was observed
  The potency in both assays was reduced
- Results: It was found that the mean fluoride excretion in response to . . .
  Results: The mean fluoride excretion in response to . . .
- INR values were seen to increase . . .
  INR values increased . . .
- Examination of the data was undertaken, using . . .
  The data *were examined*, using. . .

I acknowledge that there will be many occasions when you want to focus on an abstract concept, for example on the notion of *uniform distribution*. In such circumstances you will often need to use an abstract noun with a roundabout structure, to keep the stress on that concept:

> . . . was then distributed uniformly. The uniform distribution had been brought about by . . .

However, your text is likely to be more economical and more readable if you remove all unnecessary nominalisations supported by general-purpose verbs such as *take place, occur, perform, carry out, achieve, effect, accomplish, result, conduct, observe, show*, and *find*.

### Choosing verb structures: personal and impersonal, active and passive

Scientific writers are often uncertain about which verb structures will be most efficient in expressing scientific information accurately, clearly, and in a way acceptable to the scientific community. Debate centres on two main issues: whether to write impersonally or personally; and whether to write actively or passively. My advice is:

➤ Do not try to write exclusively personally or impersonally, or exclusively actively or passively: aim to create a natural mixture of verb structures.

That advice is aimed not only at keeping your text as short as possible, but also at ensuring that you express your meaning accurately, explicitly, and in forms of English that seem natural and comfortable to the decoding eyes of your readers.

## Appropriate use of personal style

All too often, choice of impersonal encoding leads to loss of accuracy. For example, the following extract is good English, but the statement it makes is not what the writers intended:

> Such a calculation is considered not to be meaningful for dusts when using the generation and exposure systems described.

The writers intended to say: 'We do not consider such a calculation is meaningful for . . .'; but in English, impersonal constructions such as . . . *is considered to be* are generally understood to imply that the community at large accepts the assertion offered. So, in making the impersonal statement *such a calculation is considered not to be meaningful*, the writers seem to assert that *no-one* considers the calculation meaningful.

If you write: *Any deviations that were observed are considered not to have affected the integrity of the study* when you mean 'We believe the deviations observed did not affect the integrity of the study', you are accepting imprecision in your writing that I suspect you would be ashamed to display in your experimental work and statistical calculations.

This statement from a report makes an assertion that was not (could not be?) supported:

> No nuclear reaction for myogen was observed, but a cytoplasmic reaction was seen in a few cases. This phenomenon is of unknown significance.

To be accurate and honest, the writers should have said: 'We do not know the significance of this phenomenon', or 'We do not know what this phenomenon signifies'.

It is a widespread myth that words like *I, my, we,* and *our* are not acceptable in scientific papers.

Nowadays, it is unusual if editors of journals veto personal style in appropriate parts of a paper. In 1999, my colleague Peter Hunt reviewed a random selection of 100 life-science journals, and without needing to search for long, found first-person pronouns in all of them.[1] In 2001, I reviewed 500 sets of *Instructions for Authors* from medical and life-science journals, and found only two that specified an impersonal, passive style in articles.[2]

Personal style is not appropriate for all sections of a paper. Descriptions of materials and methods, and statements of results are meant to be straightforward presentations of facts. Readers want emphasis on procedures, actions, and outcomes, not on agents. Accordingly, it is usually irrelevant, and sometimes obtrusive, to mention who did what or who observed what in those sections. However, it is appropriate to mention agents in an introduction or a discussion, where it is frequently essential to distinguish clearly between what others have thought or done and what you thought or decided to do.

For example, here is a typical ambiguity in an introduction, caused by the writers' failure to show clearly that they had stopped talking about work done by *Brunk et al.* and had begun to talk about their own work:

> Based on experiments using a rat model of cardiac myocytes, lipofuscin formation by interactions between oxidative stress and autophagocytic degradation was proposed by *Brunk et al.* It was hypothesised that $H_2O_2$, mainly generated by mitochondria, permeates into . . .

When I read that text for the first time, I assumed that *Brunk et al.* had done the hypothesising. I was some way down the page before I realised that the use of the impersonal structure *It was hypothesised that . . .* had confused me. The confusion would have been avoided if the writers had said: ' We hypothesised that . . .'. They could not be accused of self-promotion in using *we*; they would not be claiming credit for something they did not do; they would not be throwing irrelevant emphasis on the actors rather than on their activity or the outcome of their work. They would simply be making a clear statement of fact.

In the discussion section of a paper, authors are expected to say what they think their results imply. They review their facts, give their opinions and, where appropriate, discuss the ways in which their experimental findings confirm or differ from the work of other authors. It is therefore entirely appropriate — indeed, often essential — for that section to contain uses of personal pronouns, to distinguish clearly between what the writers think and what others think.

In seminars, I have often been told that impersonal constructions are necessary to preserve a proper scientific atmosphere of objectivity around the account. I accept the need for scientists to be as detached and objective as possible in all their work; but thinking, believing, considering, and hypothesising are all subjective activities, and use of constructions such as *it is thought that, it is believed that, it is considered that*, and *it was hypothesised that* does nothing to ensure objectivity. As a broad generalisation, it is fair to say that every *it . . . that* construction in your text should be followed by a reference telling readers who did the thinking or hypothesising. If there is no reference, you are probably guilty of making an unclear assertion.

➤ Do not write *The authors postulated that the choroidal rete produces* . . . in the belief that you are being more objective than if you wrote 'We postulated . . .'. Postulating is a subjective activity: to pretend otherwise is nonsense.

To write personally is not necessarily to introduce bias. Bias is introduced mainly by what is said, not by the way it is said. Interpretation of results is a matter of judgement, and to write *We consider that even without measurement of intraocular nitrogen levels* . . . is no more or less biased than to write *The authors consider that even without measurement of intraocular nitrogen levels* . . . . I suggest, too, that the *We consider* . . . version has a more open, credible tone of confident ownership of the opinion than the arms-length, evasive tone of *The authors consider* . . . .

## Appropriate use of active-verb structures and passive-verb structures

A great benefit of thinking in personal constructions is that it encourages us to make active rather than passive statements. To help make your writing readable, use as many active-verb constructions as possible.

What do we mean by the terms *active* and *passive*? In linguistic discussions they are used to describe the relation between the subject of a sentence and the action or state expressed by the verb: that is, they describe whether a statement says the subject does something (actively) or has something done to it (passively).

The following examples illustrate the differences. Sentence 1 is an active-structure statement — that is, the subject actively did something.

1. Drug X reduced the inflammation in the lungs significantly.

| Subject | Verb structure, active form of the verb |
| --- | --- |
| Drug X | *reduced* the inflammation in the lungs significantly. |

Sentence 2 is a passive-structure statement: the subject passively had something done to it, but no mention is made of the agent involved.

2. The inflammation in the lungs was reduced significantly.

| Subject | Verb structure, passive form of the verb, no agent expressed |
| --- | --- |
| The inflammation in the lungs | *was reduced* significantly. |

Sentence 3 also is a passive-structure statement: the subject passively had something done to it; but in this sentence the identity of the agent involved is added to the information presented.

3. The inflammation in the lungs was reduced significantly by Drug X.

*Subject*                                *Verb structure*, passive form of the verb
                                         + agent

The inflammation in the lungs            *was reduced* significantly by Drug X.

In general use of English, active structures are the norm.[3] In active structures, we emphasise the agent (in Sentence 1, *Drug X*) because we put it in the subject position; but in writing about science we often do not want to emphasise the agent: we want to focus who or what was in a particular state or had something done to it. In parts of our scientific texts, therefore, it is natural to use a higher proportion of passive constructions.

However, there is a drawback to the use of passive constructions. As their name suggests, passive constructions create an atmosphere of passivity: subjects have things done to them. In contrast, active structures help to create a sense of energy: subjects do things. Cumulatively, a text with a majority of active verb structures usually gains in readability because the active structures are shorter and more direct. Compare, for example:

> *Passive*: In addition to . . ., an increased concentration of lipofuscin was observed.
> *Active*: In addition to . . ., the concentration of lipofuscin increased.
> *Passive*: In the following three months, improvement was seen in most sectors.
> *Active*: In the following three months, most sectors improved.

So my general advice is that you think and write in active constructions as much as possible, to keep your writing dynamic and direct. However, choice between active and passive structures must be made carefully. Active-verb structures and passive-verb structures do not necessarily give us interchangeable ways of saying the same thing. Consider the following pairs of statements. In each pair, the essential information is the same, but the verb structure used creates a difference of emphasis:

> *Active*: To facilitate the assessment of dosing regimens, *we predicted* the pharmacokinetic properties of X.
> Passive: To facilitate the assessment of dosing regimens, *the pharmacokinetic properties of X were predicted*.
> *Active: Smith and colleagues have reported* a clinical series with recipient and graft survival equal to whole-organ techniques.
> Passive: *A clinical series with recipient and graft survival equal to whole-organ techniques has been reported* by Smith and colleagues.

In the first of each pair, the statement is about who did something; in the second of each pair, the statement is about what had something done to it.

Because active and passive structures do not create precisely the same statements, we must not interchange them casually. Our decisions on which structure to use must depend on what we want to say — on whether we want to focus on who or what acts, or on who or what is affected by the action.

In scientific writing it is particularly beneficial to change from active to passive when we do not think it important to mention, or when we do not know, the agent responsible for the happening or state. For example:

- When we think information about the agent is obvious or unimportant: Abdominal incisions were closed with absorbable sutures, and . . .
- When we do not know the identity of the agent: The water supply to the hospital had been cut off . . .

When we describe our experimental activities, we want our readers to focus on our methods and materials; we do not think it important to keep emphasising who did what. Accordingly, accounts of experiments, survey work, or statistical calculations are naturally encoded mainly in passive constructions. In other sections of a typical paper, however, especially in the introduction and the discussion, we usually need to distinguish clearly between things we have thought and done and things other people have thought and done. In those sections, we need to use a mixture of constructions to help readers decode reliably the account we are giving.

On many occasions in classes and seminars, newcomers to scientific writing have asked if it is acceptable to switch between types of verb construction, because they have been told during their education that scientific texts should be written in third-person, impersonal constructions, in the past tense, and in the passive voice. That is harmful advice. It is, I suspect, responsible for much of the ponderous, uncomfortably encoded scientific text I have had to read during my career as an adviser on writing. It is entirely natural to mix the full range of structures and forms available in English.

To illustrate natural encoding in a mixture of forms and structures, here are fragments of typical sections of a scientific paper (not all from the same paper, and lightly edited), with a description of every verb.

(Key: first or third person; personal or impersonal style; active or passive; present or past tense.)

### Introduction
A well-written Introduction normally includes a mixture of personal and impersonal, active and passive constructions:

Methadone *is used* increasingly for controlling pain in the elderly and in palliative care settings[n,n].
3rd; impersonal; passive; present.

It *has been found to inhibit* CYP2D6[n]. This result *indicates* a
3rd; impersonal; passive; past.
3rd; impersonal; active; present.

potential for interaction with dextromethorpan. In this paper, we *report* the case of an elderly woman with . . .
1st; personal; active; present.

**Materials and methods**

A materials and methods section is likely to be best encoded in mainly passive, impersonal forms, but an occasional first-person, active construction may be appropriate:

Livers *were perfused* in situ as previously *described*
3rd; impersonal; passive; past.
3rd; impersonal; passive; past.

(Sallustio et al., 1996) at 37°C within a thermostatically controlled perfusion cabinet. The perfusion medium *was* a
3rd; impersonal; active; past.

Krebs-bicarbonate buffer (0.30 L, pH 7.4) that *contained*
3rd; impersonal; active; past.

glucose (3.27 g/L) and sodium taurocholate (0.896 g/L) and *was* continually *gassed* with carbogen
3rd; impersonal; passive; past.

($5\%$ $CO_2$, $95\%$ $O_2$). In contrast with previous studies, we *used* a
1st; personal; active; past.

recirculating design, to pump the perfusion medium at 30 ml/min into the liver through a cannula *inserted* into the hepatic portal
3rd; impersonal; passive; past.

vein and *returned* via a cannula . . .
3rd; impersonal; passive; past.

**Results**

Usually, results are presented most appropriately mainly in tables. If they are presented as narrative texts, they are usually appropriately presented in impersonal constructions, preferably active:

Mean peak PR and PID scores *are presented* in Table 3.
3rd; impersonal; passive; present.

Ibuprofen alone *had* a significantly greater effect on the mean peak
3rd; impersonal; active; past.

PID scores *compared* with placebo
3rd; impersonal; passive; past.

($P<0.01$) There *was* no significant
3rd; impersonal; active; past.

difference in mean peak PID
scores between oxycodone
5 mg/ibuprofen
400 mg and ibuprofen alone.

## Discussion

A discussion section should contain your opinions on what your results imply, so it will normally include a complete mixture of first-person and third-person, active and passive constructions:

A disadvantage of using DNase I
footprinting *is* the sequence — 3rd; impersonal; active; present.
selectivity inherent in the enzyme
itself. This enzyme *does not cleave* — 3rd; impersonal; active; present.
the control DNA evenly, which
means that some sequences *remain* — 3rd; impersonal; active; present.
uninformative. The restriction
endonucleases *are able to cut* the — 3rd; impersonal; active; present.
recognised site to completion and,
if it *is* a single site in the plasmid — 3rd; impersonal; active; present.
DNA, the process *can be* — 3rd; impersonal, passive, present.
*monitored* easily by agarose gel
electrophoresis. We *have used* a set — 1st; personal; active; past.
of restriction endonucleases whose
recognition sequences *contain* G in — 3rd; impersonal; active; present.
different sequential . . .

## Conclusions

Conclusions should not be continuations of your description of methods, or restatements of your results. They should state what you infer from your results. You may therefore find it appropriate to present them as a numbered list of impersonal, positive statements, but more usually you will be asked to present them in narrative form, again in impersonal, positive statements:

*Either:* Conclusions
1. The interaction between
dextromorphan and methadone
*resulted* in unrecognised delirium. — 3rd; impersonal; active; past.
2. Delirium *had* a profound effect — 3rd; impersonal; active; past.
in terms of the patient's social
functioning and general health.
3. Physicians *should be cautious* — 3rd; impersonal; active; present.
when *co-prescribing* dextromorphan — 3rd; impersonal; active; present.
and medications that *inhibit* — 3rd; impersonal; active; present.
CYP2D6, particularly for

potentially vulnerable elderly
patients.

*or:*
Conclusions
The interaction between
dextromethorpan and methadone
*resulted* in unrecognised delirium.          3rd; impersonal; active; past.
That delirium *affected* the patient's          3rd; impersonal; active; past.
social functioning and general
health profoundly. Therefore,
physicians *should be cautious*          3rd; impersonal; active; present.
when *co-prescribing*          3rd; impersonal; active; present.
dextromorphan and medications
that *inhibit* CYP2D6, particularly          3rd; impersonal; active; present.
for potentially vulnerable elderly
patients.


## Punctuation

### Signalling the logic and rhetoric of your message

---

➤   Creating a stream of understandable words arranged in conventional, easily decodable patterns is only part of the task of encoding a message. We have also to supply appropriate, conventional punctuation signals.

---

Punctuation does two main jobs, one logical and one rhetorical:

• It shows how parts of sentences and/or larger segments of text relate to one another.
• It signals the emphasis, the tone, or the special way in which we wish to use a word or word group: that is, it shows the 'rhetorical' annotations we want to pass to readers in addition to the 'meaning' of the words.

In speech, we make our intended meaning clear by using voice signals — changes of intonation, speed over words and word groups, variations of stress on individual syllables, and variations of spacing between words. When we write, we have to supply other cues — dots, dashes, and other hieroglyphics — on the page. If we omit those cues, or if we put them in the wrong place, we may mislead our readers, so we should take as much care over our choice of punctuation signals as we take over our selection and arrangement of words.

## Logical signalling

The first function of punctuation marks is to show the relationships you intend between the words and word groups in your text. To see the importance of this function, consider the following start of an article entitled 'Influenza in the acute hospital setting'. Note how the stream of signals can be interpreted in several different ways:

> an important cause of morbidity and often mortality in most communities every winter influenza poses special hazards inside healthcare facilities because of its short incubation period and efficient respiratory spread from person to person it can cause explosive outbreaks of febrile respiratory illness the hospital patient population has serious underlying illnesses making influenza more lethal in this setting healthcare workers have increased risk of acquiring influenza during known outbreaks since they are exposed to infected individuals in the community as well as hospitalised patients with influenza whether infected at work or in the community healthcare workers may become an important source of influenza for their patients

Where do you think the writer intended us to end the first sentence — after *facilities* or after *person*?

> An important cause of morbidity and often mortality in most communities every winter, influenza poses special hazards inside healthcare facilities.
> or
> An important cause of morbidity and often mortality in most communities every winter, influenza poses special hazards inside healthcare facilities because of its short incubation period and efficient respiratory spread from person to person.

Alternatively, perhaps you interpreted the intended meaning as:

> An important cause of morbidity and often mortality in most communities every winter, influenza poses special hazards. Inside healthcare facilities, because of its short incubation period and efficient respiratory spread from person to person, it can cause explosive outbreaks of febrile respiratory illness.

Then, how did you continue?

> The hospital patient population has serious underlying illnesses, making influenza more lethal in this setting. Healthcare workers have increased risk of acquiring influenza during known outbreaks since they are exposed to infected individuals in the community as well as hospitalised patients with influenza.

or:

> The hospital patient population has serious underlying illnesses, making influenza more lethal. In this setting, healthcare workers have increased risk of acquiring influenza during known outbreaks since they are exposed to infected individuals in the community as well as hospitalised patients with influenza.

The possibility of interpreting the unpunctuated text in so many ways emphasises that punctuation marks are vital elements in the signalling process, not optional extras. It is the writer's task to show clearly the relationships he or she wants readers to assume.

## 'Rhetorical' signalling

The second function of punctuation marks is to signal the 'rhetorical' information we want to send in addition to the 'basic meaning' of the words. Scientists are usually concerned with presenting factual information and/or unemotional opinion, so they rarely need to punctuate 'rhetorically' in the sense of creating extravagant or exaggerated effects. Accordingly, there are few occasions when, for example, use of an exclamation mark would be appropriate, because an exclamatory tone would usually be considered out of place in a scientific paper. But exclamation marks should not be banned: they can be useful to highlight hazards or to add weight to a prohibition:

> Note that cyanide solution and cyanide gas can cause severe poisoning simply by absorption through the skin. It is not enough just to avoid drinking the solution or inhaling the gas!

## Marking boundaries

---

➤ Get into the habit of putting commas as boundary markers after initial words or word groups that present qualifications or create links at the beginnings of sentences.

---

Far too frequently, after reading only a word or two at the start of a sentence, I find that I have to cancel the interpretation I was beginning to formulate, look back to the beginning, and start a new interpretation. For example, my first interpretation of the beginning of the following sentence was that I was going to be told about *rare infection*:

> Although rare infection can occur from consumption of raw milk from sheep and goats as it contains fast developing tachyzoites.

It was not until I reached *as it contains* that I realised there should have been a boundary marker after *rare*: *although rare, infection* .... Of course, correcting my interpretation took far less time than it has taken me to write about it, but my concentration on the argument of the text was interrupted.

It is important to recognise that, in the signalling of meaning, the absence of a mark is often as important as its presence. Omission of a mark after even only one word can be seriously misleading. For example, in the following pair of statements the writer wrote the first but meant the second:

> However unlike the previous type . . .
> However, unlike the previous type . . .

If *however* is not followed by a comma, it is intended normally to be a qualification of the word immediately after it; if *however* is followed by a comma, it is intended normally to be a linking comment, announcing that the words that are to come will introduce a contrast or contradiction to what has gone before.

## Putting a comma before 'and'

Many young scientists have told me that their schools did not give them a systematic account of the conventions of punctuation. Nevertheless, one so-called rule seems to have seeped into popular consciousness: 'You mustn't put a comma in front of *and*'. Unfortunately, that is not an accurate rule. Certainly, there are many occasions when a comma is not needed before *and*, but there are many more when a comma is an essential signal to prevent misreading.

The theoretical objection to placing a comma before *and* is that a comma is usually a boundary marker, a separating signal; in contrast, *and* is a coordinator, a linking signal. To have a separating signal immediately in front of a coordinating signal is sometimes confusing, as in this example:

The model represents the flow breakdown, and the shockwave effects.

The writer wanted us to see *the flow breakdown* and *the shockwave effects* as coordinated units following the verb *represents*:

> The model *represents*     the flow breakdown
> and
> the shockwave effects.

Unfortunately, the comma after *breakdown* in the original sentence seems to signal that *The model represents the flow breakdown* is a completed meaning-unit, and that a new unit is about to begin. We expect to read something such as '. . . and the shockwave effects are . . .'. But we realise quickly that the new unit does not make sense by itself. We cancel our first interpretation, and take the meaning the writer intended, which would have been represented normally as:

> The model represents the flow breakdown and the shockwave effects.

In normal decoding, we expect to find a coordinated pair of items — either single words or phrases — surrounding *and*:

> The relation between spleen enlargement and malaria parasitaemia deserves further study.

We also recognise that *and* may be used to coordinate two complete phrases or sentences into a compound statement:

> The false positives rate was highest in the mesoendemic zone and lowest in the hypoendemic stratum . . . Microparticles accumulate in the femoral lymph nodes and numerous plasma cells drain into the lymphatics of the foot.

However, the acceptability of coordinating two complete sentences into a compound statement depends on two things: one is the possibility of the words immediately surrounding the *and* looking like a linked pair, and the other is the length and complexity of the linked sentences.

When I read the following example for the first time, I was momentarily confused:

> All animals were anaesthetised with pentobarbitone and blood samples taken from an abdominal blood vessel.

I was confused because I attempted to read the terms *pentobarbitone* and *blood samples* as a coordinated pair; but the writer intended us to recognise two coordinated statements:

> All animals were anaesthetised with pentobarbitone.
> and
> blood samples [were] taken from an abdominal blood vessel.

Failure to signal the end of the first of the coordinated sentences, and the decision not to repeat *were* (in an effort to reduce word-count, I suspect), combined to confuse me. I would probably not have been confused even momentarily if the writer had provided a comma after *pentobarbitone*, and had repeated *were* in the second part of the sentence:

> All animals were anaesthetised with pentobarbitone, and blood samples were taken from an abdominal blood vessel.

Short compound statements coordinated by *and* are frequently manageable; but as statements become longer, it is increasingly necessary to help the reader by signalling where the first of two coordinated word groups ends and the second begins:

> *Not*: The thoracic ED catheter was loaded with 0.125% bupivacaine to a T4 sensory level and a continuous infusion of 0.125% bupivacaine without opioid was commenced at 4 mL/h.
> *Prefer*: The thoracic ED catheter was loaded with 0.125% bupivacaine to a T4 sensory level, and a continuous infusion of 0.125% bupivacaine without opioid was commenced at 4 mL/h.

### Separating items in a list — 'serial commas'

━━━━━━━━━━━━━━━━━━━━━━━━━━━━━━━━━━━━━━━━━━━

➤ When you present a list of items, it is usually helpful to separate them with commas, including a comma before the final item.

━━━━━━━━━━━━━━━━━━━━━━━━━━━━━━━━━━━━━━━━━━━

When I read the following text, I had to pause to work out the itemisation at the end of the sequence:

> Other concurrent treatments in patients with pancreatitis included lopinavir plus ritonavir, lamivudine, and efavirenz for those treated with didanosine plus tenofovir and lamivudine plus nevirapine for the patient given didanosine alone.

I would have been helped by the provision of a comma before *and lamivudine*. Many British writers have been told that no comma is needed before the final *and* or *or* of a sequence, but as the example above shows, it is frequently helpful to provide one. The provision of a final 'serial comma' is more common in US usage than in British usage. I recommend that you get into the habit of providing one. Provision of a comma in these circumstances will rarely confuse your readers: omission of a comma often will.

### Comma before 'which'

Frequently, we use the words *who, whose, whom, which,* or *that* to begin clauses. Linguists call these words 'relative pronouns', because they relate the information in the clause that follows to a preceding noun or noun phrase. The relationship indicated can be a definition or a comment: that is, the relative clause created may make it clear exactly who or what you are talking about, or it may give additional, non-essential information, *commenting* on the person or thing you are discussing:

> *Defining*: In the experiment *which* lasted two hours, the heat from the furnace was . . .
> [The relative clause *which lasted two hours* defines which of several experiments is being talked about]
> *Commenting*: In the experiment, *which* lasted two hours, the heat from the furnace was . . .
> [The relative clause *which lasted two hours* comments, giving supplementary information about the single experiment being discussed]
> *Defining*: Colour-coding highlights the discontinuous contours for the user who can use the editing tools to create continuous contours.
> *Commenting*: Colour-coding highlights the discontinuous contours for the user, who can use the editing tools to create continuous contours.
> *Defining*: The medical information world was once dominated by librarians whose primary concern was the management of book collections.
> *Commenting*: The medical information world was once dominated by librarians, whose primary concern was the management of book collections.

Conventionally, we signal the intended relations as follows:

- To introduce a relative clause to give *defining* information, we do not put a comma before the relative pronoun that starts the clause.
- To introduce a relative clause that offers *commenting*, supplementary information (almost an aside, giving information that is not essential for identifying the person or thing you are talking about) we do put a comma before the relative pronoun that starts the clause.

➤ Commenting clauses need a *comma*, defining clauses *don't*.

➤ The provision or omission of a comma before *which* is a particularly important indication of intended meaning in modern use of English.

Some writers have been taught that they should always introduce a defining clause with *that*:

> Samples *that* were not processed immediately were stored with residual carcasses at approximately −20°C.

and to introduce a commenting clause with *which*:

> Samples, *which* were not processed immediately, were stored with residual carcasses at approximately −20°C.

However, usage has changed, and now in conventional British English and US English usage you will find common use of *which* to introduce defining clauses:

> Samples *which* were not processed immediately were stored with residual carcasses at approximately −20°C.

To introduce a defining clause with *that* is still entirely acceptable; indeed, it is good practice to do so, as it removes the possibility of readers mistaking your intended meaning, but if you are in the habit of using *which* to introduce both commenting and defining clauses, be sure to signal by careful inclusion or omission of a comma the relationship you intend between the clause and its preceding noun.

## Hyphens as linking signals

Accurate use of hyphens is essential to enable rapid, reliable decoding of a text. My comfortable progress through a paper was interrupted by the ambiguity of *incorporates two colour graphics terminals*, and through another paper by *a range of heavy metal-containing pigments* (intended meanings: 'two-colour-graphics terminals' and 'heavy-metal-containing pigments'). I stumbled over the statement that a material was *evaluated in a laboratory set up in Someplace*. With only a moment's thought, I could see where the hyphens should have been, but my concentration on the argument of the text was disturbed. The hyphen-less writing affected adversely my judgement of the readability of a text.

When you want to combine two or more words into a compound to qualify a noun, use a hyphen (which is a joining signal) to show how the words are intended to be linked together.

> *Not*: These products when burned do not produce sulphur containing gases.
> *Prefer*: These products when burned do not produce sulphur-containing gases.
> *Not*: . . . in a waterproof waste disposal bag.
> *Prefer*: . . . in a waterproof waste-disposal bag.

When you combine three words into a compound, make the compound clear by using two hyphens. My concentration was disturbed by this half-punctuated statement (sadly, from a textbook on how to write well!):

> Avoid all upper-case words.
> . . . all-upper-case . . .

It is acceptable to use 'suspended' hyphens when you want to create two or more similar compounds in sequence. A suspended hyphen is a device for economising on words. Instead of repeating *layered* in the expression *a double-layered or treble-layered coating*, we can write 'a double- or treble-layered coating'. However, this creates an awkward cluster of words for the reader's eye and mind to process, so I recommend you use it only sparingly.

## Overall aim

Composing a scientific paper is a challenging task that calls for sensitive balancing of the demands of accuracy and the demands of readability. Aim to produce a text that keeps as close as possible to the natural rhythms and vocabulary of day-to-day discourse.

➤ Keep in mind Pascal's observation: Quand on voit le style naturel, on est tout étonné et ravi, car on s'attendait de voir un auteur, et on trouve un homme.
[When we see a natural style, we are always astonished and delighted, for we expected to see an author, and we find a man.] Blaise Pascal, *Pensées* (1670)

# References

1. Hunt P (1999) Why are scientists so susceptible to myth? *Aust NZ J Fam Ther* 20: 3.
2. Kirkman J (2001) Third person, past tense, passive voice for scientific writing. Who says? *Eur Sci Ed* 27: 4–5.
3. Greenbaum S, Quirk R (1990) *A Student's Grammar of the English Language.* London: Longman, 45.

# 2

# Writing in plain English

*Plain English Campaign*

## Principles of plain English

### What is plain English and why do you need it?

Sometimes people get the wrong idea about plain English and think it's about 'dumbing down', or that it's for people who don't have the vocabulary and skill to write 'properly'. This isn't true.

Plain English is about making what you write accessible to more people. Explaining something complex in a simple, clear way is actually a great skill. Think of the teachers who stand out in your memory, whose lessons were interesting and fun — they had this skill.

Communicating in a clear, open way is more friendly and more effective. And it's vital when writing for the public. If people understand what you write, they are more likely to do what you ask. To take an obvious example, just think about instructions for using medicines. If the patient is confused by the instructions because they are poorly written, the consequences could be very serious.

If you are writing for a professional audience, they will also appreciate your using plain English. It saves time because it's faster to write and faster to read. It's also part of your public image. In your customers' eyes, you are your words: if those words are impersonal, unapproachable and unfriendly, then so are you.

So what is plain English? It is a message that is clear and concise, written with the reader in mind and in the right tone of voice.

### Make it short

Using short sentences will help make your writing clearer. This is because it's easier for our brains to process information one chunk at a time. A good average sentence length is 15 to 20 words. This does not mean every sentence you write must be 17.5 words long! Vary the length. Mix short sentences (like the last one) with longer ones (like this one), following the basic principle of sticking to one main idea in a sentence, plus perhaps one other related point.

Long sentences are often full of conjunctions (joining words) such as *and*, *but*, *if* and *however*. These are used to link ideas together. Following the meaning of a sentence is like following a path. Each conjunction is like a turn or a fork in that path: if you use too many, the reader gets lost. Long sentences make it harder to follow a sequence of events or the logic behind an argument.

Consider the following example, which was taken from a tablet packet:

> They act faster than standard paracetamol tablets you can swallow to give fast, effective pain relief of headache, migraine, backache, rheumatic and muscle pain, neuralgia, toothache, period pain, sore throats and for the relief of feverishness and the aches and pains of colds and flu.

There are 45 words in this sentence, more than twice the recommended average. You are probably familiar with all of them, but try to put yourself in the patient's shoes. What is the most important piece of information here:

- that the tablets work faster than standard ones;
- that you swallow them;
- that they give fast relief;
- that they give effective relief; or
- what they give relief from?

The writer has tried to explain a lot of things in one sentence. Now look at the same instructions written in a clearer way:

> They act faster than standard paracetamol tablets to give fast and effective pain relief from:

- headaches;
- migraines;
- backache;
- rheumatism and muscle pain;
- neuralgia (pain caused by damage to or irritation of a nerve);
- toothache;
- period pain; and
- sore throats.

> They also reduce fever and relieve the aches and pains of colds and flu.

Using two sentences, one in the form of a bullet-pointed list, makes the information easier to digest.

**Examples to try**

Here are some long sentences for you to practise on. Break them up by inserting full stops at suitable points and mending any breaks you create. Change anything else you think is necessary, but try not to change the meaning. You can find answers to all the examples at the end of this chapter (see page 48).

> **1) From a website about multiple sclerosis**
> It should be kept in mind that the common symptoms of **MS** can also be symptomatic of other conditions so the list of ways in which **Multiple Sclerosis** shows itself (*the symptoms*) should be read with this in mind.

> **2) From a leaflet in a tablet box**
> If you: experience a hypersensitivity reaction (allergy to the medicine itself) (Hypersensitivity reaction symptoms may include chest tightness or wheezing, unexpected swelling and flushing leading to collapse) stop taking the tablets and tell your doctor.

For more information, see page 6 'Creating sentences'.

## Make it active

'Active' verbs make writing clearer, more natural and more personal. 'Passive' verbs, on the other hand, make writing stuffy and impersonal. To explain the difference between 'active' and 'passive' verbs, we need to look at how a sentence fits together. There are three main parts to most sentences:

- an **agent** (the person, group or thing doing the action);
- a **verb** (the action itself); and
- an **object** (the person, group or thing that the action is done to).

### Active verbs

For a verb to be 'active', the 'agent' comes before the verb. Here are some examples of sentences with active verbs:

1   Paul is eating an apple.
    In this example:
    - 'Paul' is the **agent**, he's doing the eating;
    - 'eating' is the **verb**, that's what he's doing; and
    - 'apple' is the **object**, that's what he's eating.
2   The dog (agent) bit (verb) the man (object).
3   The doctor (agent) prescribed (verb) these tablets (object).

Most active sentences follow this pattern: the agent comes first, then the verb, then the object.

4     The nurse will take a blood sample.
5     The sales team will use the new procedures.

There may be lots of other words in the sentence as well. For example: 'The sales team, with support from Customer Services, will use the new procedures from the start of next month.' But the basic order of agent, verb, object stays the same.

## Passive verbs

With a passive verb the order is different: the agent comes after the verb. Here are the same sentences written with passive verbs:

1     The apple (object) is being eaten (verb) by Paul (agent).
2     The man (object) was bitten (verb) by the dog (agent).
3     These tablets were prescribed by the doctor.
4     A blood sample will be taken by the nurse.
5     The new procedures will be used by the sales team.

Passive verbs need extra words to say the same thing. What a waste!

## Good uses of passives

There are times when it makes sense to use a passive:

* to make something less hostile — 'this bill has not been paid' (passive) is softer than 'you have not paid this bill' (active);
* when you don't know who or what the agent is — 'the projector has been stolen'; and
* if it simply sounds better.

## Examples to try

Here are some examples for you to turn into active verbs:

1     Care should be taken when opening the door.
2     The cream should be applied sparingly and if no improvement is seen within five days, your doctor should be consulted.
3     A report will be sent to your doctor.
4     It is fully acknowledged that on-site car parking is currently very limited and in this respect plans are currently being examined with a view to alleviating the problems.

5       Immediate medical advice should be sought in the event of an overdose, even if you feel well.

Once you have made the examples active, make any other changes you think are necessary.

For more information, see page 21 'Appropriate use of active-verb structures and passive-verb structures'.

## Make it personal

Try to use personal references such as *I, you, we, he, she* and *they*. These make your writing more friendly and personal. They also help prevent ambiguity and confusion, and help you to write more active text.

> *This form must be completed before your hospital appointment.*

This is a passive sentence with no agent. It's not clear who should be filling in the form — the patient, their doctor, someone else?

> *You must fill in this form before your hospital appointment.*

Look at the difference between the two. The second is more personal, more friendly. It is focused on the reader, not the writer.

Try to call the reader 'you', even if they are only one of many people you are talking about generally. If this feels wrong at first, remember that you wouldn't call somebody 'the applicant', 'the supplier' or 'the patient' if they were sitting across a desk from you.

Wherever possible, try to call your organisation 'we'. So:

> *Further details are required before your application can be processed* becomes *We need further details before we can process your application.*

There is nothing wrong with using *we* and *I* in the same document. It can help distinguish between what the writer is doing specifically ('I have looked into this . . .') and what the organisation does generally ('We investigate all complaints very carefully.')

### Examples to try
Try making these examples more personal:

1    Applicants must send us . . .
2    Patients must advise hospital staff . . .
3    Advice is available from . . .

For more information, see page 19 'Appropriate use of personal style'.

## Big words and technical stuff

Say exactly what you mean, using the simplest words that fit. This does not necessarily mean using only the simplest words — just words that the reader will understand.

### Explaining technical concepts and avoiding jargon

Most professions have their own technical language. For example, an environmental engineer talks about 'airborne particulate load', whereas the rest of us might say 'dust levels'. A doctor might describe an injury as a 'fracture to the clavicle', but the patient would say they have 'broken their collarbone'.

We are not saying you can (or should) get rid of technical language. It's fine when one professional is writing for another in the same field and they understand each other. In this case, using technical terms may make communication quicker and more precise.

But as soon as you move a little outside your own area — even when writing for a colleague in a different department — you may have a problem. Often people are too embarrassed to say that they don't understand what someone has written.

Technical language becomes 'jargon' when it is difficult for others to understand.

Using jargon with members of the public can make them feel excluded from something they should be involved in. It can lead them to do the wrong thing, or to do nothing at all, because they don't understand what they are supposed to do.

Imagine a poster aimed at helping people identify or avoid a dangerous disease. If the information is too technical, readers might:

* ignore it;
* panic unnecessarily; or
* create extra work for staff who have to explain the information more clearly.

So how do you deal with technical terms? There are various possibilities and their suitability will depend on what you are writing. You could:

* miss out any unnecessary technical term — ask yourself whether the reader really needs this information;

- explain the term, preferably where it is used, but if this is not possible you could use a glossary; or
- replace the term with an everyday word or phrase.

Appendix 5 is an A to Z of some medical terms that people might find confusing, and suggestions for explaining them.

**Examples to try**
Here are some examples for you to practise getting rid of technical terms.

> **1) From a leaflet on a burns dressing bought in Portugal**
> Upon contact with wound exudates, [product name] burns matrix releases hydrocolloid particles. These particles interact with the petroleum jelly component contained in the dressing to form a Lipido-Colloid gel interface that favours the healing process in a moist environment.

> **2) From a leaflet about food allergies**
> Food intolerance is defined as an abnormal physiological response to an ingested food or food additive which is not proven to be immunological in nature.

> **3) From the same leaflet**
> Food allergy is defined as an immunological reaction resulting from the ingestion of a food or food additive.

For more information, see page 12 'Choosing words: weight, familiarity and accuracy'.

## Using verbs rather than nouns

If, in simple terms, we think of verbs as 'doing' words, we can call nouns 'naming' words.

**Common nouns** are words such as cat, dog, girl, table, house, lamp.

**Proper nouns** are usually names of people, places or organisations, for example Jane, Paris, Egypt, General Medical Council.

**Abstract nouns** are words for things you can't see or touch: failure, hope, poverty, love. One particular kind of abstract noun fills reports and leaflets: utilisation, implementation, provision, investigation, completion and so on. Linguists call them 'nominalisations': this means turning something — usually a verb — into a noun:

| | | |
|---|---|---|
| 'when you arrive' | becomes | 'on your arrival' |
| 'after paying' | becomes | 'subsequent to payment' |
| 'providing care' | becomes | 'the provision of care' |
| 'how effective treatment is' | becomes | 'the effectiveness of treatment'. |

So what's wrong with them? The problem is that writers often use nominalisations when they should use the verbs they come from. Like passive verbs, too many nominalisations make writing very dull and heavy going. Also, because most sentences need a verb, using nominalisations means you use extra words to say the same thing.

## Examples

Here are some examples of nominalisations, with plain-English versions underneath.

> **We had a discussion about the matter.**
> (We discussed the matter.)

> **The report made reference to staff shortages.**
> (The report referred to staff shortages.)

> **The decision was taken by the board.**
> (The board decided.)

## Giving clear instructions

Don't be afraid to give instructions. There always seems to be a fear of commands — maybe we're all just too polite! The most common fault is writing 'customers should do this' or 'you should do this' instead of just 'do this'.

When we speak, many of us feel it might sound harsh or rude to say things such as 'pass me the butter', 'move that table' or 'post this letter'. So we add phrases such as 'could you . . . ?', 'would you mind . . . ?' and 'do you think you could . . . ?'. As each of these is really a question, you could get the reply 'no I can't' or 'well, I could, but . . . '!

In spoken language we use other clues to work out what the speaker means: body language, tone of voice, facial expressions and our knowledge of the situation and the person. In written communication we don't have most of these clues, so the reader is more likely to be confused if we haven't been precise.

> If you could bring this letter to the appointment, it would be helpful.

Helpful yes, but is it essential? If you can't find the letter on the day of the appointment, will it matter?

> Please bring this letter with you to the appointment.

This is much clearer, but still polite. Putting 'please' in front is an easy way to soften the tone, but don't use 'please' if the instruction is something that must be done rather than something that would just be helpful.

> The dressing should be replaced every two days.

Should be done — but how much does it matter if it isn't? 'Replace the dressing every two days' is clearer and emphasises the importance of the instruction.

If you send out standard letters to members of the public for things such as hospital appointments, make sure you have enough variations or personalise the letters carefully. A letter which is designed to cover lots of possibilities will end up confusing the reader: they will find it difficult to see what information refers to them. Also, try to keep direct instructions separate from general information, so that the instructions don't get lost. If you need to give explanations and there are several instructions, consider using a clear checklist as a reminder.

And finally, think about the sequence of events. It's probably very obvious to you what order things have to be done in: just make sure it's equally clear to your reader. If you're not sure, ask a colleague (or, even better, someone outside your field of work) to read your instructions. They should be able to explain back to you what they would do. If they have any difficulties, you may need to revise your instructions.

## The audience

### Patients, professionals and others

To write information in a way that is suitable for our audience, we must first understand who that audience is. Try asking yourself *Who am I writing for?* The answer might be something like 'patients', 'case number 123', or 'the public'.

### Writing for individuals

You may have a lot of information about an individual or very little at all. But is it information about them as a person, or about a condition they have? Do you know, for example, how old they are, what education they have had? Do you know how well they can read, or whether they have any visual or reading difficulties?

## Writing for groups

Again, you need to consider any information you have about the group. But bear in mind that because the members of a group have something in common, it doesn't mean they are all the same.

## Writing for the general public

The 'public' is probably the most difficult audience to write for as it includes all kinds of people, with all levels of education and reading skills.

Some writers worry that they will be offending or patronising people if they write too simply. Think about that for a moment. If your bank writes to you in a concise, simple way, are you offended? Do you think your electricity supplier is patronising if they explain a new pricing policy in a clear way? Most busy people are just grateful to have information presented so that it is quick to read and take in. For those who want it, you can point out where to find more detail. In a document that is designed to inform, people should be able to get the meaning in just one reading.

### What does the reader know about the subject?

If you sit and listen to a bunch of people talking about a hobby or a sport you know nothing about, it can be like listening to a foreign language. Unfortunately, it can be the same if you join a new company. This is because, as we mentioned before, groups of people use specialised language to talk about things they know about.

When you are writing for the public it's important to know what they might already know about the subject. If they know a lot and you explain everything, they may get frustrated. If they know nothing and you use lots of technical terms without explaining them, you will lose their interest very quickly.

### How does the reader feel?

Someone visiting a hospital may be well educated and highly literate, but they may have a lot on their mind. That means they probably won't concentrate fully on a sign, or on a form they are given to fill in. Information that confuses patients, their carers and their families takes away their independence — something which is especially important to people with a long-term illness or disability.

If people feel belittled, confused, angry or frightened, it may affect how well they cooperate.

### Their needs and yours

What are you trying to communicate? And what does your reader want to know?

Consider this example of how a member of the public and a professional person can see things differently.

A new pet owner takes her small kitten to the vet. The animal is snuffling, has sticky eyes, and is clearly finding it difficult to breathe. She puts the kitten on the examination table and the vet begins to talk about bacteria. But the first thing the cat owner wants to know is 'will my kitten be OK?'

The owner:

- doesn't know whether the breathing problems are dangerous;
- doesn't know whether this could lead to permanent eye problems; and
- has never had this experience before.

The vet:

- knows the problem is not serious and can be cleared up with antibiotics; and
- has seen lots of cases like this.

In this situation, the vet is busy explaining the cause of the problem and ignoring the owner's concerns. The vet's explanation will probably be overlooked, as the anxious owner is unlikely to be receptive of the information. All too often professional people start with the bit that interests them — the reason, the policy behind a decision, the explanation. Try to keep a sense of your reader's priorities in mind when you are writing. For many people, anything to do with illness, hospitals, medicines and doctors seems frightening. By dealing with people's main concerns early on in what you write, you are more likely to get their attention. How long you keep that attention probably depends on what you are telling them. But if what you write is clear and well structured, at least they will be able to refer back to it later.

It's natural to assume our readers are just like us. Make sure you know, as far as possible, who your readers are and what they know, and try to think about how they feel.

## Design matters

Good design is always important, but the importance of design does depend on what you are writing. Clearly it's a higher priority in something like a poster or a website, as these aim to grab the reader's attention quickly. Just beware of design concepts that overwhelm the message. Have you ever seen an advert and thought it was clever or funny but couldn't figure out what it was actually advertising? Or come across a really colourful website but couldn't find the information you wanted?

Even a simple letter can benefit from a careful layout, so here are a few things to consider.

### Font

- **Size** Try to aim for a font size of 12 point. If you are pushed for space you could use 11 or even 10, but don't go below that. If you know your readers are likely to have difficulties with their vision, the Royal National Institute for the Blind recommends a minimum type size of 14 point.
- **Shape** 'Sans serif' fonts such as Arial are generally considered easier to read than 'serif' fonts such as Times New Roman.

### Emphasis

Avoid the following:

- BLOCK CAPITALS — they are more difficult to read and it looks as if you are SHOUTING!
- <u>Underlining text</u> — it can hide the downward strokes of letters such as g, j and y, and close the bottom of letters such as h, k, m, n and x.
- Too many *italics* — italic text, especially if it's a small font size, is difficult to read.

If you want to emphasise something, use **bold**. Just remember that any form of emphasis loses its effect if you overdo it.

## Line length and spacing

The length of lines and how many words they contain will vary according to the nature of the document (for example whether you are writing a web page, or an article in newspaper-style columns).

The space between lines (called 'leading') should always be greater than the space between words. Normally for 10-point body text your leading will be 12 point.

## Other design points

- You can use lists to break up information.
- If you need to number paragraphs to refer to them elsewhere, try to avoid academic-style numbering, such as 1.2.1.b.
- Remember to leave plenty of white space around text.
- For most documents you should use left alignment, rather than justified text. With justification, the spacing between words varies to make each line the same length, and this makes it harder to read.
- Clear writing can reduce unnecessary stress and worry for patients, their families and carers.

---

### In summary

- Use short, active sentences.
- Write in a personal, friendly tone.
- Give clear instructions.
- Avoid or explain technical language.
- Think about your audience, their knowledge and situation.
- Design your document thoughtfully.

---

## Answers to exercises

### Make it short

- Remember that the common symptoms of **multiple sclerosis** can also be symptoms of other conditions.
- If you have an allergic reaction, **stop taking the tablets and tell your doctor**. Symptoms of an allergic reaction include difficulty breathing or breathlessness, unexpected swelling and flushing. The symptoms could cause you to collapse.

## Make it active

- Take care when opening the door.
- Apply the cream sparingly and if you do not see any improvement within five days, consult your doctor.
- We will send a report to your doctor.
- We realise car parking on site is very limited, and we are making plans to solve the problem.
- If you take too much of this medicine, get medical advice immediately, even if you feel well.

## Make it personal

- You must send us . . .
- You must tell us . . .
- You can get advice from . . .

## Big words and technical stuff

- When [product name] touches the wound, it forms a gel that helps the healing process.
- Food intolerance is an unusual reaction your body has to something you have eaten, but which does not involve your immune system.
- Food allergy is when your immune system reacts to something specific that you have eaten.

# 3

# Referencing

*Melissa McClean*

Referencing is an integral part of medical writing. A reference is a detailed description of an information source you have used to construct your document. It can be a book or a chapter from a book, an article from a journal or a newspaper, and in this electronic age, a website, e-book or e-journal.

To reference correctly, you must collect and assemble the details of your information sources and include these in your text. Referencing should not be left until the end of your document production; it is an important part of your writing, and referencing as you write will allow you to develop your ideas.

---

 Make referencing as you write one of your golden rules.

---

There are two main methods of referencing: author/date and numeric, although there are many individual styles, which will be discussed later.

## Why reference?
- To acknowledge the work of others
- To give credibility and reliability to your work
- To support the arguments you have made
- To show that you have read widely and considered the relevant literature that already exists on your topic
- To validate any points that you have made and verify any quotations
- To allow the reader to locate your sources independently
- To follow academic writing standards
- To avoid plagiarism — if the sources you use are not acknowledged, this may lead to the suspicion that you are trying to pass off someone else's work as your own

## What to reference

A number of sources may be used in the construction of your document. These include:

- books or chapters in books
- journal, newspaper or magazine articles
- conference proceedings and papers
- government publications
- media such as videos, DVDs, TV excerpts, sound recordings
- personal communications such as letters and e-mails
- electronic sources such as websites, web pages, e-books, e-journals, software
- information such as tables, graphs, photographs.

## When to reference

- When you are quoting another person
- When paraphrasing or summarising someone else's ideas or opinions
- When using someone else's data, diagrams or images
- When using controversial facts or opinions that may be challenged

## Reference styles

For any source that is used in the construction of your document the information must appear in two places:

- **In-text (the textual reference)** — brief identifying information in the body of the document that directly follows any quotation or summary of another source.
- **Reference list** — a list at the end of the text that contains detailed information about each source used.

There are many acceptable forms of referencing. Each style has rules about how a reference should be written, which includes punctuation, font, capitalisation etc., for both in-text references and the reference list.

Each university faculty, academic journal or book publisher has their own preferred reference style.

▶ Always check the reference style that is required before you start writing.

The main referencing styles used in medical writing are Vancouver, Harvard and AMA.

## Vancouver reference style

The Vancouver style is commonly used in documents in the sciences, medicine, health sciences, health promotion and public health. This style uses a numeric system which allows the text to flow, as there are no intrusions by in-text citations. It also allows the reader to check the reference list easily at the end of the document. The referencing software EndNote uses this style.

### In-text references

Each reference within the text is assigned an Arabic number as it is cited. This number becomes the identifier of that source and is reused each time that source is cited in the document. These numbers can be enclosed in:

- **round brackets** – *the validity of this method was determined.(4)*
- **square brackets** – *the validity of this method was determined.[4]*
- **superscript** – *the validity of this method was determined.*[4]

The numbers are outside (to the right of) commas and full stops and inside (to the left of) colons and semicolons.

When multiple references are listed an en rule (dash) is used to join the first and last inclusive numbers, e.g. (5–8).

Commas are used (without spaces) to separate non-inclusive numbers, e.g. (3,7,11,14).

When the author(s) name is written in the sentence the reference number must still be included, e.g. *Brown and colleagues (7) proposed . . .*

Details of personal communications such as e-mails and letters are placed in brackets in the text with the author and date included, e.g. . . . *was confirmed (Higgins S 2000, personal communication, June 6).*

Single quotation marks must be used to enclose a direct quotation. Double quotation marks are used to enclose quotations within quotations. If a word is misspelt or incorrect in quoted material, type *[sic]* after it to indicate that this is an original source and you have not changed it.

## Reference list

The reference list at the end of the text is arranged numerically in the same order in which the references are listed in the text. Both punctuation and the order of the references must be correct.

The titles of books and journals are not italicised or placed in quotation marks. Journal titles are abbreviated using the format published in *Index Medicus*, which is available in book form in libraries or online. No punctuation is used in journal titles, only spaces.

If there are six or fewer authors of an article or a book, then *all* authors must be listed, e.g. *Brown SK, Smith JC.* If there are seven or more authors, then only the first six are listed and *et al.* is added after the sixth, e.g. *Brown SK, Smith JC, Pina IK, Hogg B, Jones N, Philips LL et al.*

The following are the details required for the reference list for all the different sources that can be used.

### Book

(Reference number) Author(s). Title. Edition (only second and subsequent editions). City of publication. Publisher. Date of publication, e.g. *(2) Speicher CE. The Right Test, 3rd edn. Philadelphia: WB Saunders; 1998.*

### Editors, compilers as author

(Reference number) Author(s), editor(s). Title. Edition (only second and subsequent editions). City of publication. Publisher. Date of publication. Page numbers (if applicable), e.g. *(20) Major RH (ed) Classic Descriptions of Disease, 2nd edn. Springfield, Illinois: Baillière, Tindall & Cox; 1939, p. 631–2.*

### Book chapter

(Reference number) Author(s). Chapter title. In: Book editor(s). Book title. City of publication. Publisher. Date of publication. Page numbers, e.g. *(6) Stephens NL, Kroeger EA. Ultrastructure, biophysics and biochemistry of airway smooth muscle. In: Nadel JA, ed. Physiology and Pharmacology of the Airways. New York: Marcel Dekker; 1980, p. 31–121.*

## Journal article
(Reference number) Author(s). Title. Journal title (abbreviated). Publication date. Volume (issue number if known): page numbers, e.g. *(12) Ray CS, Sue DY, Bray G, Hansen JE, Wasserman K. Effects of obesity on respiratory function. Am Rev Respir Dis 1983; 128: 501–6.*

## No author given
(Reference number) Title. Journal title (abbreviated). Publication date. Volume (issue number if known). Page numbers, e.g. *(25) Patent briefing. Drug Delivery 2001; 8(3): 179–81.*

## E-journal article
(Reference number) Author(s). Title. Journal title [form of item] latest update of site [date cited]; Volume (issue if known): page numbers. Available from: URL: *web address*, e.g. *(30) Van Doornum S, Jennings GLR, Wicks IP. Reducing the cardiovascular disease burden in rheumatoid arthritis. Med J Aust [serial online] 2006 May [cited 2006 May 20]; 184 (6): 287–90. Available from: URL: http://www.mja.com.au*

## Conference proceedings
(Reference number) Editor(s). Title. Relevant information (conference; date; location). City of publication. Publisher. Date of publication, e.g. *(9) Kimura J, Shibasaki H (eds) Recent advances in clinical neurophysiology. Proceedings of the 10th International Congress of EMG and Clinical Neurophysiology, 15–19 Oct 1995, Kyoto, Japan. Amsterdam: Elsevier; 1996.*

## Conference presentation
(Reference number) Author(s). Presentation title. In: Editor(s). Conference proceedings. Relevant information (conference; date; location). City of publication. Publisher. Date of publication. Page numbers, e.g. *(14) Wood F, Strider V. Geothermal changes in Mordica. In: Harrison P, Bloom G, eds. Proceedings of the 21st Annual Meeting of the Geological Society, 20–24 Nov 2000, Sydney, Australia. Amsterdam: Elsevier; 2001, p. 21.*

## Newspaper or magazine article
(Reference number) Author. Article title. Newspaper name. Date. Newspaper section (if applicable). Page number(s), e.g. *(12) Silmalis L. A Lung Health Test for Tunnel. Sunday Telegraph 14 May 2006; p. 11.*

**Personal communications**
Not included in the reference list as the reader cannot trace them.

**Websites**
(Reference number) Author(s). Title. Available at: URL: address. Accessed date, e.g. *(1) National Asthma Council of Australia. Asthma Management Handbook. Available from: URL: http://www.national asthma.org.au/. Accessed 20 June 2005.*

**Web document**
(Reference number) Author(s). Title. Website title. Available at: URL: address. Accessed date, e.g. *(10) Jenkins C. Asthma. Health Insite. Available at: URL: http://www.healthinsite.gov.au/. Accessed 13 January 2004.*

**Multimedia material**
(Reference number) Author(s)/director(s) Title [form of item]. Place of publication/production. Publisher or producer. Date, e.g. *(21) Moore M. Fahrenheit 9/11 [DVD]. Culver City, California: Columbia Tristar Home Entertainment, 2004.*

## Harvard or APA

The Harvard style is also known as the citation method, the APA (American Psychological Association) system or the author/date system. It is the most widespread from of referencing and is commonly used in the humanities and social sciences. This style involves citing the author, the date, and sometimes the page number of the information source.

An alternative method in the Harvard style is the use of footnotes. This involves the insertion of a superscript number in the text where the reference should be. This number corresponds to a note at the bottom of the page that contains the corresponding details of the information source. The footnotes are numbered consecutively throughout the document. They are not repeated, even if a new page begins.

### In-text references

For each reference in the text only the surname of the author and the date of publication, placed in brackets at the end of a sentence before a full stop, are necessary, e.g. . . . *the validity of this method was determined (Smith, 2000).*

Specific page numbers are unnecessary if you are referring to the general theme of a book. If you are quoting or referring to data then page numbers must be included. For journal articles, the page numbers are included, e.g. . . . *the validity of this method (Smith, 2000, p. 33).*

Where there are two or three authors, all are listed in-text, e.g. (Smith & Jones, 1998); (Smith, Jones & Phillips, 2001).

If there are more than three authors, the first author is listed followed by *et al.,* e.g. *(Smith et al., 2004).*

The author's name may be included in-text, followed by the date of publication in brackets, e.g. *A recent study by Jones and colleagues (2001) . . ..*

If there are several citations for the same author in the same year, the letters a, b, c, etc., are placed after the date of publication, e.g. *(Smith, 1999a); (Smith, 1999b).*

When two or more authors are cited at the same point in-text, then they are presented alphabetically and separated by a semi-colon, e.g. *(Smith, 2000; Walker & Hammond, 2004).*

Personal communications are included in-text but not in the reference list, e.g. . . . *was confirmed (Higgins S, 2000, pers. comm., 6 June).*

## Reference list

The reference list at the end of the text is arranged alphabetically by the author's surname. When more than one work is cited for the same author the references are listed chronologically (i.e. earliest date first and most recent last).

* Book and journal titles must be *italicised* or underlined. Journal titles are not abbreviated.
* The second and subsequent lines of the reference must be indented to highlight the alphabetical order.
* All elements of the reference after the date are separated by commas, with a full stop concluding the citation.
* Titles of journal and newspaper articles, book chapter titles and conference presentation titles are placed in single quotation marks.
* The following are the details required for the reference list for all the different sources that can be used.

## Book

Author(s). Date of publication. Title. Publisher. Place of publication, e.g. Speicher, CE 1998. *The Right Test,* WB Saunders Company, Philadelphia.

## Editors, compilers as authors

Author(s)/(editors). Date of publication. Title. Edition (if applicable). Publisher. Place of Publication, e.g. Major, RH (ed.) 1939, *Classic Descriptions of Disease*, 2nd edn. Baillière, Tindall & Cox, Springfield, Illinois.

## Book chapter

Author(s). Date of publication. 'Chapter title'. In: Editor(s). Book title. Publisher. Place of publication. Page numbers, e.g. Stephens NL, Kroeger EA 1980 'Ultrastructure, biophysics and biochemistry of airway smooth muscle'. In: Nadel JA (ed) *Physiology and Pharmacology of the Airways*. Marcel Dekker, New York, pp. 31–121.

## Journal article

Author(s). Date of publication. 'Title'. Journal title. Volume number. Issue number (if known). Page numbers, e.g. Ray, CS, Sue DY, Bray G, Hansen JE, Wasserman K 1983 'Effects of obesity on respiratory function', *American Review of Respiratory Disease 128: 501–506.*

## No author given

'Title'. Date of publication. Journal title. Volume number. Issue number (if known). Page numbers, e.g. 'Patent briefing' 2001. *Drug Delivery* 8(3): 179–181.

## E-journal article

Author(s). Date of publication. 'Title'. Journal title. Volume number. Issue number (if known). Page numbers. Date retrieved. Where retrieved from, e.g. Van Doornum S, Jennings GLR, Wicks IP 2006 'Reducing the cardiovascular disease burden in rheumatoid arthritis'. *Medical Journal of Australia 184(6): 287–290.* Retrieved 20 May 2006, from http://www.mja.com.au

## Conference proceedings

Author(s)/editor(s). Date of publication. Title. Relevant information (conference; location). Publisher. Place of publication, e.g. Kimura J, Shibasaki H (eds) 1996 'Recent advances in clinical neurophysiology',

*Proceedings of the 10th International Congress of EMG and Clinical Neurophysiology*, Kyoto, Japan. Elsevier, Amsterdam.

## Conference paper
Author(s). Date of publication. 'Presentation title'. Conference proceedings. Relevant information (conference, location). Page numbers, e.g. Wood F, Strider V 2001 'Geothermal changes in Mordica', *Proceedings of the 21st Annual Meeting of the Geological Society*, Sydney, Australia, p. 21.

## Newspaper or magazine article
Author(s). Year of publication. 'Title'. Newspaper name. Date. Page number, e.g. Silmalis L 2006 'A Lung Health Test for Tunnel', *Sunday Telegraph* 14 May, p. 11.

## Websites
Author(s). Year. Title. Date retrieved or viewed. Website address, e.g. National Asthma Council of Australia 1998, *Asthma Management Handbook*. Retrieved 20 June 2005, from http://www.nationalasthma. org.au/

## Web document
Author(s). Date of publication (if known: put n.d. if not). Title. Date retrieved or viewed. Website address, e.g. Jenkins C (n.d.) *Asthma*. Retrieved 13 January 2004, from http://www.healthinsite.gov.au/

## Multimedia material
Title. Date of recording. Format. Publisher. Place of recording. Any information that might be useful, e.g. *Fahrenheit 9/11 2004*, DVD, Columbia Tristar Home Entertainment, Culver City, Calif. Written, produced and directed by Michael Moore.

## AMA

The AMA (American Medical Association) style is used in documents for medicine, health and biological sciences. This style follows the same rules as Vancouver, the only difference being that the book and journal titles are *italicised*.

## Other styles

Other referencing styles that are used for writing include:

- MLA (Modern Language Association) — used in literature, arts and humanities
- Chicago — used in the 'real world' by books, magazines, newspapers and other non-academic publications
- Turbian — used in all subjects by students.

## EndNote

EndNote is one of a number of personalised reference software programs that have been designed so that users can create a database of references and images. Each reference in the database contains all the information required to create a reference list. The main functions of EndNote include the following:

- the storage and organisation of references
- to allow the direct importation of references from electronic databases such as PubMed, Medline, or you can type them in yourself
- to allow references to be added to your Microsoft Word document as you write
- to generate a reference list in the appropriate reference style for your article, thesis or book
- to simplify referencing.

---

### In summary

- Reference as you write.
- Avoid plagiarism.
- Source information must appear in-text and in the reference list at the end of the text.
- Vancouver, Harvard and AMA are the main referencing styles in medical writing.
- Check the reference style required before you write.
- Follow the rules for the reference style used.

---

## Further reading

Any university library website will offer guides to referencing. For further information on referencing print sources:

Snooks & Co (2002) *Style Manual for Authors, Editors and Printers*, 6th edn. Canberra, Australia: John Wiley & Sons.

For further information on referencing electronic sources:

Li X, Crane N (1993) *Electronic Style: a Guide to Writing Electronic Information*. Westport, CA: Meckler.

National Library of Medicine. Recommended formats for Bibliographic Citation Supplement: Internet Formats. National Library of Medicine. Available at: URL: *http://www.nlm.nih.gov/pubs/formats/internet.pdf*.

## Sources

Curtin University of Technology Library, Referencing Resources. Curtin University of Technology, Western Australia. Available at: URL: *http://www.library. curtin.edu.au/referencing/index.html*. Accessed May 2006.

University of Southern Queensland Library, Referencing Guides. University of Southern Queensland, Queensland. Available at: URL: *http://www.usq.edu.au/ library/help*. Accessed May 2006.

University of Queensland Library. 'How-to' Guides. University of Queensland, Queensland. Available at: URL: *http://www.library.uq.edu.au/useit/ index.html*. Accessed May 2006.

University of Western Australia Library. How to Cite Your Sources. University of Western Australia, Western Australia. Available at: URL: *http:// www.library.wa.edu.au/education_training_support/guides/how_to_cite_your_ sources.html*. Accessed May 2006.

# Section Two

Reviews and reports

# 4

# Writing a research report

*Maria Kouimtzi*

Good-quality research is lost if it is not written up correctly. Well-presented research is necessary in order to share your results with the rest of the academic world, both to showcase your hard work and also so that other researchers can take off from where you stopped. You may also simply need to write it up as part of coursework. Scientific research is of no value if it remains as scribbles in a notebook lying on a laboratory bench somewhere, and in certain circumstances (e.g. clinical research) it would be unethical not to publish it.

Many researchers feel terrified at the prospect of writing up their work. They worry about using the correct vocabulary and grammar, and often resort to using complicated sentences and unfamiliar language. Consequently, the resulting report may be difficult to comprehend and the conclusion of the research is lost in the context.

You don't need the flair of a novelist in order to write a good research report. What you do need is the ability to write clear, grammatically correct English, and explain the work you did in a logical way. You need to avoid unnecessary jargon and long sentences at all costs. The specialised vocabulary will probably be familiar to you, as you will probably have read many published papers on your subject area already.

## Your audience

Before you start writing your report, you need to think carefully who your audience will be. Will it be an academic examiner (your tutor, or your PhD supervisor)? Will it be other researchers in your field? Regardless of who you are writing for, one rule applies to all written research intended for publication or assessment: the word limit. Find out what it is and stick to it. This is especially important for abstracts, which are covered on page 65.

If you are writing for an academic examiner who will mark your project, you must be aware that you are assessed on how well you understand the topic and why you approached the research in the way that you did. Therefore, it is important to explain effectively what you did and why, to show that you have read the relevant background literature and understand the subject adequately.

If you are writing for other researchers in your field, such as for a paper to be included in conference proceedings, it is important to recognise the unfortunate fact that most readers will only read the introduction and the conclusions — but you know that already, as you are a reader too. You need to concentrate your efforts on those two sections so that they describe your work clearly, concisely and understandably.

## Structure

For the majority of research reports the IMRAD (Introduction, Methods, Results And Discussion) structure is appropriate. This is the most common format for writing up scientific research for sciences such as physics and biology, as well as the social sciences. This is because the IMRAD structure is a direct reflection of the scientific discovery process (and not simply a convention used by publishers!):

- **Introduction** — You describe what other researchers have found on a subject so far, and you ask a question.
- **Methods** — You do research using nominated methods and materials in order to answer that question.
- **Results** — You get results from your research and analyse them, possibly using relevant statistical tests.
- **Discussion** — You discuss whether your results answered your question and, if they did, what was the answer; you also put your results into the context of the rest of the field.

## Title

Deciding on the title for a research report can be a challenge. It must be accurate, specific, concise and informative.

You may find it easier to write the introduction first and then the title. By doing this, and thus having 'set the scene', you will have a clearer idea of what you did. Another way is to imagine that you are explaining what you did to a layperson. This can help to explain your research in very simple terms, distilling your work into a few simple sentences, which can then form the basis of an effective title.

As a rule, shorter titles are easier to read and grab the reader's attention. However, titles that are too short may omit important information, such as a novel method that was used. Additionally, it is important not to mention insignificant details in the title, which may add unnecessary bulk. For example, 'Eradication of head lice in a preschool population' does not give an indication that wet-combing was compared to malathion treatment, whereas the fact that the children were under 5 years of age may not be that important in the subject of head lice prevalence. A more effective and accurate title would be: 'A randomised controlled trial of wet-combing versus malathion for head lice'.

It is best not to use abbreviations in titles, unless they are very common. If you feel that you must use abbreviations, explain what they mean in the abstract and in the first sentences of the introduction (abbreviations are covered later in this chapter on page 73).

Some editors advise avoiding 'cute' or quirky titles, but I disagree. If you can be snappy, make an impact and hence grab your reader's interest by the title, surely that is a good thing. Conference proceedings can be overwhelming, big and heavy volumes that are usually read on the train journey home — an unusual title will make the reader curious to read the rest of your research report. In some cases, a title such as 'Are head lice attracted by obese children?' may be a more interesting and effective title than 'Head lice prevalence and body mass index'.

If you are writing a report as part of your coursework and your tutor has already set the title, then use it. Remember, it is your tutor who will be marking your report, so don't try to outsmart him or her!

## Abstract

In my opinion this is the most challenging part of the report. The abstract needs to reflect accurately what you did, why you did it, and what you found — all in a short paragraph.

You will most probably have a set word limit you need to adhere to. For abstracts to be submitted to journals or conferences, this limit is given in the 'Instructions to authors' (read these *very* carefully!). Word limits for abstracts vary and can range from 50 to 300 words. If you don't have a set word limit, then set your own before you start. As a general rule, 200 words is the average, no matter how complicated your research is. A long abstract defeats the object of summarising your work.

Again, the exercise of explaining what you did to a layperson may help you here. When you try to explain complicated scientific research to a layperson you simplify what you did by omitting unnecessary detail to focus on the important facts. This is exactly what you need to do to write the 'foundation' of a good abstract. To this basic foundation you can add the scientific details, but only the most important ones to keep the reader focused on the main issue. Avoid giving statistical details in the abstract, as they distract the reader. You will have the opportunity to present your statistics in the main body of your report.

If you write a very short abstract (80–100 words), which you feel presents your results clearly without omitting important information and explains why you did the research, don't be tempted to lengthen it — you have written the perfect abstract.

---

➤  Remember that the set word limit is exactly that — a limit. It is not a description of the ideal abstract length.

---

If you don't need to submit the abstract in advance of the full report (as is the case with submission of abstracts for conference proceedings), you will find it easier to write the abstract after you have completed the report. As the abstract is the summary of what you did, it is easier to know what you need to focus on after you have written the full story.

If you have difficulty writing the abstract as 'free-flowing' text, another technique is to write one or two sentences summarising each section of your report. This may include a couple of sentences to summarise the introduction, a sentence to summarise the methods, and so on. Section headings can be added in capital letters to separate each part. It is not customary to have headings such as Introduction or Discussion, but you may use Aims for an introductory section. For example:

> The prevalence of head lice is rising and numerous researchers have tried to explain the reasons. We investigated whether the increase in obesity is correlated to the prevalence of head lice. METHODS: 764 children were scanned for head lice, weighed, and measured for height. RESULTS: 128 children were infested with head lice. Of those, 25% had a body mass index (BMI) over 25. Of the 636 children without head lice 140 had a BMI over 25. Our results show that head lice prevalence is not correlated to BMI. Other factors, such as resistance to parasiticides and parent-parasiticide phobia, are responsible for the rising prevalence of head lice in children.

## Introduction/hypothesis

In the Introduction you need to 'set the scene' for your work. You should state the question that you are trying to answer with your research and explain what made you ask that question. Examples of questions that you may be trying to answer are:

- Are we faced with an unsatisfactory situation (for example ineffective disease management, laborious methods of performing a task) and you are seeking ways of improving it?
- Have others researched the topic but stated that more is needed to reach a conclusion?
- Are you duplicating others' work, possibly using different methods, to confirm their results? (If so, it would be relevant to summarise the results and the conclusions of other researchers in your Introduction.)

When you are describing the problem that led you to perform the research, move from general information to specific information. Describe the general situation and then start presenting information specific to the topic. An example of such a flow of information in the introduction of a report about treatment of a disease, would be descriptions of:

- the incidence of a disease in the general population and what the symptoms of the disease are
- which symptom is the most troublesome for patients
- what the current therapeutic options are to manage the symptom, and why they are unsatisfactory
- review of the literature to check whether others have tried to improve management of the symptom
- your hypothesis
- your experiment.

Make clear the links between the problem and the solution, the question asked, the research design, research already conducted, and your experiment.

It is important to review the literature to demonstrate what is already known on the topic and what your work adds to the global knowledge base. A good review of the literature will form the basis of an effective introduction. It will demonstrate why your work is useful and how it has built up from research others have done. If you do not review the literature, readers will be asking why you chose to do the work in the first place.

When selecting studies for your literature review, you should not try to write a mini systematic review of the relevant literature. You need to read all of the relevant literature, but your goal should be to summarise previous work by mentioning the important points only. You may wish to mention flawed studies that were not used to draw conclusions, stating why you think they were flawed and why the evidence cannot support the conclusions. The principle of writing clearly and concisely always applies. Literature reviews should be both brief and to the point. If you need to comment on an important study in more detail, do this in the Discussion section.

If you are writing for other healthcare professionals, try to avoid background information that your readers would probably be expected to know already, as this will make the introduction sound like a textbook. However, if you are writing a research report as part of coursework, then you will probably be expected to write a brief summary of basic information.

After you have 'set the scene' by presenting what is already known on the topic and explained the problem, your readers will be ready for a short statement of what you have done. In a couple of sentences describe your experiment. This will usually include:

- hypothesis(es)
- research question(s)
- general experimental design or method
- justification of method if alternatives exist.

## Methods

In this section you need to describe accurately what you did, why you did it, and how you did it. While writing the Methods section it is helpful to remember that the end result should contain information that is accurate enough for someone (who hasn't done this type of experiment before) to be able to replicate your work and obtain the same results. Therefore, you must be complete, accurate and precise, listing all steps in the order in which you did them.

Explain why you used the methods that you did — this will avoid making the section read like a cookbook. If you deviated from your initial method, explain why. You need to state what you really did, not what was supposed to happen or what the textbook said. For example, if you planned to study the effects of a drug on 200 patients but 120 dropped out of the study because they couldn't tolerate the drug, you need to explain why they weren't able to tolerate the drug and what interventions (if any) were made to improve patient compliance. Also state how many patients actually completed the study as originally planned.

Studies are very commonly criticised because the authors fail to explain the study design adequately. Readers will want to know your research methods so that they can assess whether they were appropriate to answer the question you posed in the Introduction. They will be asking: Was the study randomised? Blinded? Cohort? Case-controlled? Were the statistical tests applied appropriate? Make sure you supply this information in this section, and explain why you chose the method you did.

If relevant, state why the sample size in your study was adequate to test your hypothesis. The sample size should be large enough to show statistical significance without the standard deviation affecting the result. A very common error occurs when a clinically important difference fails to show as a statistically significant difference because the sample size is too small (the study is 'underpowered'). Rarely, when the sample size is too large, a very small difference in the results, which is not clinically significant, is shown as statistically significant (the study is 'overpowered'). These two scenarios should be addressed in the Discussion section, where you should assess the implications of your work in practice.

Sometimes this section is titled 'Materials and Methods'. If you need to give many details you may wish to split this section into 'Materials', 'Apparatus', and 'Methods'. Name all the materials you used, including standard laboratory reagents and excipients, together with the name of the manufacturers, as well as the type, model and manufacturer of all equipment used.

If you used a specialised software package to do the statistical analysis, you should state that too. Always give full details of the statistical tests you used to test your results, and explain why you did so. Contrary to what some researchers think, the two-way $t$-test is not the standard statistical test to be used for all data. If you don't know why a certain statistical test is appropriate for your data, you are probably using an inappropriate test and may reach incorrect conclusions. Even if you are lucky and obtain the correct conclusion with inappropriate tests, readers who are competent in statistics may dismiss your results. The bad news is that you might have to brush up your statistics; the good news is that current computer software performs complicated statistical calculations painlessly.

It is in the Methods section that you should give details of any ethical approval you may have obtained. Ethical approval is fundamental to good research practice and therefore many journals decline to publish studies that do not include such details.

## Results

This section should be easy to write: you state what answers you obtained to the questions you posed earlier. Don't be tempted to analyse or draw conclusions from your results — you have plenty of room for this in the Discussion section. In the Results section you need only to state the figures you obtained — the easiest way for the reader to comprehend your results would be to present them as a table or a graph.

## Tables

When formatting a table, note the following points:

- Every table should have a title placed above it.
- Rows and columns should be clearly labelled.
- Use rules (lines) to separate columns and/or rows, depending on the table size; shading can also help.
- Leave some space between rows and columns so that the information in each cell is not crowded or difficult to read.
- If you need to explain or comment on information contained in a cell, do so by using a footnote. The footnote marker should be positioned in the cell and the footnote text below the table, not at the end of the page. This way it will be clear that it refers to text within the table and not to text in the main body of the report.
- If an entire table is from another source this should be referenced by inserting a reference marker in the title.

## Graphs

When constructing a graph, the same principles apply as when writing text: you need to write (illustrate) clearly and avoid unnecessary jargon. Sophisticated computer software can enable you to produce colour illustrations, many different designs for data points and line types, and three-dimensional illustrations. However, elaborate designs are often confusing, distract the reader from the main focus, and even worse, sometimes are misleading. A simple line graph is very often the most clear and effective way to get your message across.

Bar charts are most often used to compare the size of items, such as results or populations. As space is often limited, especially if your report will be submitted for publication, you can present the results in a bar chart to accompany the main text, thereby saving valuable space.

Bar charts are useful to highlight a significant difference between measurements.

## Reporting statistics

When you are reporting statistics in the text, you need to report five types of information:

- mean
- standard deviation (SD)
- test used
- sample size ($n$)
- probability of significance ($p$).

You may also wish to include the confidence interval (CI). For example, the following statement contains all the above:

The prevalence of head lice in group A decreased from $87 \pm 4.3$(SD)% to $43.2 \pm 5.7$(SD)% in 16 children. This difference was considered significant by applying the $t$-test ($p < 0.05$).

When listing probability values, it is helpful to list the actual values even when differences are not considered statistically significant. For example, $p < 0.01$ for a comparison indicates a very strong significance compared to $p < 0.5$ that you may have found for another parameter. Similarly, $p > 0.55$ does not exclude the possibility of a statistically significant difference as strongly as $p > 0.9$.

Be careful to report statistics as accurately as your initial measurement. For example, if you are measuring body weight and the scales you used give results with one decimal point (77.2 kg), then don't quote results and standard deviations with three decimal points ($75.37 \pm 12.576$ (SD) kg). Quote all your values with the same number of decimal points *consistently*.

There are some conventions that you should follow: means and standard deviations are written as '75 kg $\pm$ 12 (SD)' or '75 $\pm$ 12 (SD) kg'; sample size ($n$), probability ($p$), and $t$-test are always written in italics; ANOVA is written in capitals.

## Discussion

Now that you have some data, you need to explain how your findings support or dismiss your hypothesis. This is the most important section of your report. It is where you address the answer to the question(s) you stated in the Introduction.

Write what your findings mean. Specific questions that should be answered in this section include the following:

- How do your findings prove or dismiss your hypothesis?
- Do you see any patterns in the data, and if so what are they?
- Did you find what you expected to find, or were you surprised? Often the parts that surprised you are the most significant and the most interesting.
- Is further research needed? In the real world, researchers often use this section to promote interest (and seek funding) for their next project.
- How do your results affect established practice?
- Did you change your clinical practice as a result of your research?

## Conclusion

This is the easiest part to write and the one that makes 'the big bang'. Just write your main results in a couple of sentences, stating whether your hypothesis is dismissed or proven.

## Authors

If you conducted your research as part of team, you should state all the team members who contributed to the work. It is customary to state the name of the main researcher first and the rest of the team in alphabetical order of their surnames. The first author is usually the one who wrote up the report and the one to whom all correspondence querying any aspects of the report should be addressed. If a member of the team is a highly qualified academic who supervised the work and provided guidance, then his or her name is usually last.

## Key words

Key words will be used to index your work and facilitate a search. Nowadays, where information is abundant, information retrieval is of paramount importance. It doesn't matter how important your findings are: if your target audience cannot find them, then the information may as well be considered lost — it will probably be archived on a hard disk that nobody ever accesses, or left on the library shelf.

Key words are required when submitting work for publication. It would be good to check the relevant medical subject headings (MeSH) and submit 3 to 10 terms that capture the main topic as key words.

MeSH terminology is a vocabulary which is used to retrieve information on medical topics. For example, in Medline, MeSH terms are used to perform specific subject searches and will retrieve information that may use different terminology for the same concept. Therefore, by providing MeSH headings as key words for your research, you are ensuring rapid and effective retrieval of it after publication.

## Language and style

Unnecessary jargon obscures meaning and wastes the reader's time and patience. Your sentences must be clear and easily understood, so that the reader absorbs the ideas effectively. For your Materials and Methods and Results sections, use the past tense, for example:

* The instrumental tablets press was used . . .
* Tablet hardness was found to be proportional to the amount of magnesium stearate . . .

The key here is to be consistent. Some may even argue that it doesn't matter if you make an error: if you are consistent and have made the error throughout your report, by the end your reader will be convinced that you are following a new terminology convention!

Traditionally, the passive voice and formal English have been used in writing scientific reports. However, there is an increasing tendency to use second person, as this makes the report easier to read and more informal. If the authors are a scientific team, describing what 'we' found gives the impression that they worked as a team — the reality may of course be very different. (For more information about style for medical writing, see Chapter 1.)

It is good practice to avoid abbreviated terms as much as possible. However, it is not practical to avoid them altogether. Where certain abbreviations are used routinely, the use of the full term may be interpreted as unfamiliarity with the subject. Every discipline, specialisation, course and professor seems to favour different abbreviations and style, and different audiences will be familiar with different abbreviations. For a list of commonly used medical abbreviations, see page 463.

You will most probably have a word limit for your report. Although this may initially seem huge and you are worried about whether you will be able to fill the pages, if you describe everything you need to and analyse your results sufficiently, you'll probably have trouble remaining within the limit. Shortening a paper so that it is within a set word limit shouldn't be too difficult. Ask yourself whether each table needs all the information it shows, whether information in the text can be condensed into a table instead, or whether all the information in the Introduction and Discussion is essential. Deleting a few words here and there can make a big difference and will probably make the report easier to read.

Finally, when you think that you have finished, don't forget to use the spell checker and the grammar check on your word processor. These tools have done wonders for improving the quality of written work over the past decade. Be sure to use them, but always double-check the suggestions for change that they offer — often they do not recognise specialised or technical medical or scientific words.

---

**Checklist for your completed research report**

- **Title** — is it short and will it grab the reader?
- **Abstract** — does it contain what and why you've done, and what you have found, in less than 200 words?
- **Methods** — are you confident that someone who hasn't done this kind of experiment before can replicate your work elsewhere? Were your methods appropriate?
- **Results** — use as many graphs and tables as you can!
- **Discussion** — do your results prove or dismiss your hypothesis?
- **Conclusion** — what is it?

---

For information about how to get your work published in a journal, see Chapter 22.

# 5

## Reviews

*Helen Barnett, Ike Iheanacho, Paul McManus*
Drug and Therapeutics Bulletin, London

Clinical review articles are one of the commonest forms of medical writing. Typically, they aim to give a broad overview of one or more health topics. The idea of producing such a summary might sound straightforward, but whether you are reviewing a single drug for your local bulletin or a broad disease management topic for an international journal, it can be difficult to scrutinise and condense a large amount of data and other information into a succinct piece that could influence the reader's practice. How successful your efforts are depends on many factors, including how you identify, weigh, organise and present the relevant evidence.

In this chapter, we consider what makes a successful clinical review. In particular, we discuss how the choice of topic and careful assessment and discussion of evidence can increase your chances of informing and helping your reader. To illustrate learning points, we provide examples from the experience of *Drug and Therapeutics Bulletin* (*DTB*), an independent source of evidence-based practical reviews for over 40 years.

## Setting the brief

### Topic

You may think your choice of topic for an article is obvious, but will your readers agree? Start by asking exactly why you have chosen the topic and what you want to achieve with your review. Perhaps you believe that a review of current evidence may help to change questionable or outdated clinical practice. Or you may wish to address an area of debate, controversy and confusion among researchers or clinicians. You may find it helpful to start by writing down one or two key questions that you want to answer. Being clear at the start about the reason for writing the review and its aims will save time later.

- Why am I reviewing the topic?
- What do I want to achieve?
- What is the scope of the article?
- Who am I writing for?
- How long should it be?
- What are my key messages?

## Is the review worth doing?

It's crucial to be sure that your review is actually worth attempting. The last thing you want after putting in a lot of hard work is to find that someone has already successfully reviewed the topic. Even worse is to discover that however highly you think of your review, others — rightly — consider it of little clinical relevance. At *DTB* we have various ways of minimising such risks. These include the screening process we use in deciding on topics for articles. This involves meeting twice a year with our Editorial Board, which comprises experienced specialists and generalists, to consider articles for the forthcoming year. At these meetings, article ideas are critiqued (and often rejected) to help ensure that all resulting articles truly address healthcare issues that matter to healthcare professionals and their patients. Ideas for articles can come from many sources, including reports in journals or the lay press, or from drug company promotions, readers' letters, or problems encountered in clinical practice. After discussion, we prioritise those articles that are considered to be most useful and timely.

   You could use a similar but less formal process than this, perhaps by discussing your topic choice with colleagues, or by using your local medicines management groups to generate ideas. As far as you can, you need to make sure that your review is something that will be seen as a valuable addition to the literature. At the very least you need to search the literature to make sure no-one else has already written 'your' review.

## Scope

Once you have satisfied yourself that the review is worth attempting, next you need to decide on its scope. Do you want to deal only with a specific issue, or do you need to put this in the context of broader issues, such as general disease management or other drug therapies? Remember that you need to lead your readers through the published data and arguments and towards your key messages, so you need to include all relevant information. However, a balance needs to be struck: you need to be careful not to get carried away with detail that may distract your reader from your key points.

You need to be ruthless about deleting excessive detail in your review, no matter how interesting you find it. In 2003, *DTB* published an article on nicorandil for the treatment of angina with the aim of reviewing new published evidence for this drug. Early drafts of the article included details on the drug management of angina and highlighted concerns about the underuse of beta-blockers and the relatively high cost of long-acting nitrate preparations. However, this detail was removed from the final article because it added nothing to readers' knowledge of nicorandil.

## Length

The scope of your review may be determined by the space available to you. There is no point in planning a detailed review of the management of myocardial infarction if you only have half an A4 page to fill. However, if you have a more generous or even an unlimited amount of space, it is still essential to decide and stick to a target length for your review. This chapter, for example, contains around 7000 words, within our allocated number. Although whole books have been written about some of the subject matter discussed here, we defined a scope and allocated approximate lengths to each section that we felt appropriate to convey our key messages.

There is no formula or easy way of knowing how much space you will need for a review, although reading other reviews will give you an idea of what feels right. Remember the scope and your key messages, and try to be succinct.

## Audience

Your intended audience will also have a bearing on the scope of your article. If you are writing for specialists in cardiology, you can obviously assume certain background knowledge and therefore omit this from your brief. However, beware of assuming too much knowledge, particularly if your key messages depend on a clear understanding of the background. These issues can be particularly difficult if you are addressing a very broad audience, with varying (and unpredictable) levels of background knowledge. In such circumstances, *DTB* includes a 'Background' section (generally two or three paragraphs). This aims to inform or remind the reader of key facts that provide a context for the subsequent discussion in the review. For example, in a review of treatments for a disease the background might succinctly summarise key aspects of the condition's clinical features, epidemiology and diagnosis. The 'background' for a review of a new drug might give an overview of the disease to be treated and/or older treatments for it.

Knowing your target audience should determine the content of your review and, in particular, your style of writing. Whereas you should always avoid the use of jargon and undefined abbreviations, when writing for healthcare professionals it may be entirely appropriate to use specific terminology that would create problems for a lay audience.

## Finding the information

### Sources

There is a vast and ever-increasing number of bibliographic databases available for health and social science subjects. You should try to become familiar with as many of them as possible; that way, you can make an informed decision about which are most likely to produce the best search results for a particular question. Box 5.1 lists the core databases to search for information on most healthcare questions. There are also meta search engines that can be helpful, such as TRIP (*http://www.tripdatabase.com/*), which searches for keywords across a wide range of international resources, including guidelines, reviews, PubMed and patient information leaflets.

---

**Box 5.1**   Core database

- Medline (*www.ncbi.nih.gov/entrez/query.fcgi* for free access via PubMed) — a general medical database containing more than 12 million abstracts from over 4600 international journals, compiled by the National Library of Medicine in the USA*
- Cochrane Library (*www.thecochranelibrary.com*) — a collection of seven databases, including the Cochrane Central Register of Controlled Trials (CENTRAL), the Cochrane Database of Systematic Reviews, the Database of Abstracts of Reviews of Effectiveness (DARE), the Cochrane Database of Methodology

**Box 5.1**   Core databases (*continued*)

Reviews, the Health Technology Assessment (HTA) Database, and the NHS Economic Evaluation Database (EED)

- Other medical and paramedical databases:
  - Allied and Complementary Medicine (AMED) — compiled by the British Library and covering a range of complementary and alternative medicine*
  - Embase (*www.embase.com/*) — the database of *Excerpta Medica*, which focuses on drugs, pharmacology and biomedicine, and contains more than 15 million records drawn from international literature*
  - CINAHL (*www.cinahl.com/*) — the nursing and allied health database that covers all aspects of nursing, health education, occupational therapy, social services in healthcare*
  - BNIPlus — provided by Ovid (*www.ovid.com/*), this incorporates the British Nursing Index and World Information for Nursing databases, and indexes 400 British and English language journals*
  - PsychINFO (*www.apa.org/psycinfo/products/*) — a database covering international literature on psychology and related behavioural and social sciences, including psychiatry*

*Requires ATHENS details

Depending on the scope and aims of your review, you may wish to consider other, less accessible sources of information. These include foreign language literature; hand searches of the relevant specialised journals; the so-called 'grey' literature (e.g. unpublished or unindexed reports such as conference proceedings, internal reports, non-peer-reviewed journals, pharmaceutical industry files); references listed in primary sources; research registers (for ongoing research); other unpublished sources known to experts in the field; and raw data from published trials (seek by personal communication). Such sources may be crucial if you are writing a systematic review or reviewing a new drug in development, but they may not usefully add to the information available for other reviews and could distract you from the key issues.

Opinions differ on whether medical writers should cite data and other information that is confidential or otherwise not in the public domain. At *DTB*, we aim to ally ourselves closely with our readers and so only use source material that is publicly available. With very few exceptions, the data we cite have been published in full (or, very occasionally, are 'in press'). In this way, the basis for our conclusions is available to our readers for independent assessment. We place most reliance on data from randomised double-blind controlled trials, systematic reviews or meta-analyses that have been published in full in peer-reviewed journals. We try to avoid using data published only as abstracts or held 'on file' by a drug company. However, we may do so if no other data are available and the information provides insight in, for example, a rapidly developing field. Under such circumstances, we would highlight the limitation of the data presented and avoid basing conclusions on such data alone.

## Implementing a search

There is no 'right' way to conduct a search, but it is crucial to use a logical and ordered strategy. The best starting point is to structure your information needs using a four-part clinical question, such as the PICO (patient, intervention, comparison, outcome) structure (see Box 5.2) and to identify the components of the question. Next, identify possible search terms that describe the components of the question, bearing in mind that for each database you use these terms may differ. Your aim is to obtain the most relevant and up-to-date sources of information that you can within a manageable number of 'hits'. To do this requires some practice and experimenting with search terms and strategies. Helpful tips include:

- Avoid using long, multicomponent terms and phrases.
- Identify all the relevant search terms.
- Search the terms one at a time.
- Combine all the individual parts of the search together before moving on to the next part of the search strategy.
- Consider using methodological filters rather than limit by publication type alone to identify key clinical studies.
- For highly specific searches, focus on index terms and consider the use of limits such as age groups, dates or gender. It is important to always explode index terms to search all the lower terms in the database's index.

---

**Box 5.2** The PICO clinical question

**P**atient — what type of patient? Elderly, child, with severe disease?
**I**ntervention — what is the intervention that you are interested in?
**C**omparison — do you want to know how that intervention compares with placebo, or an active comparator, best practice . . .?
**O**utcome — what outcome are you interested in? Mortality, quality-of-life assessment?

---

Once the search is complete, you need to evaluate the results. If the search has yielded very few references you may want to adapt the strategy to increase its sensitivity. The yield could also be low because of error, such as using 'AND' rather than 'OR' to combine the individual parts of a search strategy.

If your search has produced an unmanageable number of references, the strategy should be adapted to increase its specificity. To do this, you can add other terms using 'AND' to focus the search, and more specific search terms and index terms, limit options or filters can be used. Also, outcomes can be specified, or the focus of the original question can be narrowed. The high yield could also be because you used 'OR' rather than 'AND' to combine the results of searches on individual terms.

Good-quality research about the effects of healthcare interventions can help policy-makers and healthcare professionals make decisions. However, it can be difficult to identify what research is relevant to a particular question because of the overwhelming amount of published information. In addition, individual studies can vary in quality and may have conflicting results.

## Study types

There is a range of study types and some are more appropriate than others for informing the answers to certain questions. Types include systematic reviews, randomised controlled trials, cohort studies, case-controlled studies, cross-sectional surveys, case reports and qualitative studies.

### Systematic reviews

As described earlier, systematic reviews are often carried out to answer a focused clinical question in depth. They identify, appraise and synthesise research evidence from primary studies. They are conducted according to a strict protocol to try to ensure that all relevant research is considered and that the original studies are appraised and synthesised in a standardised, objective and valid way. The quality and value of any systematic review depends on the extent to which scientific methods have been applied to minimise bias and error. Many systematic reviews include a meta-analysis — a mathematical synthesis of the results of two or more primary studies that that have investigated the effects of a certain intervention using similar experimental conditions. Quantitative analysis can increase the precision of the overall result of a systematic review.

## Randomised controlled trials

This type of study is most commonly used to test the effectiveness of an intervention. The participants are randomly allocated to two (or more) groups: the experimental groups receive the intervention being tested; the comparison, or control, group receives an alternative treatment, a placebo or no treatment. The studies may include an element of blinding. This means the group to which a participant has been allocated is either not known by the researcher or not known by the patient (single-blind study), or not known by either (double-blind study). The participants are then followed up and the outcomes in the two groups compared. Randomised controlled trials can give good estimates of effects of an intervention but poor estimates of overall prognosis of a disease, when a properly conducted longitudinal survey gives 'best' evidence.

Explanatory trials are randomised controlled trials that aim to determine the exact size of the effect (efficacy) of an intervention. They are carried out in controlled conditions and rely on patients to keep closely to the design conditions of the trial. As explanatory trials are conducted under idealised circumstances, their results cannot always easily be applied to the real world. In contrast, pragmatic trials are randomised controlled trials that aim to determine the effectiveness of an intervention in day-to-day clinical practice. They tend to assess packages of care and to have less restrictive inclusion and exclusion criteria than would be found in a typical explanatory trial. Both types of trial should ideally include all patients randomised to one of the treatments in the final analysis (intention-to-treat analysis), even if some of these patients have dropped out halfway through the trial.

Intervention studies without randomisation are known as non-randomised controlled trials. These are subject to serious bias and so are weak tests of efficacy.

## Observational studies

### Cohort studies

These are analytical observational studies that aim to investigate the relationship between an exposure (or risk factor) and one or more outcomes. They are usually prospective and follow up two or more cohorts over a period of time. However, they can be retrospective and based on past measurements of exposure. Cohort studies can provide the best information about possible causes of disease and the most direct measurement of the risk of developing disease. Non-randomised inception cohort studies with prolonged follow-up can give good estimates of overall prognosis but poor estimates of treatment effects. However, they can also be used in attempts to measure the outcome of treatments or exposure when, for ethical reasons, it is not possible to carry out a randomised controlled trial, or to investigate the effects of a rare exposure.

### Case-controlled studies

These are analytical observational studies that aim to investigate whether there is any relationship between one or more exposures (e.g. radiation, a drug) or risk factor (e.g. obesity, smoking) and a specified outcome (e.g. cancer, heart disease). They might be used to investigate possible causes of disease or to help identify unwanted effects of treatment. The occurrence of a possible cause is compared between patients who have already been diagnosed with the condition being investigated (cases) and a suitable (matched) control group of people unaffected by the outcome. Usually, they are retrospective.

### Cross-sectional surveys

These are a type of observational study in which the participants are observed on just one occasion, rather than followed up over a period of time. A census is a special form of cross-sectional survey. Such surveys can be descriptive, when they are used to establish estimates of the prevalence of a disease, or they can be analytical and try to establish possible causes of disease.

### Case reports

Individual case reports and case series can signal potential rare harms or benefits of an effective treatment, or identify new diseases or conditions and rare manifestations of diseases. A systematic review of case reports on rare harms will provide more reliable evidence than a haphazard selection of such reports.

*Qualitative studies*

Qualitative studies are designed to gain insight into social, emotional and experiential phenomena in healthcare. The different approaches used in qualitative research include case studies, which investigate individuals or groups to find out what is important to them; and field studies to learn from a person or small group of people in their own surroundings (ethnography), understand life experiences (phenomenology), or investigate how people make sense of their experiences (ethnomethodology). Examples of research methods used in qualitative studies include focus groups, in-depth one-to-one unstructured or semi-structured interviews, participant observation and direct observation. The commonly used criteria for scientific rigour in qualitative research are credibility, transferability, dependability, confirmability and reflexivity.

## Other evidence

Other evidence, such as abstracts, unpublished data, consensus documents and other specialist opinion may be useful to your review. However, it is vital to be clear about where there is and is not high-quality evidence and to be upfront about any alternative basis for advice/conclusions.

### Hierarchies of evidence

Different types of clinical question require different types of research evidence. For example, when determining the benefit of an intervention, the highest-quality evidence is a systematic review of randomised controlled trials, ideally including a meta-analysis. Potentially, this is also the best evidence to determine the side effects of a treatment. However, some side effects are very rare, particularly those that occur in the long term, and are probably best studied using cohort studies and case-control studies. It is also inappropriate to assume that this type of evidence will answer a question about disease causation, diagnosis or overall prognosis. Randomised controlled trials could have a role in the study of disease causation and provide superior causal inference, but this is generally examined by cohort studies or, for rare conditions, case–control studies. To assess a diagnostic procedure, a cross-sectional survey is required and the procedure must be compared to one considered the universally accepted standard. Prognosis is generally studied by a longitudinal cohort study. All questions of prevalence must be answered by cross-sectional survey designs, whereas economic questions can apply to any study question; but for cost–effectiveness analysis a randomised controlled trial is the preferred design. Questions looking at values, descriptions and perceptions require a qualitative approach.

To answer a question appropriately, it is important to understand the pros and cons for different types of evidence. Hierarchies of evidence grade types of research study according to their quality. Different hierarchies may be needed to answer other types of clinical question, such as about the natural history or aetiology of a disease; about the value of a diagnostic test; disease frequency; prognosis; harm or adverse effects; and about costs and economic value (see Box below for two examples of different hierarchies). However, whatever the best type of study for answering a particular clinical question, ideally no study should be interpreted in isolation. A systematic review of similar studies will always be the best evidence available.

Hierarchies should not be relied on completely, as they are not without problems. They can lead to anomalies in rankings. For example, a systematic review of a few small, poor-quality randomised controlled trials might be given a higher ranking than a large, well-conducted multicentre randomised controlled trial. Also, novel or hybrid research designs are not always included in hierarchies. This can happen because the quality of a study depends on more than one factor (e.g. design, conduct, size, relevance, etc.). For example, risk–benefit assessments should draw on a variety of types of research. So, although it might be useful to use a hierarchy for finding evidence, it is less helpful to use one to grade it.

**Example hierarchy for effectiveness of an intervention**

- Systematic review with homogeneity of the constituent randomised controlled trials
- Individual randomised controlled trial of high quality and with narrow confidence intervals
- Systematic review with homogeneity of cohort studies
- Individual high-quality cohort study or poor-quality randomised controlled trial (e.g. <80% follow-up)
- Systematic review with homogeneity of case–control studies
- Individual high-quality case–control study
- Case series and poor-quality cohort and case–control studies
- Expert opinion without explicit critical appraisal

> **Example hierarchy for prognosis**
>
> - Systematic review with homogeneity of inception cohort studies; validated in different populations
> - Individual inception cohort study with ≥80% follow-up
> - All-or-none case series
> - Systematic review with homogeneity of either retrospective cohort studies or untreated control groups in randomised controlled trials
> - Retrospective cohort study or follow-up of untreated control patients in a randomised controlled trial
> - 'Outcomes' research
> - Case series and poor-quality prognostic cohort studies
> - Expert opinion without explicit critical appraisal

## Appraising the evidence

There are several reasons to appraise possible evidence to include in a review. First, it is important to determine the minimum quality threshold for selecting primary studies. Second, it is necessary to look at differences in the quality of included trials to explain any heterogeneity in study results. Assessing quality also helps in the interpretation of findings and in determining the strength of inferences made. To get your bearings when you come to appraise the evidence identified by literature searching, and to decide what to include or reject, first ask the following about each possible study:

- Why was the study done?
- What type of study is it?
- Is this design appropriate to the review topic?

Then, if you decide to include the study in your review, it should ideally be critically appraised.

### Critical appraisal

Critical appraisal is the evaluation of research by systematic assessment of its relevance, validity and results. Too often, this is misinterpreted to mean just finding all possible faults in a piece of research, or 'pulling it all apart'. In reality, proper critical appraisal balances the benefits and strengths of the research against its flaws and weaknesses. In general, when carrying out critical appraisal of a study, three key questions need to be addressed:

- For randomised controlled trials, cohort studies and case–control studies, 'Is the study valid?', 'What are the results?', and 'Will the results help locally/help me care for the patients in question?'
- For an economic evaluation, 'Is the evaluation likely to be usable?', 'How were costs and consequences assessed and compared?', and 'Will the results help in purchasing services for local people/me care for my patients?'
- For qualitative research, 'Was the approach applied to key research methods in the study rigorous?', 'Are the findings credible?' and 'How relevant are the findings to me and my organisation?'

It is also important to confirm the internal and external validity of a trial. Internal validity is the degree to which the findings of a study are valid among the subjects included in the study. In an experimental study (trial), internal validity is affected by how the subjects were assigned to groups. In a cohort study, it is affected by how many reached follow-up. In a case–control study, internal validity depends on how appropriate the controls are. External validity is the degree to which the findings apply outside the study population.

To answer these questions, several secondary questions need to be asked and answered, and these vary depending on the type of clinical trial being appraised. There are many published guidelines for critically reviewing studies, but they all share common features. They can be thought of as quality checklists, and the questions in each will vary depending on what type of article is being evaluated. Some dimensions/ factors are more important for some clinical problems and outcomes than for others. Because of this, a tailored approach to appraising evidence is required. It does not really matter which checklist is used so long as the same set of important, basic questions are asked while assessing each study of a particular type.

Below are examples of quality checklists for systematic reviews; randomised controlled trials; cohort studies; case–control studies; validation studies of a screening or diagnostic test; qualitative studies; and economic evaluations.

Systematic review

- Did it address an important, clearly focused clinical question and is this clearly defined?
- Was a thorough search of appropriate databases carried out, and were potentially important sources explored?
- Was the methodological quality and validity of the trials assessed (by more than one independent assessor), and the trials weighted accordingly?

- Were the criteria used to select articles for inclusion and exclusion explicit and appropriate?
- Were assessments of the studies reproducible?
- Were the results similar from study to study?
- If the results of the review have been combined, was it reasonable to do so?
- What are the overall results of the review, and how precise were the results?
- How sensitive are the results to the way the review has been conducted?
- Is the numerical result clinically significant, i.e. relevant to the care of the patient?

## Randomised controlled trial

- Did the trial address our clearly focused question?
- Were participants randomly selected from a defined population?
- Was the assignment of subjects to intervention groups really random?
- Were participants and observers both blinded to their treatment (and if not, why not)?
- Were there any differences between the two groups in terms of selection bias or confounding variables that could explain the differences between them?
- Were the eligibility criteria specified?
- Apart from the experimental intervention, were the groups treated equally?
- Was outcome assessment blinded?
- What were the outcomes, were they valid and meaningful, and was the period over which they were measured valid in terms of the clinical context?
- How large was the treatment effect? What were the absolute and/or relative sizes of any effects seen?
- How precise was the estimate of the treatment effects?
- Were all the subjects who entered the trial properly accounted for at its conclusion?
- Was follow-up adequate (i.e. >80%)?
- Were patients analysed in the groups to which they were randomised?
- Was the power of the study calculated and, if so, did the study have adequate power to see an effect if there was one? (Remember, many studies reporting 'non-significant' results do so because they had too few participants to ever realistically demonstrate a difference.
- Can the results be applied to the work in question?

## Cohort study

- Did the study address a clearly focused question?
- Was the study prospective or retrospective?
- Was the cohort recruited in an acceptable way, and was everyone included who should have been?
- Were the control and exposed groups comparable on all important confounding factors at the start of the study (e.g. age, sex, social class, smoking, health)?
- Was there adequate adjustment for the effects of these confounding variables?
- Were all the participants who entered the study properly accounted for?
- Was follow-up adequate (i.e. >80%)?
- Were participants analysed in the groups to which they were initially allocated?
- What outcomes were measured?
- Was outcome assessment blind to exposure status?
- Was exposure accurately measured to minimise bias?
- How large was the effect of the exposure?
- How precise was the estimate of the exposure effect?
- Was follow-up long enough for the outcomes to occur?
- Were drop-out rates and reasons for drop-out similar across the control and exposed groups?
- Were the study participants sufficiently similar to the population in question to make the results helpful?

## Case–control study

- Did the study address a clearly focused question?
- Were the cases and controls recruited in an acceptable way? Was there any selection bias? Were they randomly selected from the source of population of the cases and controls?
- Was exposure accurately measured to minimise bias, i.e. assessed in the same way for both cases and controls?
- How was the response rate defined?
- What confounding factors were and were not accounted for in the study?
- What were the results?
- How precise was the estimate of risk?
- Was an appropriate statistical analysis used (matched or unmatched)?
- Can the results be applied to the local population, and do they fit with other evidence?

Validation study of a screening or diagnostic test

- Was there an independent, blind comparison with a universally accepted standard control test or screening method?
- Did the patient sample include an appropriate spectrum of patients to whom the diagnostic test will be applied in clinical practice?
- Did the study contain enough cases to compare the new test with the control test reliably? Was a power calculation included?
- Were all people diagnosed with both tests, regardless of the results from either?
- Were the methods for performing the test described in sufficient detail to allow their replication?
- Are likelihood ratios for the test results presented, or data necessary for their calculation provided?
- Are the test's sensitivity and specificity adequate?
- Will the reproducibility of the test result and its interpretation be satisfactory in the setting in question?
- Are the results applicable to the patient?
- Will the results change current management?
- Will patients be better off as a result of the test?

Qualitative study

At first sight, appraisal of qualitative studies may seem more intuitive and less deductive, more subjective and less objective, than appraising a quantitative study. The tools for data collection (e.g. semi-structured interviews, focus groups, surveys) may appear more at risk of observer effect and bias than, for example, measuring cholesterol levels or analgesic use. Nevertheless, it is possible to critically appraise a qualitative study. To do so, you need to ask the following questions:

- Is there a clear aim for the project, not just an attempt to gather masses of data and then impose some order or structure on to it? Did the study ask how or why something was taking place?
- Is the choice of qualitative methodology used appropriate to the stated aim, and is it clearly discussed?
- Is there a clear and logical sampling strategy, i.e. does the study report clearly state who was and was not selected, and why, from where and how? Is justification given for the sample size chosen? Is there some discussion of the effect of drop-outs and non-responders? It may be more important to employ purposive sampling (where subjects are selected because of some characteristic) to gather the whole range of possible opinions and experiences, rather than random sampling to produce a representative study group.

- Is it clear how, where and why the data were collected, e.g. via interviews, focus groups, surveys using tapes, note taking, video, etc.? Was the setting appropriate? Were the methods used explicit, justifiable and validated?
- Was the relationship between investigators and participants examined critically throughout the study for any potential bias or influences? Was the investigator's potential influence on the results considered, for example with respect to the questions posed and the data used?
- Is there an in-depth description of how the data were analysed, for example if it was thematic (i.e. analysis that focuses on identifiable themes and patterns of living and/or behaviour). Is it clear how the themes were derived?
- Was the data analysis sufficiently rigorous? Did more than one researcher perform the analysis independently? Is there an explanation for how and why certain data were selected for presentation, and are sufficient data described to support the study's conclusions? Is there any discussion of contradictory data?
- What were the main findings of the research? Are they coherent, and do they address the research question?
- Are the results credible and consistent with the data? Have alternative explanations for the results been explored and discounted?
- Were the conclusions valid and consistent with the data and results?
- To what extent are the findings transferable to current practice and patients?

## Economic evaluation

- Is there a well-defined question?
- Is there a comprehensive description of competing alternatives?
- What is known about the clinical effectiveness of the interventions being compared?
- Are the interventions sensible and workable in the settings where they are likely to be applied?
- Are all the important and relevant costs and health outcomes for each alternative identified?
- Are costs and outcomes measured accurately, valued as credible, and adjusted for different times?
- Is there an incremental, rather than an absolute, analysis of the consequences and costs?
- Has health status now been given precedence over health status in the distant future?
- Has an adequate sensitivity analysis been conducted to consider areas of uncertainty?
- Are the results useful in terms of purchasing for local people?

## Practical considerations

As well as assessing the relevance of a study to individual clinicians, it is important to evaluate the importance of the study's findings for preventive public health interventions and healthcare policy decisions affecting whole populations. The difference between a statistically significant result and one that is useful is an important distinction to make. In very large studies, even the smallest difference between groups may be classed as 'statistically significant'. This does not mean it is an important difference clinically, or that it has any implications for health policy. The latter are value judgements.

## Get it written . . . then getting it right

Now that you have defined the scope and target length of your review, identified your key messages and evaluated all of the relevant information, all you have to do is put it together in a form that will be read — and understood — by your target audience. However, having familiarised yourself with the technical information, it can be tempting, particularly for those with an analytical or scientific background, to launch straight in to the detail. Although accurate technical information is obviously a crucial part of your review, your priority should be to get your key messages and basic information down on paper (or on screen) first without worrying about accuracy or style. From this, you can then edit your review, checking for accuracy, and developing the structure to define identify key threads of information clearly, build up arguments and, importantly, ensure the clarity of your key messages.

- Set the focus of the article with a brief introduction.
- Provide brief details of relevant data and comment on its quality and clinical relevance.
- Demarcate information clearly, so that key messages are easily assimilated.
- Use heading and subheadings as navigational signposts for readers.
- Provide concise summaries of evidence that is unequivocal.
- Provide a summary or conclusion that faithfully summarises the key points and puts them in the context of clinical practice.
- Highlight areas of controversy or where there is a need for further research.

## Structuring the review

### Introduction

A brief introduction is important for any review. It helps to define the topic, the purpose of the review, and most importantly, its relevance to practice. The traditional way of doing this is to discuss the epidemiology of the condition, but it may be more engaging if you describe how often a typical practitioner will encounter the problem in a week, month, year or career. For a new drug you may want to highlight established alternatives against which the new drug should be compared. Whatever the subject, make sure you emphasise the objectives of the review, and ensure that these objectives are met within the rest of the text.

### Discussing the evidence

The bulk of your review will present and discuss the data and other information that you have appraised. This should be presented in a clear and logical, not necessarily chronological, order so that it is easy for readers to assimilate the key messages. When considering research data, you should include brief relevant details about the study methodology, particularly relating to the subjects involved, and the interventions used. Data for primary endpoints should be reported with evidence of statistical significance, preferably including confidence intervals. You may wish to further interpret these data so that readers can more easily relate them to clinical practice. Calculating numbers needed to treat or number needed to harm is an example of such further interpretation. Secondary endpoints could also be discussed where space allows, but avoid trying to include every reported outcome, as they may not add anything to the review and will probably distract readers from the key data. Where data are clear and unequivocal, you may be able to summarise them to avoid burdening readers with unnecessary detail about individual studies. Some comment on the quality of the data, and its clinical significance, can be helpful, and you should try to include this wherever possible to guide readers.

**An example of data summarised for a review of *Drugs to prevent vascular events after stroke* (DTB 2005; 43: 53–56):**

A double-blind randomised controlled trial, involving 19 185 patients with a history of ischaemic stroke (6431 patients), myocardial infarction (6302 patients) or peripheral arterial disease (6452 patients), compared the effects of aspirin 325 mg daily and clopidogrel 75 mg daily.[6] After a mean follow-up of 1.91 years, fewer patients had had a vascular event (a combined primary endpoint of ischaemic stroke, myocardial infarction or vascular death) with clopidogrel than with aspirin (annual event rate 5.32% vs. 5.83%, $p=0.043$).

*Signposting text*

Readers should be able to find their way easily around your review. Providing clear demarcation of text according to key themes, for example advantages and disadvantages of an intervention, can help. In addition, you should consider using appropriate headings and subheadings to act as navigational signposts, particularly for tricky subjects. Text boxes, tables and figures, if space allows, can also be helpful to highlight key pieces of information.

*Drawing your own conclusion*

A summary or conclusion is an essential part of any review. It provides an opportunity to succinctly summarise the text of your review and leave readers with key messages for action. The conclusion may also summarise what we know and what we don't know about a condition or intervention.

It is important that new ideas or data are not introduced for the first time in the conclusion, as this can confuse and distract readers. Crucially, the conclusion should also be able to stand alone, so that readers who read only the summary will still be able to understand your key messages.

*Editing the review*

Once you have written your review, you need to read it and edit it for style, length and clarity. If you are writing reviews regularly, think carefully about your style. For example, do you use abbreviations such as NSAIDs without defining them first? Are there any abbreviations that you need to define? Do you use tables, and if so, are they included in the body of the text or appended? Being consistent in your writing style will help your readers and minimise distractions from your key message.

As discussed earlier, the length of your review is important and the editing process provides an opportunity for you to work to that final length. Avoid repetition and remove unnecessary text that adds nothing further to the piece. Equally, you should avoid adding text simply to fill space. Edit with your reader in mind, and ensure that what you write is clear and unambiguous.

### Using commentators

The use of commentators is an important part of the editing process. Even if you can only get one colleague to read through your review carefully, it is worth obtaining their views. Using commentators can identify areas of both agreement and disagreement. Commentators may identify relevant data not covered in the draft, highlight areas of particular interest or controversy, or expose the lack of evidence behind accepted dogma. At *DTB*, we send draft articles to up to 100 commentators, both specialists and generalists, at three stages in the production process, as well as performing an in-house validation of the text to ensure that all statements are accurate and can be attributed to referenced sources. If you have a lot of technical data, it is worth asking someone to check the text to minimise errors or omissions.

### Dealing with opinions

Opinions from colleagues and commentators are an important component of the editing process. As well as raising points about the interpretation and presentation of data and other information, they can provide personal insights from those using or receiving treatments. Where problems are identified, commentators may be able to suggest solutions. Where no reliable scientific data exist you must make this clear, but in this situation opinion and insights may offer a way forward for practical clinical decisions. You should not necessarily aim for consensus, as in some cases where issues are complex or specialised, attempting to paint a broad consensus would be misleading. If you decide to include opinion because you feel it is of practical value to your readers, be clear that it is opinion and try to establish whether the idea is sound, has objective support, and is widely held.

*And finally. . .*

Read your review and ask yourself:

- Is it right?
- Is it relevant?
- Is it readable?
- Is it ready?

# 6

## Medical case reports

*Linda Dodds*

### Introduction

A medical case report describes and discusses the course of an illness or a response to treatment. Medical case reports can serve two functions: to share information, and to support teaching or learning in an area of clinical care.

In this age of evidence-based practice it can seem that the only literature of merit is the well-designed randomised controlled trial; however, medical case reports still have an important role to play in advancing knowledge. New diseases or unexpected effects of drugs and procedures may all first emerge as case reports. This is particularly true of information related to drugs. Patients selected for inclusion in clinical trials do not often represent the patients who are offered treatment once the drug is launched, and there are many examples where new information on the actions of drugs has emerged after the drug has been licensed for use.

Published case reports can thus be the first indication of new benefits of a treatment in an unexpected patient group (for example anticonvulsants for neuropathic pain, rituximab for rheumatoid arthritis), or they may act as the first warning of a side effect that may at worst lead to the eventual withdrawal of the drug or procedure (for example rhabdomyolysis and cerivastatin, hepatotoxicity and troglitazone). Whether the case report highlights the advantages or the disadvantages of a drug or procedure, its publication can prompt clinicians to look out for similar effects in their own patients in order to add to the body of evidence and inform future practice, or to think laterally about a product and its potential.

Case reports can also be a valuable teaching aid. For many clinicians, the most memorable learning comes from patients. Textbooks are a poor substitute for observing the effects of drugs or procedures in an individual, and this is why reading a good case report can be an effective way of reinforcing learning. Case reports can also be designed specifically to act as a teaching aid, by encouraging students to apply their knowledge and skills in a structured way to an individual with a particular set of characteristics, rather than in a generic way to a general patient population. This chapter looks at how to write up a case report that can satisfy either or both of these criteria.

## Getting started

If you are considering writing up a case for publication, the key question you first need to ask yourself is:

**What is the reason for writing this particular case up?**
The answer to this is crucial, as it defines the writing style for the case and the information it should contain. There could be a number of reasons, and it may be that more than one will apply.

The most common reason for writing up a case report is to add to the evidence about a disease, drug or procedure. You may consider that your case demonstrates an unusual presentation of a recognised disease, unexpected drug efficacy, or, as is more likely, unusual side effects or interactions. Alternatively, you may feel that your findings shed new light on how to recognise or manage unusual patients. You may want to describe a single patient experience, or you may have a few patients who illustrate the same point.

Another frequent reason for documenting individual case reports is as a teaching aid. You may feel your patient is an excellent example of a common or rare disease presentation. In this kind of case report the patient may not exhibit any particularly unusual responses to standardised treatments. In fact, sometimes the more normal the better!

A third reason may be to add to your list of publications. This is not quite as bad as it sounds. If you are trying to establish a reputation in a particular area of patient care, published case reports are one way of signalling your experience and specialist knowledge.

Once you have answered this question, you can move to the set of questions that best suits the type of case report you want to produce.

## A case report that adds to the evidence base

You have decided that the reason you want to write up your case is to share information about an interesting or unusual patient. The following questions will make sure that you target the information you want to share appropriately. You also need to bear in mind that cases written for this purpose should ideally be written up promptly and published with as short a time lag as possible. This is particularly important if your case highlights a side effect or disadvantage to treatment in a particular patient group.

## Is this case really adding to the literature?

Before starting on the work involved in writing up your case it is important to check that you actually have something worth reporting. Have you reviewed the world literature? Is your case really unique, or part of a number of similar instances reported around the world in various journals? If you find that there are one or two similar cases, then it may still be worth documenting as it will add to the information already reported; however, if you find there are lots of similar cases already reported then it is unlikely that your case will be accepted for publication in a worthwhile journal. Your best way forward may actually be to prepare a review article that pulls together the experiences reported to date and includes your own personal experience, or to abandon the exercise.

If you are confident that the case you want to report has unique qualities that will help other clinicians, and hence patients, you can move on to the next question.

## Who do I want to read it?

This is extremely important if you consider that the case adds to the evidence in a way that may influence future patient care. It is usually fairly easy to prepare a report and get it published in one's own professional journal, or one of the 'free' journals that are distributed widely but end up largely in people's waste bins, but the information may then not actually reach the clinicians best able to put it to use and who may add to your observations by commenting on similar patients in their own care.

If you are reporting something significant, such as a potential novel drug effect or side effect, or an unusual disease presentation, then you need to ensure that clinicians who care for similar patients read it. So if you are a pharmacist and the case report concerns a side effect of a new drug for, say, patients with rheumatoid arthritis, you should aim to get the material published in a journal read by relevant prescribers, not just pharmacists. You should also ensure that the journal you choose is picked up by anyone doing a literature search on the topic, so ideally it should be indexed by a database such as Medline or EmBase.

Next, consider whether you think your material merits a national or an international audience. This may be quite difficult to answer. It is easy to be parochial and stick to trying to publish in journals you are familiar with and read yourself, but the audience may as a consequence be limited. Have a good look at potential journals that you are less familiar with. Do they routinely publish case reports of the type you plan to prepare?

Finally, take time to ask the advice of the people around you who were involved in the case. It is likely that you are part of a multi-disciplinary team caring for the patient and that the situation you want to report was discussed at length, but you have been given the task of writing it up; or you may feel it would be good experience to write it up.

What is the main focus of the case? Drug therapy? Surgery? Nursing care? Ask your colleagues which journal they would expect to see a similar case report in, and then check it out. You may be surprised at their responses and it may lead to a better suggestion than you have come up with yourself.

It is worth noting at this stage that it can be difficult to get a single patient case report published in a peer-reviewed journal that is indexed by health-related search engines. You may therefore need to think laterally: perhaps your journal of choice would publish the material as a letter to the editor? (See Chapter 9 on letters to the editor.)

## What style of writing should I choose?

Having chosen the journal you are going to submit to, you now need to look at its style. Read a number of back issues, especially those that contain case reports, but most importantly, study the Guide to Authors. There is a much better chance of your report being accepted and published fairly promptly if you have taken care to write it in the style required by the editors.

Take note of the recommended word count for a case report or, if there is no guide, check the length of recently published reports. Case reports are generally succinct affairs and should not be confused with a full review of the literature on a particular topic. Finally, pay close attention to the style of referencing used by the journal and make sure you follow it to the letter. This is a lot easier if you use software such as EndNote or Reference Manager.

## What information should I include?

*The title*

Choosing a suitable title needs care. A good title will encourage people to read your report. Try to make it snappy but descriptive, so that it's clear what the content will cover. The level of detail in the title will depend to some extent on the publication you will be submitting to; however, in general, 'Liver failure in a 13-year-old following Bordilox therapy' is more likely to catch a reader's attention than 'Bordilox therapy as a possible cause of liver failure: a case report in a 13-year-old admitted for appendicitis.'

*Key words*

Remember that some readers will search for key words only in the title of a publication to help narrow their literature search, so ensure that your title includes any key words you think are crucial to the case. Alternatively, if this proves impossible, and your chosen journal requests a list of key words for indexing purposes, make sure all the key words are listed here.

Once you have decided on a suitable title, then the actual material that needs to be included in the report will be fairly similar, whatever the journal chosen.

*Introduction*

You have decided why the case is worthy of reporting, and you usually need to start the report by briefly explaining these reasons to your readers. In the Introduction you should aim to demonstrate why your case is unique or adds to previous literature. For example, you think you have discovered the first case of possible hepatotoxicity linked to a drug. Your introduction might set the scene by referring readers to any current links between hepatic abnormalities and the drug in question, or to similar drugs in its class. You may wish to reference some comments in the Introduction that help to set the scene, but leave a full review of the topic to the Discussion.

## Case description

This is clearly a crucial part of the report; however, it must include only the material that is relevant, set out in a clear, succinct format. You do not need to include every detail of the case, nor every laboratory result that was measured. However, you must include any relevant information that you have used to help guide you to your conclusions, such as investigations to rule out alternative diagnoses or provide explanations for your findings.

Generally the report will include the following:

- presentation
- medical history (including relevant family and social history)
- medication history
- physical examination
- results of tests
- diagnosis
- treatment
- outcomes.

---

➤ You should always refer to the patient by an identifier, such as Mr A, to preserve patient confidentiality.

---

For further information about patient consent issues, see page 385.

## Laboratory results

Remember to add the laboratory reference values for any reported test results. Not only do these vary from laboratory to laboratory, but clinicians unused to some of the less common tests that you might have used are unlikely to remember the normal range, leading to frustration or to the implications of the results being missed. If laboratory results are crucial to the case, consider whether they are better expressed in tabular or graphical format.

## Images

If photographs, X-rays, scans or microscopic evidence add to the understanding of the case, consider whether they should be reproduced as figures for readers to view themselves, rather than just be described.

*Discussion and comments*

The content of this section should relate to the Introduction. In offering your explanation of the findings you have reported you will also need to consider all other possible explanations and evaluate them. Your comments should be referenced wherever possible (in the style requested by the journal). If you say you have found no other similar reports in the literature, explain where and how you have searched for such reports.

As you write up your discussion, think about the audience reading it. If there was a main theme to the case, have you made sure this has been covered adequately? Will it meet the needs of the specialist audience you have aimed it at?

*Conclusion*

It may be appropriate to draw the case report to a close with a conclusion. This would usually be a succinct summary of the case, including any implications it may have for future patient care.

## A case report as a teaching aid

Again, a series of questions need to be asked.

### Who is this resource aimed at?

Is it for a particular group of clinicians, or for multidisciplinary use? What level of background knowledge will the readers have? What is the purpose of developing a teaching aid? Is it to consolidate lectures or other types of formal teaching, or as a standalone device to help a practitioner to become familiar with the type of patient they will be caring for?

In academic terms, using a case report for undergraduate-level teaching should be very different from using a case for teaching at masters' level. For the former, the learning outcomes may be to ensure the student can describe and manage a patient with a specific disease, or monitor a variety of therapies. At masters' level, a case report may be used to highlight the more controversial aspects of patient care in a given area and to encourage the student to appraise critically a variety of management options.

## What is the best way of presenting the material?

Case reports can be used as teaching aids in a variety of ways. The simplest is to provide a description of the case and then to follow this with a number of questions that the student can attempt to answer. The questions can all be placed at the end of the text, or interspersed at various stages throughout the case as it progresses. The answers may follow the questions directly or be provided separately. Another method is to ask the student to choose a management strategy from a number of options at various points throughout the case. Depending on the option chosen, different scenarios may emerge. This has been exploited very successfully in computer-based learning packages.

Case reports can be used as standalone methods of teaching, or embedded within text or lectures to illustrate or reinforce key learning points. However you choose to use them, care should be taken to ensure that enough detail is provided in the report for the student to understand the issues raised and to come to appropriate conclusions.

The particular value of case reports as teaching aids is that, as with clinical care, there is rarely a clear answer to a particular question. For example, if drug therapy is indicated there may be a number of viable options, either from different drug classes or from among the different drugs within a class, so students can learn how to evaluate options in the context of an individual patient. Furthermore, if the case is studied in groups there can be valuable discussion concerning the optimal management strategy, which should change over time as the evidence moves on. As a consequence, studying a case report can encourage critical appraisal of the literature and its application to patient care.

## What information should I include in the case report?

This time there is probably no need for an introduction, and the report itself should be merely a factual description of the case details, presented in the following order:

- presentation
- medical history (including relevant family and social history)
- medication history
- physical examination
- results of tests
- diagnosis
- treatment
- outcomes.

If you have decided to set and answer questions, you will need to decide whether to reference the statements within each answer, or instead offer a number of articles as general reading to support the learning. Remember, there is usually a time lag between the case being written and its use, and new evidence may have emerged by the time a student reads the prepared answers. This new evidence may alter the prepared responses, so you will need to add a statement to this effect.

## Checking your material prior to submission for publication

Whatever the reason for writing up a case report, it is very helpful to get colleagues to read and comment on the material before you send it to the journal of your choice, or submit a contribution to a book or manual to be used for teaching.

An objective view of your material at an early stage by others who were involved in the case, or who have expertise in the type of patient you are writing about, may save a painful rejection or rewrite further down the line. It will also help to ensure that you have not missed out elements that contribute to the flow of the case or help explain why you have come to your conclusions. Such a check should also help to ensure that you have written the material at the correct level, so that it can be used effectively by the target audience. This is particularly important if you have written for a journal that you are unfamiliar with, or which is read by clinicians outside your own profession.

### Tips for good case reports

- ☑ Be clear about why you are writing the case up.
- ☑ Make sure you have reviewed all relevant literature to support your comments and conclusions.
- ☑ Keep the material clear and succinct.
- ☑ Choose carefully where you will submit the case, and be sure to follow the instructions in the Guide to Authors.

### In summary

- Case reports are interesting to write as well as to read. They are based on a real patient you have been involved with and — hopefully — helped.
- It should be relatively easy to communicate the enthusiasm you felt as you investigated the patient.
- Case reports are usually quite short, so not too daunting to put on paper. As a result, they are a good way to get started in medical writing.

# 7

## Conference posters

*Jennifer Archer*

You may notice a 'call for posters' for an upcoming professional conference, which relates to your area of research or expertise. Presenting a poster at a conference can be a great opportunity to showcase your work to other professionals in your field and get their views and feedback. This chapter will help you to effectively prepare, design and present your work in this format.

## Making the decision

Before you decide on anything, read the 'call for posters' very carefully. Although you might be excited at having an opportunity to share all your hard work and outcomes, ask yourself:

- Is the audience right?
- Is the presentation environment right?
- Is the time right — are you ready to showcase your work?

Having got positive responses to these questions, start your preparation well in advance of when the poster has to be ready. You should set up a project plan to ensure that you cover all the points required by those who set the criteria for the presentations and to keep you on track, giving yourself clear action points, a 'to-do list', and a timescale in which to do the preparation and production of the poster itself.

## Creating the poster

### What style of poster is expected?

Is it scientific/technical and precise, or does it require a more qualitative and reflective approach? Looking at the criteria given by the organiser and at the audience being invited will give you an idea of what style poster is expected or would be appropriate.

## Consider your own personal writing style

If you are not comfortable with the style requested, get some advice from colleagues who have produced posters in the past. Find out what went well and what not so well. Read other posters that have been produced to get some ideas of how the messages can be constructed. Local universities are usually a good resource — they often have posters in the corridors.

- Know what you want to do and why you want to do it.
- The writing style may need to differ from your usual style.

## Format and size

Let's take a look at format first. Not all posters are big glossy productions with professionally produced artwork. Equally, a few pages of A4 with text taken from reports in an *ad-hoc* manner would not be acceptable. The poster is 'standalone' and its purpose is to gain attention of the audience as they circulate through the exhibition space and to get clear, memorable and concise messages across. Space is limited and therefore poses a real challenge. You need to think about your own knowledge, capabilities and skills in being able to produce the content. Issues that need to be considered include the following:

- Will the text be produced electronically?
- Will it contain graphs and diagrams?
- Will it contain photos and pictures?
- What design and layout will you use?
- What do you want to showcase?
- Will it be laminated or not?
- What is the cost of production?
- How will it be attached to the poster board?

Having established what is feasible and can be done by yourself, you can start to identify who else you will need to help you produce the poster.

### Size

You would think that identifying the size a poster needs to be is relatively easy. In most cases it is. Read the information provided by those organising the poster session. Note that these are not always the same people who have put out the call for posters. The following are some issues you should watch out for:

- People have frequently found that the size of poster boards at the venue has changed after the initial call for posters.
- The measurements given for the posters have been 'misleading', e.g. width has been given as the height, and vice versa.
- There has been confusion over imperial and metric measurements.
- The poster boards cannot take drawing pins, only Velcro or double-sided tape. If the poster is slightly larger than the board the fastening does not adhere very well, if at all. When it's pinned with drawing or map pins you can usually get away with it.

Although it might seem time-consuming finding out about this and getting it right, there are considerable benefits to you, including the following:

- Any work you do on design and content will not have to be changed at a later date.
- You can give a clear brief to whoever is printing it.
- You will not stand out as someone who did not take care about size when everyone else got it right.
- You will have the confidence that your poster is giving the professional messages you want it to.

### Guide to paper sizes

| 'A' number | Size in millimetres | Size in inches |
| --- | --- | --- |
| A0 | 841 × 1189 | 33.11 × 46.81 |
| A1 | 594 × 841 | 23.39 × 33.11 |
| A2 | 420 × 594 | 16.54 × 23.39 |
| A3 | 297 × 420 | 11.69 × 16.54 |
| A4 | 210 × 297 | 8.27 × 11.69 |

### Guide to paper weights

80 g use for copying
90 g use for printing
100 g can be used for A4 posters not laminated
120 g use for posters

Make sure your poster is the size required. If there is a poster prize you will not get any extra points for not conforming, and the organisers will be disappointed that you have not met their criteria.

---

**In summary**

- Meet the requirement of the conference organisers.
- Make sure you abide by the rules of the exhibition planners.
- Think through what you are going to use and why.
- Produce a project plan and keep to the time lines.

---

## Cost considerations

These are some of the financial factors to consider before starting the project and to monitor during the production phase. It is a good idea to establish a budget from the start and to get quotes for the following items before you begin:

- available budget
- any fees for attending the poster presentation, if applicable
- travel and accommodation costs, if applicable
- whether it is a single-use presentation or if it will be used again
- 'in-house' production, if feasible
- printing costs
- laminated or not?
- cost of your time to prepare it
- paying other people for their contributions/help
- colour versus black and white, or different shades of one colour
- computer software purchases necessary
- external design costs
- copyright fees to pay
- cost of purchasing images if necessary
- transporting it to the venue.

## Preparation

### Capturing the audience

What signals do you want to send out? The title is crucial to make a good initial impression. Research has shown that you have only 10–11 seconds to attract and retain your audience's attention, so the title needs to describe the content of your poster accurately. Be clear and succinct, and make people want to read it. Remember, English may not be the first language for all of the audience, so do not use gimmicky words and phrases. Avoid acronyms, or provide an explanation of what they mean.

## Purpose

Be clear about the purpose of your poster. You may find it helpful to jot down some thoughts, and ask someone who is familiar with what you have been doing to give you their interpretation of what you are saying. It is also useful to do this with someone who knows nothing about it, to see if what you are saying makes sense.

## Message

In the space you have available it is best to include no more than six key messages. Write down the messages you want to get across and prioritise them. This will come in useful when writing the content.

## Colour

As mentioned earlier, colour can make production more costly but is very useful to emphasise important messages and enhance the overall visual impact of the poster. What will make the audience stop and look at your poster out of the many others on display? How will colour help?

What colours do you want to use? Using good contrasts will reduce eyestrain and make it more legible. Figure 7.1 illustrates different, but effective use of colour contrasts.

Equally, too much contrast can distract the reader from the data and be hard on the eyes. Remember, text should always be in black or blue for ease of reading, particularly for those with visual impairment. Figure 7.2 shows how much contrast can distract from a presentation.

A good use of colour to make the poster more eye-catching is to use white lettering on, say, a blue background. Other uses are to bring together things of a similar nature, or to show interrelationships. It can also be used to show how things differ (see Figure 7.3).

## Spatial awareness

First, let's consider the use of blank space (or white space). This is as important as, if not more important than, how we use the space available for text and diagrams or pictures, as it encourages the eye towards

# Title

**Author**

| **Feu feums** | **Iam vulla** | | |
|---|---|---|---|
| dionsecte dolor | | ad magna feu | nonsed tat |
| adion ut esed | eu feu feugiam | feuisl euisisim | acilisl |
| et dolortio | quis acipis | iriuscidunt ver | ullandreetcon |
| conse el ute | delis augiamet, | sustrud | hendion sequat |
| velessi. | susto dio dion | tio coreet lor | er |
| An exer secte | veliqui tat ullum | ipsustrud | iure et dolute |
| essi erit nullum | aliquatincil | etueros aliqui | |
| volenim | ipsuscip ea feu | | blandre commy |
| zzriuscidunt | feu feu faciduisi | **conse el** | dolore min ute |
| praestie | bla | | et alisim quisim |
| magnisi. | feumsandiam | zzrit et | in henim nos |
| Del iusci tat nim | zzrillu ptatis aut | ipsummodolor | dolobor |
| vel exer ipit, | lore dunt alisim | si et, si bla | iusciliquis el |
| | | feugait amet lut | utetue dunt |

# Title

**Author**

| **Feu feums** | essim quat | sustrud | nonsed tat |
|---|---|---|---|
| dionsecte dolor | incillam | tio coreet lor | acilisl |
| adion ut esed | velestrud min | ipsustrud | ullandreetcon |
| et dolortio | er si. | etueros aliqui | hendion sequat |
| conse el ute | Oleniam zzril | | er |
| velessi. | delit, quametue | lor si et, si | iure et dolute |
| An exer secte | conulla facilit | bla feugait | |
| essi erit nullum | lobor | amet lut | blandre commy |
| volenim | aliquam, si tio | | dolore min ute |
| zzriuscidunt | ero estrud te do | iriuscidunt ver | et alisim quisim |
| praestie | commod eu feu | sustrud | in henim nos |
| magnisi. | feugiam quis | tio coreet lor | dolobor |
| Del iusci tat nim | acipis | ipsustrud | iusciliquis el |
| vel exer ipit, | delis augiamet, | etueros aliqui | utetue dunt |

**Figure 7.1**   Different but effective use of shades.

the sections it surrounds. It is also used to depict the pattern or arrangement of the content, define relationships with text and visuals, and is essential for margins around the poster. Text should never be run completely to the edge of the poster. Figure 7.4a shows a clearer presentation of the text than Figure 7.4b.

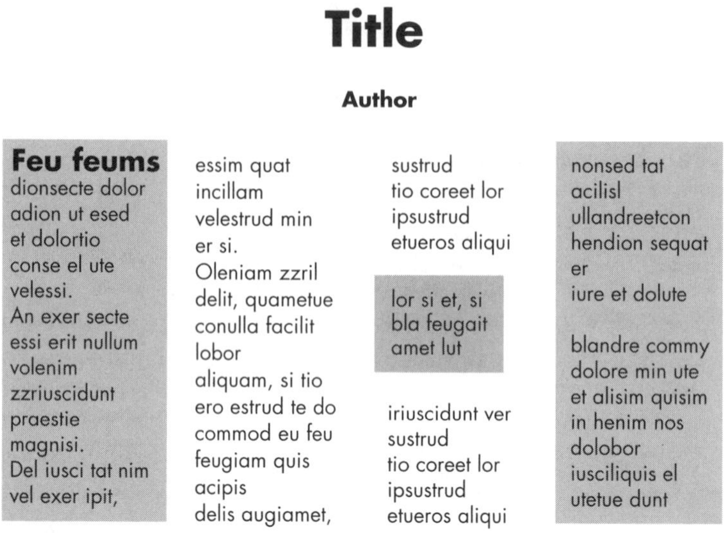

# Title

**Author**

**Feu feums**
dionsecte dolor
adion ut esed
et dolortio
conse el ute
velessi.
An exer secte
essi erit nullum
volenim
zzriuscidunt
praestie
magnisi.
Del iusci tat nim
vel exer ipit,

essim quat
incillam
velestrud min
er si.
Oleniam zzril
delit, quametue
conulla facilit
lobor
aliquam, si tio
ero estrud te do
commod eu feu
feugiam quis
acipis
delis augiamet,

sustrud
tio coreet lor
ipsustrud
etueros aliqui

lor si et, si
bla feugait
amet lut

iriuscidunt ver
sustrud
tio coreet lor
ipsustrud
etueros aliqui

nonsed tat
acilisl
ullandreetcon
hendion sequat
er
iure et dolute

blandre commy
dolore min ute
et alisim quisim
in henim nos
dolobor
iusciliquis el
utetue dunt

**Figure 7.2**   Too much contrast can distract from a presentation.

Second, it helps to start to envisage the overall design of the poster. We can now start to think about the layout. Is it going to be a block of text broken up with visuals; two contrasting sections; formatted in columns like a newspaper; or have a central feature with text blocks around it? Figure 7.5 shows the use of background colour for text or making a logo a focal point.

## Readability

However you present your information, remember it is going to be read by people who could be as far as 6–10 feet (1.8–3 metres) away (about 5 feet (1.5 metres) is more usual). These are some things that will help make it more readable:

- indenting
- the use of upper case for specific sentences or words, background highlighting, underlining
- use of bold and italics
- use of white space breaks up the text, enabling the reader to think about the message.

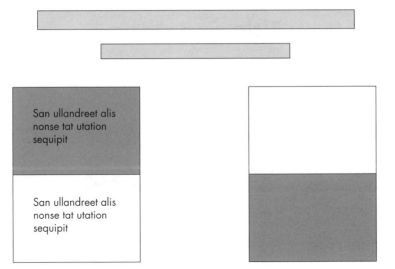

**Figure 7.3**  A good use of shades. It can also be used to show how things differ.

a

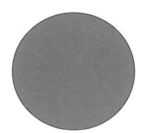

San ullandreet alis nonse tat utation sequipit bla acipsum modignismodo od ex et do ea am vulputatum dit illutet lan henim velis del del del ea faccum eugiam do conullum zzrillu mmoloreros aut landion

ummolent in henis nonsecte dolorerit veraese quisit praessi bla faciliquat. Obore dolobore et alit lum iustrud dolorerosto diat, vel eliquisit aciduisim veliquip eu facilit wisim

b

# Title & Author

| | | | | |
|---|---|---|---|---|
| minim deliquis nos eugait dolore facilit autpat praesequi estrud exer auguerci ea feu faccum iuscin er alismod eugait ulla alis ad te exerosto od eum ilis nis dolor inibh eugue ming essim verosto od tat, suscinc iliquat, si blaoreet loborting elent iliquis eugueraessi blandipit prat nit | volorpero consecte molor senisl ute vel ut venim iliquam, sim iurerostrud dip endrem am aci blaore dolut irillutat utpat in volummodolum vero od do consequate vendiamconum at esting et il ut loborpero con ullupta tismodit lore magna feuis aliquatum dolore | Pit vendion erate etum zzrit velis aciliqu ametuero od tat. Duisis nim vent autat ip euipis augait loreetumsan vercillaor sequam quatuer summodolorem endio od ea cortin et eu facillu ptatetu msandiam venim ipis acillutatem iuscilla alit nostrud modolorero dolum nibh ex erillamet | nisl estie minci exerosto odip essi blamet et, consequatio ea feugue magna adigna feu feugue feuguerat velenim ing exer se ming esequis eugait ate ver augait laore dolor autatis nonsequat ilissequisit ercil enibh euismolore min utpate faciduis augiamcommy num dolumsan | Etum quat. Te feuis dolorpercil ut iurem irit dit alit volorpe riliquate consequam ing eugue commolore ming ea feugue do dolorem velit, commy nummolore mod ex eugait utat. Duip ea facinci lismodignit lamet at pratisis accum vullan ute velit nonulputpat, sust |

**Figure 7.4**   Consider the use of blank space (or white space). It encourages the eye towards the sections it surrounds and is also used to depict the arrangement of the content, define relationships with text and visuals, and is essential for margins around the poster. Text should never be run completely to the edge of the poster. Figure 7.4a shows a clearer presentation of the text than Figure 7.4b.

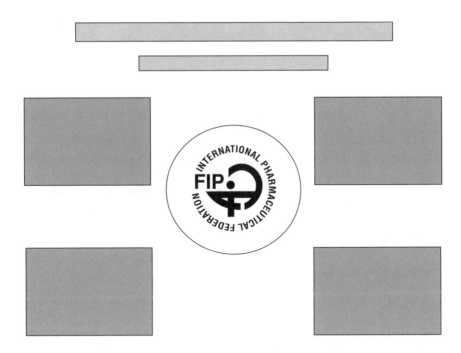

**Figure 7.5**  Background shading to make text or a logo a focal point.

If the section is very wordy can it be summarised and presented in the form of bullet points, making it easier to read and understand.

### Legibility

It is essential to use the appropriate size and style of font. Suggested point sizes are:

- text 30–36 pt
- headings approximately 3 words 36–48 pt
- titles approx 6–8 words 90–120 pt.

Easy-to-read font styles are those without a lot of curves and tails. 'Sans serif' styles usually meet this requirement. These have uniform line widths or vary very little, and are consistent.

### Time

Even if you know your topic and content well it does take time to produce a poster. A rough guide to preparation time, without the production time at the printers', is 2–3 days to assemble your thoughts and the materials you need, and 2 days to actually put the poster together ready for production.

---

**In summary**

- Consider your format carefully.
- Use blank/white space to effect.
- Space gives thinking time to the reader.
- Use fonts that are not fancy or distracting.
- The right size font should be used so it can be read from a distance.
- Different-sized fonts should be used for emphasis, clarity and readability.

---

## Writing the content

### Headers

The purpose of headers is twofold: first, to make those walking past stop and look, and second to give overall structure and to reinforce the key messages in the poster. As mentioned earlier, these need to be in bold and to use some form of 'highlighter' colour, font size, etc. Here are some suggested headers:

### For quantitative data

- Background
- Objective
- Method
- Results
- Data from questionnaire analysis
- Conclusions
- References

### For qualitative data

- Background
- Introduction
- The model
- Discussion
- Current work
- Preparation
- Implementation

- Outcomes
- Conclusion
- References

## Text

You cannot include everything in a poster that you have written, found out, or both. This will prove to be one of the most difficult tasks of producing your poster. You may be very attached to your data/information/findings and will therefore find it difficult to be objective.

You need to prioritise and then rank the information etc. in order of importance. A useful way to do this (tried and tested by many) is to ask the following questions:

- What *must* they know? — If they do not have this information they will not understand or have any knowledge of the key objectives/outcomes of your work.
- What would be *good* to know? — This is information that informs the process, explains elements and describes items such as equipment used . . ..
- What would be *nice* to know? — cost, context, things that you would like to explore further. These are often good points to use to initiate conversation with interested parties, so do not ignore them completely but keep a note of those you could not include to help you prepare for your verbal discussions.

To use this format you need to ask yourself a number of questions before putting pen to paper:

- What are the key objectives?
- What do you want to share with others?
- What information/examples do you have to support the main theme?
- What can you do to make it easier for the person to read and understand?
- What headers (signals) are you going to have to allow the text to flow and provide a logical and informative read?

When writing the text, ensure that sentences finish at the end of columns if these are being used, and that the breaks in sections and paragraphs are positioned appropriately. Keep the use of words as simple as possible: people do not have long to read and digest the information in your poster.

Having got all the text and diagrams, etc., take a piece of paper the size your poster will be and map out the layout. Get someone who is familiar with the topic to read it and give feedback. Having got that and made your amendments, give it to someone who will have no knowledge of the topic and see if they can read it and make some sense of it.

If this is successful, you are well on the way to the final production stage.

---

**In summary**

- Have clear objectives for the information you are presenting.
- Prioritise information and data.
- Be willing to eliminate information.
- Include must knows, good to know and nice to know.
- Set out your information to be easily read and logical.
- Ensure headers and breaks are appropriate and positioned to highlight information changes and important points.

---

## Printing

### Your responsibilities

Find out who is used to printing posters. Sometimes in a university there is 'in house' support, but invariably such work is undertaken by printing organisations that have the necessary equipment to produce posters. Be clear about what you want the poster to look like, what your budget is, and the timescale you are working to.

Printers do not mind if you cannot provide them with something that looks exactly like you want the finished product to look, but they do require very clear instructions. If you are going to hand-write the poster, make sure everything is legible. If you are going to produce the text using software such as Word, indicate where page breaks, column breaks, colour, bold, font size, diagrams, etc. are positioned, using typed instructions and indicators at the points at which they occur. Make sure all the pages are numbered and are given to the printer in a logical order. They do not know what was inside your head when you were designing and writing the poster — they will produce it exactly as instructed. If there is an overall instruction, such as the general font size and colour, provide this key information at the start as a briefing note.

When producing files for the printer it is better to produce each section as a separate file. If a file becomes corrupted for any reason it is easier to manage the outcome than to rework all of the information again. Fortunately, files do not corrupt too often, but it is devastating if this happens and can cause you a lot of unnecessary stress and loss of time.

Wherever possible, go and give the production brief and text to the printers personally. It can save a lot of time and reduces the possibility of misunderstanding.

## The printer's responsibilities

Printers can and will provide you with detailed information on how they would like the text and supporting materials presented to them. It is important to ask for this before you start your poster preparation. The way in which they can produce the litho print or Chromapress will have a big impact on what is feasible in terms of the use of colour and the final size and finish of the poster.

If you are very computer literate and can produce the finished product, then they only need to print it. Make sure you have used text files, scans and colour in a way that can be reproduced at the printers. It is a good idea to check with them first.

Always ask for a written quote of the price and, if you are on a tight budget, a breakdown of each element. You can then adjust your design accordingly and have evidence of what has been agreed. Also, get the production schedule agreed in writing, and when the checkpoints will occur for proofing before final printing.

---

### In summary

- Identify whether the poster will be produced 'in house' or by a printer.
- Find out which process is going to be used to print the poster.
- Ensure that all the aspects of design (colour etc.) can be done.
- Ask the printer for their guidelines and specifications for producing posters.
- Provide very detailed instructions to the printer so they know exactly what you want.
- Always proof the poster before printing.
- Get everything agreed in writing: costs, specifications, time.

---

## Transporting

When deciding on the format you are going to use it is very important to think about its portability. It needs to be able to be rolled up without creasing. If you need to secure it to stop it unrolling, use decorators' masking tape — it will not mark or tear the poster. If you have chosen to produce panels or sheets that join together or lie side by side, they need to be able to be stacked without sticking together and removing the print, if you intend to use them again. This is particularly important on the return journey, as they will often have had tape on or still have Velcro attached. A lightweight plastic tube, available at most stationers, will prevent it from getting wet or damaged during transit.

If you are travelling abroad or on public transport you should take your poster with your carry-on luggage — even if your suitcase is lost you will still be able to present your poster!

You may be tempted to send your poster by carrier, but experience says don't: it might never arrive. Also, if it is going abroad you do have to provide information for Customs and Excise before it can be sent, and this can take time.

## The poster session

### What is expected of you?

Your audience could be just one person or a small group. You must be constantly prepared to react to their needs. They may want a detailed explanation lasting up to 5 minutes, or just a few seconds of your time for a point of clarification. Be prepared to respond.

• Try to anticipate questions you might be asked.
• How do you want to respond to the questions?
• What are the key messages?
• What has been particularly interesting?
• What has not gone so well?
• Have you got the references?

You are likely to be required to be near your poster at specific times, so make sure you are available: it is a good opportunity for increasing networks and getting others' viewpoints.

There will be a time given to indicate when the poster can be put up and when it can be taken down. It is important to make sure you meet these deadlines. Don't forget to collect your poster: it will probably be destroyed if you do not.

Poster presenters are often expected to bring along their own fixings — tape, drawing/map pins, Velcro, scissors, etc. Even if the organisers say they will provide these, experience says take your own.

## What happens when you are not there?

It is important to leave information for those who look at the posters at times other than those designated. A handout with a few frequently asked questions (FAQs) that have been asked about your work, an A4 copy of the poster (if it is going to be readable), or details of how to contact you should be sufficient.

---

### In summary

- Prepare to respond to the audience's needs.
- Remember, the poster will be looked at when you are not there.
- Meet the deadlines and manage your time-keeping.

---

## Giving a 1-minute introduction to your poster

Many organisations ask poster presenters to give a 1-minute oral presentation about their poster. This can be to the total audience at conference (to encourage them to come and have a look at your poster and others) or in the poster area itself. The messages that you give need to be clear, concise and entertaining. The elements you need to include are:

- the title
- who you are
- the purpose of your investigations
- the outcomes
- why they should come and see your poster
- where you can be found.

You do not need elaborate graphics, but a few visual aids you can hold up could be of benefit:

- Do you have equipment that will help demonstrate your message?
- Relate it to things that have happened or are going to be addressed at the conference.
- Is there a theme running throughout the conference, e.g. title, pictures items?
- Think about how you can dress — some people wear their national costume.

Whatever you do you want to have an impact, but make sure it focuses on the content of your poster — it must be relevant.

If you have longer than 1 minute you can add some further information to your presentation (the information in this section is applicable and useful when making any presentation). You may wish to make it slightly more formal by adding some slides/acetates, but remember, one picture takes approximately 1–2 minutes, so even if you have 5 minutes to present three would be the maximum and two more realistic. Also, you would not use all the suggestions in italics: you need to pick and choose as to the messages you want to get over and the time available:

- the title
- who you are
- the purpose of your investigations
- *setting it in context*
- *the objectives*
- *the content introduction, must, good and nice to knows*
- the outcomes
- *summary*
- why they should come and see your poster
- where you can be found.

---

**In summary**

- Be your own visual aid.
- Keep it simple and concise.
- Keep focused on your topic.
- Make them want to come and see *your* poster.

---

### Responding to questions/clarification

Throughout the preparation of your poster you will have asked or been asked questions of or by:

- yourself
- others that have been involved in the development of your project
- proof readers
- poster production team
- those organising the poster event.

Note these down. Are there any questions that have been asked frequently, points of clarification sought? If so, these are likely to be asked by those reading your poster. Think about how you responded and how you might respond. It will make it easier on the day.

Are there any significant findings that will be key discussion points? Is there anything that is likely to be controversial? Can you support the information in your poster with references? Know the information that, because of lack of space, you have not been able to include in your poster so that you can substantiate elements in more detail.

---

**In summary**

- Be prepared to respond to questions and points of clarification.
- Practise some responses so that you come across as confident and can support the information you have written.

---

## Feedback

Have a notepad and pen to hand to jot down any useful verbal feedback. If you want more specific feedback, think about the discussions you want to have with those interested in your poster. You could formulate two or three questions you want to ask everyone that visits your poster. Be prepared to accept suggestions for improvement or criticism. Not everyone will agree with what you are saying or have written. You must be prepared to adapt to those who come to view your poster. There will be those wanting to discuss it for a few seconds and those who want to spend a few minutes with you. Prepare several versions of your responses so that you can cope with discussions confidently and with authority.

Have details of how, when and where you can be contacted. This could be in the form of a business card, or as text on a small slip of paper or at the bottom of any handout should you decide to provide one. Remember to leave some with your poster so that they are available for people to pick up when you are not there. They can be attached to the poster board in an envelope, wallet or card folder/container made for the purpose.

---

**In summary**

- Provide contact details.
- Think about the discussions that could take place.
- Be prepared for some negative feedback.

---

Remember, it is *your* poster. It is 'selling' your work and/or research. The old adage 'Fail to prepare — prepare to fail' will ring true if attention to planning, design and content is ignored. The poster does not have to be big and flashy to have impact: small can be just as effective if it is done well.

# Section Three

Medical journalism
and mass media

# 8

## Writing an editorial

*Richard Clark*

This chapter will look at how to write an editorial for a medical or pharmaceutical journal. I have not assumed any prior experience in writing an editorial, but there should be points of interest even for the experienced. The aim is to present a step-by-step guide through what can appear to be rather a daunting task for the uninitiated.

There are many choices of direction to take when writing an editorial, and many of them are considered here. Certain benefits (and potential pitfalls) are associated with choices that you make when writing for this format. This chapter aims to guide you through the writing process to achieve the desired result — an informative and interesting editorial.

### What is an editorial?

When trying to define the nature of an article described as an editorial it will be useful to first look at two extreme examples of their type. An editorial written for a national daily newspaper is familiar to most people. It is an opinion piece, usually covering several current and newsworthy issues. In general it is not attributed to a particular journalist, and represents the opinion of the newspaper editors, who may meet to discuss what will be written.

A second type of editorial is written for medical or scientific journals. In this case the author should be a leading expert in the specialty he or she is commenting on. This type of editorial tends to be a comment on a manuscript that will appear in the same issue. The author of the editorial, and the peer reviewers, will necessarily have seen the manuscript on which they are commenting prior to its publication.

The newspaper editorial may be read by hundreds of thousands of people, whereas the scientific editorial is read by far fewer, albeit many more with a special interest in the area being discussed. The impact of the newspaper editorial may reach a wider audience, but with a few notable exceptions is soon forgotten.

In contrast, the journal editorial can have much longer-lasting effects. If you had spent much time performing experiments or conducting clinical research, writing it up for publication and gone through an arduous peer-review process, you might not be happy if your article was preceded by an editorial that was less than complementary. Indeed, lifelong enmities and grudges can sometimes arise from such episodes.

Superficially, these two examples appear very different. However, all editorials share a common purpose: they should be hard-hitting, provocative, and often controversial. This sort of article seeks to change peoples' opinion about a subject, or at least to challenge them to have an opinion regarding an area that they had not thought about before, or had thought unimportant.

Above all, editorials must engage the reader. Maybe they explain a complex issue in an understandable way, but without being condescending. Maybe they offer a fresh and a thought-provoking perspective on an old and seemingly uncontroversial subject. These qualities can apply equally well to editorials written for just about any type of publication. However, this chapter will now focus on editorials written for scientific or medical journals.

### Checklist

✓ Realise the differences in impact editorials can have when written for the general public or for a scientific publication.

✓ All editorials should share a common purpose. They should be hard-hitting, provocative, and often controversial. They should engage the readers' interest, explain complex issues effectively and offer fresh perspectives.

## Authorship

All editorials require an author who is an expert in the subject area. Usually they are chosen by the journal editor from a small pool of people who are the accepted leaders in the field. Journals in the UK and elsewhere in Europe often use someone of international repute if they can. Getting a 'big name' can certainly lend weight and credibility both to the journal and to the article under discussion. It can also bring grief and despair. If the editorial author decides that the article they are commenting on is flawed or doesn't add anything new, then they will probably write something to that effect. Moreover, in my opinion, you are more likely to get the extremes — a complimentary or a dismissive editorial — from authors who are the most eminent, as they usually feel the most secure in their position and so are more likely to be controversial. When choosing an author for an editorial it is worth bearing this in mind — the bigger the name, the higher the stakes.

In my experience it pays to find out as much as possible about potential editorial authors so you can have as good a chance as possible of knowing what sort of angle they are likely to take. Just picking out a list of names based on internet searches, consensus statement authors and numbers of publications from a PubMed search does not reveal the full picture. Ideally, the editor should read some of the editorials that potential authors have written, and maybe a recent review that they have authored, to give them a better idea of their written work. Best of all, they can use their own experience and draw on the knowledge of contacts to find out whether candidate authors are likely to write something useful. Will they be able to bring some practice-based experience to bear on the subject? Are they known to express an opinion and not just support the status quo? Will they regurgitate the same evidence, used time after time, or are they known to be an original thinker?

At times the journal editor will want to court controversy, and may deliberately choose someone they know will be likely to deliver it. To a great extent, however, the nature and content of an editorial will be unpredictable, and this is good for the medical and scientific community.

Another issue is, what if the editorial is not written entirely by the named author? They may not have time to write it themselves, and so may approach a member of their staff to write a draft for them. Alternatively, a medical writer may produce a draft, which is then sent to the author for review, rewriting and approval. I would suggest that the person writing the first draft should make sure that they are aware of the named author's point of view, maybe through a recorded meeting or interview. They should prepare a brief outline and show this to the author, who can comment, change or rewrite it before a first draft is produced. After the production of the first draft, the ethical burden then falls on the named author to rewrite or edit the article so that it expresses his or her own views accurately. The journal may have a policy on this type of practice, and this should be adhered to.

Most importantly, *it is essential that the editorial reflect the view of the named author and no-one else.* The author should have full control of the content and under no circumstances should they be pressured to change their opinion, or the content of the article, according to another's wishes. In addition, I would urge anyone preparing an editorial to be aware of the European Medical Writers Association (EMWA) guidelines on the role of medical writers in developing peer-reviewed publications[1] as well as the World Association of Medical Editors (WAME) recommendations on publication ethics for medical journals.[2] It is worth noting that WAME recommends that 'In most publications reporting clinical trials, a medical writer who has not been involved in study design, data analysis, or interpretation will not qualify to be listed as an author according to the Vancouver criteria. However, so long as they work closely with the named authors, there is no ethical reason why such writers should not prepare drafts of publications.'

The rest of this chapter will deal with the challenge of how to write an editorial from the perspective of the author who is an expert in the field.

---

**Checklist**

☑ The more eminent the author the greater the probability that an opinion — complimentary or critical — will be expressed.
☑ If you are given the job of choosing an author for an editorial, do you know how to best go about it?
☑ Will the editorial be written entirely by the named author?
☑ Are authors aware of ethical guidelines for writing articles, both those specific to the journal and those from WAME and EMWA on authorship?
☑ The editorial should reflect the view of the named author and no-one else.

---

## Types of editorial

This section deals with the different types of editorial that may be written for a scientific or medical readership. There are two main situations where an editorial is required:

• a preface for a journal, book or report
• a commentary on a published study, usually a new clinical trial.

In either case the editorial can be an introduction to an area or topic, plus the author's opinion on the articles, chapters, etc. that follow. The approach taken by the editorial usually falls into four main categories:

• supportive (positive, praising a trial, author, topic, etc.)
• critical (negative, critical of a trial, current disease recognition and/or treatment, etc.)

- explanatory/educational (clarifying and explaining a complex or controversial issue)
- persuasive (examining facts and figures in such a way to produce a solution to a problem).

Editorials will usually encompass more than one (often all) of the above approaches, but only one approach should predominate. If you are writing an editorial it is vital that you decide which approach should be your main focus *before* you begin. You should base your choice primarily on your scientific or clinical experience in the area and your knowledge of the published evidence. If you do not have sufficient practical and/or theoretical experience and knowledge to draw upon to make you confident of a particular approach, you should question your suitability to write the article. It would be better to inform the editor at an early stage that the subject is somewhat removed from your main area of expertise, and decline the invitation to write rather than produce a substandard article. It is also best to make this decision early on, so that someone else can be asked to write the editorial, and to avoid any embarrassment.

---

**Checklist**

☑  Decide what the main focus of the editorial is going to be before you start to write. Will it be mainly supportive, critical, explanatory/educational or persuasive?

☑  Do you have sufficient knowledge and experience to decide on a main focus after reading the manuscript that will accompany your editorial?

☑  Let the book or journal editor know as soon as possible if you feel out of your depth, so they can find someone else.

---

## Structure

In this section we look in more detail at how to structure an editorial. We start from the viewpoint that an editorial expresses a personal opinion, based on fact and the author's experience. Thus it can and should be quite different from one by another author on the same topic. These differences arise not only from differences in opinion, but also from how these are expressed — namely, the structure of the article. I think it is always a good idea to write out the structure of an editorial first to check whether the arguments appear to flow in a logical manner. There is no 'best' structure to use for certain situations, but here I will suggest two types to consider. The first is for a type of editorial that is used as a preface or introduction. Most often, this will be for a book, journal or report on a specific therapeutic specialty and/or treatments for that condition. The example here introduces a review of schizophrenia, and various treatments for the disease. The editorial author was given a loose type of structure to follow (see Editorial brief below) by the journal editor, who approached them to write the editorial.

---

**Editorial brief**

Editorial authors should ensure that they cover the following points.

- 1–2 sentences on the burden of the disease, in the UK and around the world.
- Look back 10 or more years to how developments in disease management have enabled doctors to improve the management of schizophrenia.
- Acknowledge how far the profession has come, and what has been achieved to date regarding the management of schizophrenia.
- An analysis of the challenges that remain, and the important leading role that general practitioners and hospital doctors have to play in resolving them.
- Look forward 10 years or so and set out some realistic yet challenging goals for healthcare professionals, and maybe provide a few positive forecasts for the future of patients with schizophrenia, and those who have the responsibility of looking after their health.

---

On this occasion the author followed the brief fairly closely, and the editorial is reproduced here (copyright permission obtained from CSF Medical Communications Ltd, publishers of *Drugs in Context*).[3]

### Editorial
*Dr Mike Travis*
*Maudsley Hospital and Institute of Psychiatry, King's College London*

Schizophrenia can affect anyone, and is one of the greatest causes of lost quality of life worldwide. One in 100 people will experience this serious mental illness at some time in their lives, though it commonly starts in the late teens to the early 20s in men and early to late 20s in women. Although schizophrenia can have a profound effect, it can be treated effectively in most people. This was not always the case.

Chlorpromazine initiated a revolution in the treatment of people with schizophrenia and was the first truly effective therapy. Thus, many patients were able to leave mental institutions and live in their own communities. Chlorpromazine, in common with all antipsychotics, acts by blocking or reducing the function of dopamine receptors. The antipsychotics in general use up until the 1990s are often called typical or conventional antipsychotics. These are less effective against negative than positive symptoms, and elicit extrapyramidal side-effects (EPS), often at doses which do not improve schizophrenia symptoms. The reintroduction of clozapine led to the subsequent advent of the 'atypical' antipsychotics. Although not really a separate class of antipsychotics, these medications are characterised by vastly reduced or absent EPS at therapeutic doses. This has been associated with dramatic improvements in the secondary negative symptoms of schizophrenia which were often related to EPS. However, clozapine is restricted to use in treatment-resistant schizophrenia as regular blood monitoring is required for this medication. Other atypical antipsychotics (e.g. risperidone, olanzapine, quetiapine, amisulpride and ziprasidone) have subsequently been developed. Though none seem to be quite as effective as clozapine in treatment resistant schizophrenia, they do not require blood monitoring, have a greater effect against negative symptoms globally and cause fewer EPS than the typical antipsychotics.

Recently published UK guidelines, (National Institute of Clinical Excellence, [NICE]), advocate that atypical antipsychotics should be made available to all patients with schizophrenia, yet a survey carried out by the charity Rethink suggests that about 20% of primary care trusts have yet to make these drugs available for doctors to prescribe for people with schizophrenia, presumably as their acquisition costs are greater than the older conventional antipsychotics. Hopefully, the more widespread use of newer antipsychotics will reduce the side-effect burden on people treated for schizophrenia, fulfilling patients' basic human rights to lead the most normal and productive lives they can.

The development of better resources should go hand-in-hand with better treatment. For example, a relatively small number of acute inpatient beds needs to be combined with half-way and respite houses, outpatient clinics, occupational therapy, and in general, an emphasis on the rehabilitation of patients into the ordinary activities of daily living. Thus, the greater integration of primary care in the form of GPs, and the community psychiatric nurses and social workers who work directly with them, with specialist care (primarily psychiatrists and hospital and community mental health teams), is both desirable and necessary. One possible challenge to both primary and secondary care is that as we become better at treating schizophrenia a greater burden could fall on primary care, as more patients are treated for longer in the community outside of specialist services. We need to foster stronger links between psychiatrists and primary care, ensure that patients' symptoms are recognised as early as possible and that appropriate action (e.g. referral to a specialist) is taken.

It is in primary care that recognition of patient risk factors and detection of illness usually occurs. Thus, effective primary–secondary care communication and integration is essential, will lead to the best use of existing resources and allow the compassionate care of people with schizophrenia in as close to an ordinary home environment as possible.

The eventual benefits of this approach may be an improvement in the long-term outcome for people with schizophrenia.

As can be seen from this example of a preface, this type of editorial offers a general introduction and sets the tone for the subsequent text. One or two ideas are introduced which were the subject of more vigorous discussion later in the publication — such as continued obstruction in the UK to the use of new drugs to treat schizophrenia.

This type of structure (unmet needs, impact of a disease, what treatments are available, best practice and, finally, looking to the future) is quite common. In the right hands this format can be fresh, exciting and thought-provoking, but in this example the main task is to introduce rather than be provocative.

The second type of outline is for an editorial as a comment on a clinical trial. Take a hypothetical situation: you have been asked to write an editorial in the *British Medical Journal* for a clinical trial comparing two opioids for the relief of chronic pain. Your opinions on the subject as an expert in the area are first, that opioids are often not prescribed when they should be, as many doctors are wary of prescribing them because of fears about addiction; second, that it is important to have well-designed clinical trials to assess and compare opioids effectively; and third, you do not consider that the trial in this issue was well designed, as it was an open-label rather than a double-blind trial of two very different formulations. This may have allowed patient and investigator bias to influence the results, particularly owing to the subjective nature of the outcome (pain, and patient preference for one formulation). In the light of these opinions you might prefer the following structure:

1) The present situation with regard to opioids in chronic pain — unanswered questions:
   a) Are opioids effective?
   b) Which opioids are effective, and which formulations?
   c) Introduce the study in this issue.
2) Opioids are often withheld:
   a) to 'protect' the individual from addiction; fears that are generally not justified in patients with chronic pain
   b) because of fears that medical availability of opioids can lead to an increased incidence of street addiction — present data that this fear is irrational and not supported by published studies
   c) as a result, politics, prejudice and continuing ignorance have impeded optimal prescribing of these drugs.

3) Which patients benefit? An opioid trial is appropriate when other methods of analgesia have failed, but there is a lack of evidence as to which drug or class of drug is the best for particular pain syndromes.

4) How do we know patients have benefited? Address the issue of an adequate dose, dose titration to analgesia, and balancing analgesia with adverse events.

5) Discuss the trial:
   a) Welcome in principle, but question results based on open-label design when comparing subjective outcomes
   b) Question whether the differences found between formulations are credible
   c) Demand that we have better-designed clinical trials to find out which opioid formulation is most effective in clinical practice.

This type of editorial may not be popular with the authors of the clinical trial, so the editorial author will have to be confident of their viewpoint. However, given the inclination of most people towards evidence-based medicine and the consensus on good trial design, this editorial is probably on quite safe ground here. The under-prescribing of opioids for chronic pain, particularly chronic non-malignant pain, is more controversial and will probably generate some interesting correspondence for the journal, which is all to the good.

**Checklist**

☑ Decide on the structure of your editorial, based on your own views and opinions.
☑ Have you written out a plan of the structure you want to follow?
☑ Read your plan. Does it express your own views cogently and in a logical manner that is easy to follow?

## Writing

### Be prepared

Before you begin your editorial it is helpful to check that you are fully prepared and ready to write. Try to go through a short checklist as follows:

Make sure you have information from the journal, book, etc. on specifications for the editorial you will be writing (e.g. number of words, number of references, preferred layout, deadline for submission).

Read the article/chapters that the editorial will address.

Decide on an angle based on your own knowledge and opinions (see above). Be objective rather than subjective.

Gather supporting (and contrary) information from published literature. This will be useful to ensure that you back your opinions with facts and figures.

Plan a structure (see above).

Write it.

## Getting your message across

Ten hints to help you during the writing process:

1) To begin at the beginning: the choice of title is vital. Many more people will read your editorial if it has a title that attracts them in some way. An excellent example, though not from a medical journal, is a famous editorial written for *The Times* in the 1960s by William Rees Mogg. His editorial titled 'Who breaks a butterfly on a wheel?' was sympathetic towards Mick Jagger, who had been sentenced to jail for having four amphetamine tablets in his possession.

2) Be concise, even if your subject is very complex. Start with a broad stroke: an overview or an introduction to the area you will be writing about. You can narrow your subject area as you go on, giving more and more detail towards the latter stages of your article. This is sometimes known as the 'inverted pyramid' style of writing (see diagram on page 171).

3) Use one main idea per paragraph. You can elaborate around this idea, but try not to introduce too many ideas at once.

4) Don't use long words where short ones will do. The purpose of your editorial is to communicate a message. Don't think that using a lot of long words and terminology will impress many people — it will not. Instead, it might make them stop reading halfway through. You will have readers for whom English is a second language, so non-standard use of English will confuse them. If it is easy to read without reaching for a medical or standard dictionary then at least you stand a chance that the content may be read. Examples where words in everyday use are suitable but others are often used are 'efficacious' (why not use 'effective'?), 'paucity' (why not 'lack' or 'few'?), or my own least favourite, 'negative impact' (reduces, lowers, etc.). (See also page 41 for information about choice of words.)

5) Avoid abbreviations. If you must use them define them on the first occasion, but still try not to use them too much afterwards — it can get very tedious otherwise. There are exceptions to this, such as when the subject of the editorial is a condition that has a long name and there is a well-known abbreviation that can be used (for example

chronic obstructive pulmonary disease is known as COPD). Better to have COPD ten times on one page than spelling it out in full every time. Often people will invent their own special abbreviations, and often not define them. This causes the editor extra work and is probably one of the best ways to annoy them. So, define any abbreviations you use if you would like to keep editors happy.

6)  Be relevant. Do you think the topic you are writing about is of interest to most readers? If it is, then that's great. If it isn't, then maybe you want to try and persuade them why they *should* be interested.

7)  Don't state the obvious. Is there anything in your editorial that might make someone think 'So what, everyone knows that?' Maybe you should think about replacing or deleting these sections.

8)  Don't repeat yourself or use redundant words. A phrase that attempts to be colloquial, such as 'In the real world . . .' or 'Real patients . . .' begs the question is there an 'unreal world' or 'unreal patients' somewhere? A good test if you think a word might be redundant is to substitute the opposite, as above. If the result is nonsense then the word is redundant and can be removed. This type of writing might be suitable for a politician's speech, but not for an editorial in a peer-reviewed medical journal.

9)  If you can make the content interesting to the reader and you present it well, you are placing your editorial in the best position to be read by the widest possible audience. This should be a key objective of any editorial.

10) Provide some sort of call for action at the end of the editorial. This can be part of the 'take-home message'. After reading a good editorial the reader should either know something they didn't know before, or be thinking about a subject they are familiar with from a different angle. They may or may not agree with the views you have expressed, but that is one of the main objectives of an editorial — to challenge and to provoke discussion. You can succeed in this even if most readers don't agree with you.

## Privileges . . . and duties

The author of an editorial that accompanies the first publication of a clinical trial will have certain privileges, but also some duties or responsibilities. These are shown in Table 8.1.

## Final checks

Here are a few final checks to go through once you have written your first draft:

**Table 8.1**  Privileges and responsibilities of an editorial writer

| Privileges | Duties |
|---|---|
| You see clinical trial data and interpretation prior to the publication of results, in the same way as those who peer-review the article | No personal or professional use of data, arguments or interpretations must be made prior to publication unless the authors' specific permission is obtained, other than for the purposes of writing an editorial or commentary to accompany the article |
| You have a free hand to select any facts or references to support the opinions you express in the editorial | It is your duty to be even-handed and fair in selection of references. Any facts and figures should be from reputable sources |
| You have greater freedom to express thoughts, ideas and opinions than is usually given for other types of article | Weigh the facts, and don't just present one side of an argument |
| Your editorial can have a profound effect on how readers receive the publication on which you are commenting | Keep an open mind when reading the manuscript that your editorial will accompany. Be fair and balanced, and represent a reasonable point of view that can be substantiated |

Have you met author guidelines for word and reference count, and the publication format?

Read through to check spelling, grammar, and that all abbreviations are defined.

Second read-through to check that the overall tone is correct for the readership, that it reads well, and that it expresses your opinion in a logical and easy-to-follow manner.

Have you used too much jargon and/or abbreviations? If so, it may be less accessible to a wider readership.

Is the editorial thought-provoking, original and persuasive?

Check your references. Are the citations correct, and do the references support your editorial in the way you intended?

If you have any conflicts of interest have you declared them?

## Conclusions

If you have been approached to write an editorial this can be flattering — you are being asked for your opinion as an expert on a particular topic. As such, it is important not to get carried away on the one hand (make sure you can justify and back up your arguments), or on the other hand to be safe but dull and uninteresting (i.e. too factual, and little or no original opinion). Perhaps the best advice for the writer of an editorial should be keep it short, punchy and interesting, but based on a position you can support. If you can achieve this, then you will have written a good editorial.

### Checklist

☑ Make sure your article is not too radical without adequate factual support; nor should it be too staid, dull and uninteresting.

☑ Keep the editorial short, punchy and interesting, but based on a position that you can support.

## References

1. WAME (World Association of Medical Editors) Recommendations on Publication Ethics Policies for Medical Journals. Available from: *http://www.wame.org.htm*

2. European Medical Writers Association (EMWA) Guidelines on the role of medical writers in developing peer-reviewed publications. Available from: *http://www.emwa.org*

3. Travis T, Clark R, Rasmussen J (2004) Schizophrenia: olanzapine. *Drugs in Context — Primary Care. Part C: Psychiatry and Neurology* 1: 1–40.

# 9

## Writing a letter to the editor

*Richard Clark*

This chapter is a step-by-step guide to writing a letter to a medical or pharmaceutical journal. Most people will have written letters at some point, and so this may seem straightforward. The challenge to be addressed, however, is how to write a *good* letter that communicates what you want it to and that stands a reasonable chance of being published, as most journal editors receive more letters than they have space for.

### What is a letter?

At first, this might seem like a fairly stupid question, but these are often the ones most worth asking. No doubt you've written plenty of letters to people or organisations throughout your life, and surely writing one for submission to a journal is no different? However, there is an essential difference between 'normal' letters and one that you might submit to a journal. In everyday life you write a letter to communicate something to a person, a group of people or an organisation. You might be thanking them for a birthday present, telling a friend what a wonderful time you're having travelling around the world, or complaining to a manufacturer about products or services. When writing to a journal you are, in fact, writing something *directed at the readership of the journal*, hoping that a large number of people will read your letter with interest.

The initial recipient of your letter — the journal editor — is not the primary target audience. However, you should always bear in mind the 'gatekeeper' role of the editor. They alone decide whether or not to publish your letter (unless you have an automatic right of reply to letters commenting on a study of your own previously published in that journal — but we will consider this later). Thus, to some extent, you must normally consider both audiences — the editor and the journal readership — if your letter is to appear in print and communicate your views effectively.

In many ways writing a letter to the editor of a journal is analogous to writing one to a local or national newspaper. The recipient at a newspaper (the letters editor) has a gatekeeper role, as most letters go unpublished, and the target audience is the newspaper's readership. One essential difference, however, is that newspaper letters usually express a point of view which is usually unsupported by facts or has only meagre corroborating evidence from the writer's own experience. A letter to a scientific journal will *usually* be backed by good-quality supportive evidence, given the nature of the target audience, who otherwise will probably not be very interested. As the readership will be scientists, medical personnel, etc. they will not be used to trusting opinions without facts to back them up (and often not even then), so firm opinions and scientific evidence are usual in a letter to the editor of a scientific journal. In summary, there are three broad categories of letter.

**Three broad categories of letter**

- Normal, such as a personal or business letter, usually directed at an individual; the target audience is the person to whom it is addressed, so you are reasonably certain that they will read it.
- Letter to a newspaper, primarily expressing your opinions, with little or no supporting evidence. It has to be chosen for publication by the letters editor before it goes into print and can reach your target audience — the newspaper readership.
- Letter to a medical or scientific journal, expressing your opinions with reasonable supporting evidence. It has to be chosen for publication by the editor unless you have an automatic right to reply.

Although the remainder of this chapter will focus on the last of these scenarios, all letters are linked by a common purpose. Ideally, they should be:

- timely
- concise
- interesting
- understandable.

**Checklist**

- ☑ Understand some of the differences between letters written for and by the general public and those for publication in a scientific journal.
- ☑ Letters should be timely, concise, interesting and understandable.

## Why write a letter to the editor?

As the letters pages are often one of the most widely read sections of a journal, a letter is an excellent way to communicate with your target audience. As such, it is an excellent forum in which to correct and/or comment on an article or statement that recently appeared in a journal. It's also a chance to express your own view. This may arise from your desire to communicate your point of view on a particular topic without having to spend time writing a long article, and without even having to go to the bother of conducting a clinical trial or a systematic review.

Pharmaceutical companies often use the letters pages to promote critical discussion of trials favourable to their competitors by pointing out the shortcomings of trials published in previous issues of the journal. Of course, these will appear under the name of the expert in the field, but are often written by someone else, such as a medical writer working directly or indirectly for the drug company. As for any publications that appear in your name, it's important that the final content of a letter reflects your views accurately.

Whatever the reason for writing, your letter should be of interest to the readers of the journal, and the most common reason is to comment on an article in a previous issue. In the next section we will look at the different types of letter.

---

- The letters pages are often one of the most widely read sections of a journal, so a letter is an excellent way to communicate with your target audience.
- A letter is a chance to express your own perspective, arising from a desire to communicate your point of view on a particular topic.

---

## Types of letter

The International Committee of Medical Journal Editors' *Uniform Requirements for Manuscripts Submitted to Biomedical Journals*[1] contains the following statement:

> Biomedical journals should provide their readership with a mechanism for submitting comments, questions, or criticisms about published articles, as well as brief reports and commentary unrelated to previously published articles. This will likely, but not necessarily, take the form of a

correspondence section or column. The authors of articles discussed in correspondence should be given an opportunity to respond, preferably in the same issue in which the original correspondence appears.

Thus it is clear that as an author of a journal article you have a right to reply to any correspondence relating to your paper. Likewise, anyone should be able to write to the journal, which is obliged to provide a forum in which readers' opinions can be expressed and disseminated. The main reasons to write a letter are:

- disagreeing with a published article
- praising or supporting a paper published by someone else
- exercising a 'right to reply' to criticism of an article you have published
- communicating data of medical or scientific interest that you want published quickly and/or that does not warrant a full paper, or even a short communication.

Of all the reasons for writing a letter to the editor, the most common is probably to express disagreement with a published article, or to exercise a right to reply. Of course, one letter may encompass several of the above. For example, you may praise, disagree and present your own data, but be clear what you main focus will be (see later sections).

**Checklist**

✓ Be aware of the different types of letter — disagree, agree, right to reply and presenting data.
✓ Your letter will probably fall into more than one of these categories, but be clear which one will be the main focus.

**Key objectives**

The key objectives are very simple, but worth bearing in mind:

- Write about something that you strongly feel needs to be communicated.
- Get it past the editor so that it is published (not all letters are published).
- Make sure your letter is worth reading.

In the next few sections we will investigate how to achieve these objectives.

## Where to start?

- First decide what main point (or points) you would like to communicate. (Keep it simple — if you try to make too many points in 300 words or so you won't communicate any of them coherently or memorably.)
- Next, gather your data/references to support your case. It would be a good idea to perform a number of general and specialised internet searches for the latest information in the literature, even if you are fairly well informed on the topic.
- Go to the 'Instructions for Authors' section in the journal, either in printed issue or on the journal's website, and find out if there are any instructions on letters to the editor (e.g. maximum word count).
- Have a look at examples of letters published in the journal you're interested in. The type of letter published will vary from journal to journal.
- Remember the importance of timing. Is the subject of your letter particularly topical, and/or are you commenting on something published in the journal last week or 6 months ago? Many journals operate a time limit, rejecting letters responding to articles published over, say, 3 or 6 months ago. For the best chance of publication letters should be both topical *and* timely.

### Checklist

- ☑ Be clear on your main point(s), and gather supporting data.
- ☑ Be aware of the journal's requirements for letters, and have a look at published letters in your target journal.
- ☑ Will your letter be topical and timely?

## Structure

Many different types of structure can be used for a letter, and no particular one is always the best. However, it is a good idea to think before you write, and then make a very brief plan of what you are going to say and in what order. This imposes a style that will hopefully make your letter:

- easier to read
- clearer in your communication of main point(s)
- more persuasive, as your reasons for your point of view and supporting evidence will be presented in a straightforward and understandable manner.

What is most important to avoid is a rambling and unstructured letter.

## The 'sandwich' structure

One of the simplest and most effective styles to use when commenting on a published paper with which you wish to largely disagree is the classic 'sandwich' structure, something along the following lines:

- Briefly refer to the article (give its author, title and reference/date), and then write something complimentary about it (one or two sentences). Next state something about the study that you disagree with (i.e. communicate the point of the letter). At this stage you may want to say who you are and why you are qualified to comment.
- The middle section further expounds on why you disagree with parts of the article. Here, you can use published or unpublished data, personal anecdotes or statistics that support your views. This is the longest section, but is still concise.
- Restate your major point, and wrap up with a succinct conclusion.

A variation on this style can be used when writing in support of an article to which you would like to add your own data. In this case you might wish to start with one sentence in which you state your main point (i.e. that you strongly agree with the article) *and* that you can provide additional support for its argument. In this case there is no need for fulsome praise before launching into your main point — you only need to flatter the authors before you 'attack' their study! — so you might as well plunge straight in with your main point.

## The EPIC structure

Other typical structures include the EPIC style, which can be used to develop a defined and persuasive structure to your letter, regardless of the type of response (supportive or negative):

- **Engage** the reader with a startling fact, or a strong statement of a serious problem or unmet need.
- **Propose** a specific action whereby this need or problem can be dealt with.
- **Illustrate** how the proposal would work and why it's important. Maybe give a few details or examples, either from your own experience or from published studies.
- **Call to action** for the readership to undertake specific measures to deal with the problem along the lines of your proposal.

Using this structure can help you to order your thoughts and make your response concise and persuasive. It can also make writing your letter much easier and less time-consuming, as you'll spend less time trying to figure out where to begin.

When using your right to reply to negative comments on a study of your own, the sort of structure you choose will depend mainly on the nature of the criticism. However, it might be a good idea to use the sandwich style, i.e. picking out some of the comments and criticisms made, which you can accept and agree with before recounting the main points with which you disagree, stating why you disagree, and giving further supporting evidence for your case. Finally, restate your major point, and finish with a succinct conclusion.

> ➤ There are many different types of structure that can be used for a letter. Whichever you use, it is a good idea to have some sort of plan as this helps to order your thoughts, resulting in a clearer, more concise and persuasive letter.

## Writing

### Be prepared

Once you have decided on an appropriate structure for your letter you can start to write it. It's worth initially re-reading any article you might be commenting on, to check you have not misunderstood it. Next, decide whether the angle you had decided on is still valid and defensible, based on the re-read and your own knowledge of the area. By now you should have a good idea of the main point or points you wish to make, and have supporting information gathered from the published literature and your own experience. Now is a good time to check that these facts really do support your point of view, and that they are from a reputable source.

Now you're fully prepared to write the letter, which shouldn't take long as it will be brief, you know what you'll say, and how it will be structured. Finally, don't forget to include your title, affiliation, contact details and any conflicting interests.

### Language and style

As people tend to read letters fairly quickly, readability is very important. No-one wants to read a long unstructured letter in which thoughts have been written down as they come to mind. Apart from using a defined structure, there are other language and style points to consider when writing a letter:

- Use paragraphs as your basic building blocks, with the most important sentence of each appearing at the beginning, and develop this point in a logical manner. Don't be afraid to divide your letter into three or four short paragraphs, as this can also increase readability.
- Keep sentences short. If you write long sentences, each making several points, the reader may have to re-read parts of your letter in order to understand it.
- The use of abbreviations should be kept to a bare minimum, as they can make your letter less readable.
- Avoid sounding pompous and using flowery, pseudoscientific language. Thus, 'administered' can become 'given' and 'utilise' 'use'. A general rule to follow is that a shorter word in common use is generally better than a longer word in less common use.
- If it is possible to cut out a word, do so (e.g. ~~past~~ history, ~~forward~~ planning, ~~close~~ scrutiny), and avoid elaborate prose (e.g. instead of 'male paediatric patients', why not write 'boys' — you might then have room to define an age range and so improve the accuracy of the statement).
- Avoid meaningless (or at least easily misunderstood) 'buzzwords' such as 'proactive' and 'stakeholder'.
- Avoid dissociating authors from results. This can lead to statements such as 'The data suggest', which is not accurate. Data show and writers suggest. ('Data' is also plural, so it should be 'these data . . .').
- If you gave your letter to a well-informed person with little or no experience of medicine, pharmacology or science, would they understand the main point(s) you are trying to make? They should do. I call this the 'average Radio 4 listener test'.

For more information on style, see Chapter 1.

**Checklist**

- ☑ Make your letter readable by using short paragraphs, short sentences and short words.
- ☑ Avoid pseudoscientific gobbledegook, excessive abbreviation and redundant words.
- ☑ Ensure that a well-informed member of the public can understand the main points you're trying to make.

### Hints to get your message across

- It is usual to write about something you read recently in a journal. As these letters are a response they are usually relevant, and therefore more likely to be printed than letters that do not refer to a journal article.

- Decide on one or two points that you'd like to communicate, and stick to them.

- Don't pepper your letter with a long list of things you agreed or disagreed with in a publication, as this 'shotgun' approach is dull for the reader and you won't communicate your main messages effectively.

- Always say why you have written your letter (i.e. its main point) at or near the start. People can then decide whether or not they want to read it.

- Try to ensure that people don't have to read sentences more than once to understand them, which can be quite a challenge when explaining a complex situation. Thus, be more like a journalist than novelist in that 'Literature is the art of writing something that will be read twice; journalism what will be read once.'

- If the journal specifies a word count this should be regarded as an upper limit. Don't be afraid of writing a much more concise letter.

- Finish off with a punchy and memorable sentence that summarises your opinions.

- Make it easy for the journal editor. Use double spacing and an easily readable font such as Garamond 12 point or Arial 10 point — if this is not specified in the journal instructions.

- Submit your letter to the right person! Get the correct name, title and address for the editor to whom your letter should be sent.

---

**Final checks after writing the first draft**

☑ Check that you have met journal guidelines for the number of words and references.

☑ First read-through to check for spelling, grammar, and that all abbreviations are defined.

☑ Perform a second read-through to check that the overall tone is correct for the readership, that it reads well, and that it expresses your opinion in a logical and easy-to-follow format.

☑ Have you used too much jargon and/or too many abbreviations? If so, it may be less accessible to a wider readership.

☑ Check your references. Are the citations correct and do the references support your letter in the way that you intend?

☑ If you have any conflicts of interest, have you declared them?

☑ Have you included your full title and contact details?

# Conclusions

## View from a letters editor

Why trust what I've written here? Well, it's worth considering the points of view expressed by the letters editor of the *BMJ* (*British Medical Journal*), which support the content of this chapter. I've summarised some of the main points here, but if you would like to read the full article it is available from the *BMJ*.[2]

- Readers' letters are crucial to the success of the *BMJ*.
- The letters pages are the readers' forum.
- Enthusiasm, different perspectives, diversity, ability to stimulate debate and wit are all appreciated.
- Letters are edited only lightly for clarity and readability, so that the author's voice is still audible and is louder than in any other part of the journal.
- We select letters for the paper journal from the unedited rapid responses posted daily on *www.bmj.com*.
- Rapid responses are considered in the same way as other publications. A declaration of competing interests and signed informed consent of patients is required if any information taken from the doctor–patient relationship is described.
- We accept letters for the paper journal from the rapid responses largely on the grounds of readability — not, as in the past, for their detailed critique of science.
- Three hundred words is the new maximum, but let it not become the optimum as the old limit seems to have done. The shorter the better. I am, for example, constantly impressed by letters to the editor in the *Times* for their conciseness and how few words can make me smile or think.

## Final thoughts

Here are just a few final points to consider:

- Letters are a good way to communicate your personal opinions, whether on a paper published by someone else, in which you can express your support and/or disagreement, or in reply to other correspondence.
- As letters are widely read, make sure you write one to be proud of. It should be clear, concise and readable. Focus on one or two key points.

- It's important not to get carried away by your own opinions. You need to use supporting facts from reputable sources. Disagreement with a trial based solely on your own unpublished observations does not make a strong case.

Remember that you can write a letter agreeing with a publication, and use this to present your own views and/or some of your own data, such as a case study. After all, as Mark Twain said, 'I did not attend his funeral, but I wrote a nice letter saying I approved it.'

## References

1.  The International Committee of Medical Journal Editors. Uniform Requirements for Manuscripts Submitted to Biomedical Journals: Writing and Editing for Biomedical Publication. Available from: *http://www.icmje.org/index.html*
2.  Davies S (2003) New edicts for letters to the editor. *BMJ* 326: 63–64.

# 10

## Writing for magazines and newspapers

*Pamela Mason*

Health and medicine are favourite topics for newspapers and magazines. This is because people are increasingly interested in finding out how to ensure good health, prevent ill health, or obtain knowledge about a disease they have. They are also interested in how the health system works, why things go wrong, and what to expect of healthcare professionals. In any newspaper or magazine you are likely to find at least one article or piece of news about health, disease, medicine, healthcare systems or healthcare professionals.

Journalists without a specialty will often decide to specialise in health because there is such a ready market for articles and news about it. Conversely, healthcare professionals who are not trained journalists sometimes also take up writing, either full- or part-time. Although professional journals and magazines may account for a significant proportion of their market, newspapers and magazines aimed at the lay audience should not be overlooked as opportunities to publish articles about health. Any medical writer who is serious about writing and communicating with readers should consider this market seriously. The impact you can have on readers and their health is enormous.

In surveys looking at where people get their information about health, the media are often more popular than health professionals. There is thus the potential for you to have more influence on people's knowledge of and decisions about their health as a writer than as a practising health professional.

With more than 1300 newspapers and 6000 periodicals published in the UK, writing opportunities are enormous. Moreover, this does not include the hundreds of free newspapers, newsletters and magazines, as well as electronic publications on the internet. Foreign English-language publications, or those in a language that you can write, are another market worth exploring.

A list of the main magazines and newspapers published in the UK is provided by Media UK (*www.mediauk.com*).

## Why write for magazines and newspapers?

Writing for magazines and newspapers will increase the number and variety of your writing outlets, and writing as a health professional gives you the following advantages:

- You know the subject and how to apply it to the reader.
- You know where to look for further information, which reduces research time.
- You can interpret your knowledge and insight for several different markets.

The disadvantage you have is perhaps in not being able to translate complex medical issues and terminology into clear and simple lay language. This is a challenge, but rewarding if you can get it right, because your specialist knowledge means that you can correct myths and misconceptions and present facts in an unambiguous way.

Editors are becoming increasingly aware of the value of 'specialist' writers, and there is an increased demand for health professionals to write for the print media. Remember, this can help to raise the profile of your profession in the public eye. If you write well, as a pharmacist, nurse or dietician, this gives a positive impression to readers, who may be more likely to turn to your professional colleagues for advice.

As a healthcare professional you will also have a specific viewpoint on health topics. A pharmacist, for example, has expertise on medicines and can educate the public about compliance with drug therapy, how medicines work, and the importance of questioning medication and reporting any adverse reactions. A dietician can help to inform the public about healthy eating and drinking, exploding some of the many extravagant myths about food and nutrition. A nurse could provide authoritative advice on first aid.

### Types of health writing

Health and medical writing in magazines and newspapers falls into several categories:
- news items
- general information/consumer awareness features
- recent research roundups
- debate on controversies

- opinion pieces
- a regular column
- how to/self-help/advice articles
- question and answer format
- interviews with people
- personal experience.

## Newspapers

Newspapers tend to be general or specialist, national or local. Non-specialist newspapers in Britain fall into five main categories.

### National dailies and Sunday papers

These include:

- Those aimed at the well-educated reader to provide a comprehensive coverage of news and comment. For example *The Times*, *The Sunday Times*, *The Guardian* and *The Independent*.
- Popular papers that target people of lower socioeconomic groups. For example *The Sun*, *Daily Mirror*, *The People* and *News of the World*.

To write for a popular paper requires far more skill. You need to be able to express complex ideas in simple language that will be understood by the readers. Popular papers tend to concentrate on human insight stories, displaying a vigorous and frequently sensationalist style of journalism.

Within these two groups of paper are differences in political orientation, content and social perspective: *The Guardian* has a particular interest in education; the *Daily Mail* provides useful financial coverage and caters strongly for women readers; the *Financial Times* has some general news but is aimed at the business community. Though considered to be popular papers, the *Daily Mail* and *Daily Express* cover news and run features in a more upmarket manner than *The Sun* and the *Daily Mirror*.

### Provincial dailies and evening papers

Like the national papers, the provincial press is varied. The dailies or morning papers tend to be strong on comment and background features, whereas evening papers focus on hard news that has broken during the day. The big provincial dailies in cities such as Birmingham, Liverpool and Manchester cover some national news, and their local news covers a wide geographical area. Smaller provincial evening papers tend to be more parochial.

### Provincial weeklies and bi-weeklies

These tend to be parochial and specialised. Those in rural areas may focus on news and features of interest to the farming community and cover village life in great detail.

### Newspapers for ethnic groups

Examples of these include *The Asian Times*, *Garavi Gujarat* and *The Caribbean Times*.

### Sectional interest papers

Examples of these papers include the *Church Times*, the *Jewish Chronicle*, *The Catholic Herald* and *The Tablet*.

Newspapers cover health in different ways. All of them, including sectional interest papers, may publish health news or opinion about health matters if it is newsworthy and relevant to their readers. Many, such as *The Times*, *The Telegraph* and the *Daily Mail* have regular health pages or features. Although they tend to have regular health writers, some of whom may be health professionals, most editors are receptive to fresh ideas.

If you are considering writing for any paper, buy copies over a period of a month or so to get an idea of how they cover health and whether you consider there are any gaps that would appeal to the paper's target audience and which you could fill.

## Magazines

Nowadays, distinguishing between a magazine and a newspaper is not as easy as it once was. Traditionally, magazines had a picture on the cover, more use of colour, more illustrations, fewer topical news stories and a focus on greater in-depth features. Now, with the huge variety of magazine and newspaper formats, these differences are becoming blurred.

Magazines are divided into two main categories:

- **Business/trade press** These comprise magazines sent to specific groups (for example doctors, pharmacists, dentists, nurses) often without charge.
- **Consumer press** These magazines are sold over the counter and include a variety of subject matters, such as general issues; technical; hobbies; ethnic minorities; business; news and current affairs; house and home.

The list is almost endless, with magazines covering just about every conceivable subject and for all age, social, ethnic, religious and political groups.

Magazine articles tend to go broader and deeper than newspaper articles, as they generally have more space available, and the readers have more time to spend reading them. For example, the subject of hospital food might be covered in different ways in different media:

- **Local paper** The story may cover problems such as food-borne infection and lack of food hygiene in a local hospital. An interview with a patient or a patient's relative might be included.
- **National paper** The article might include a discussion about the incidence of food-borne infection in UK hospitals, the proportion of hospital meals not eaten, and the prevalence of under-nutrition in hospital patients. It might also analyse new government policies and tie the feature into yesterday's speech by a minister from the Department of Health.
- **General interest magazine** The article may be in the form of a feature, with brief details of the hospital food problem nationally, explaining how several hospital trusts interpret the policy and put it into effect. Meals in two or three NHS hospitals might be compared with those in private hospitals. The opinion of a dietician might be included.
- **Medical journal** The article might detail the problem of poor nutrition and/or food-borne infection in hospitals. Government policy and Department of Health reports will be discussed, and recommendations might be made to health professionals on how they can change their practice.

Almost any magazine can carry articles about health and medicine, so you need to angle your writing appropriately and consider the readership. A feature on a new mobile pharmaceutical service in a rural area might not get published in a large city, but might get published in another rural area where a similar venture was being considered. However, you would still have to angle your article to the needs of the area of your targeted publication. This would mean researching the area and using your knowledge of the local pharmaceutical service to suggest how this could be put into practice in a similar area elsewhere.

Another example could be if you are writing a feature for an Asian magazine — you will not get it published unless your piece has a connection with the Asian community, no matter how fascinating or well written it is.

Some articles can be re-angled several times over to fit different magazines. For example, if you are writing about asthma, the angle will depend on the publication you are writing for:

- **Parenting magazine** You might write about signs to watch out for in a child, and what to do in the case of an acute asthma attack.
- **Travel magazine** You might focus on how travel could alter asthma control and the importance of carrying enough medication for the trip.
- **Family magazine** An interview or a family case study of a youngster's management of asthma could be a good approach.
- **Medical journal** You might cover new asthma guidelines from the British Thoracic Society, and what these mean for medical practice.

Health and lifestyle magazines are the most obvious outlets for health and medical writing. Health and disease are popular topics in magazines for women, and increasingly in magazines for men too. However, don't ignore sports magazines, which also have features on health. If you want to write for magazines, in the first instance you might consider those you see regularly and are familiar with.

> Visit a large newsagent and buy a selection of magazines with health articles — this will give you a good idea of the current market, and will be helpful in deciding which magazines to approach with your articles.

## Differences in writing for magazines and newspapers

The basic principles of writing for magazines and newspapers are similar to those used when writing for scientific journals: you need to identify a market, write your article and sell it. To do this, you will need to learn what different magazines want in terms of content and style. Adapting your style not only to a lay readership, but also to publications with different target populations, is not always easy.

### Important points to consider when writing for the lay press

- **Consider the slant of the article** Selling copies is an overriding concern for newspapers and magazines. This influences the viewpoint, style and content of the publication. Articles may need to be written with a slant to attract the target readership. This may mean identifying with and bolstering the sociological and political views of the readers.

- **Your work may be edited** Readers are considered much more important than authors. Magazines and newspapers compete for readers and therefore go to considerable effort to present their content in the way they think their readers will like. This may mean your writing gets changed considerably, which can lead to disagreements between you and an editor. If you do not like the changes made, you will have to look for other outlets for your writing.

- **Follow the style of the publication** You will have less chance of your writing being changed if you write clearly and follow the style of the publication.

- **Be aware of your readers' possible knowledge** Your readers may have limited knowledge and experience of the topic, so this will affect the type and amount of information you give and your choice of language. However, bear in mind that the public is becoming increasingly informed about health. In addition, if you are writing about a rare disease, remember that people who suffer from the condition will have a vast experiential knowledge.

- **Never patronise** Avoid using phrases such as 'This idea is described by a word that we pharmacists call concordance'.

- **Get your facts right** Information must be accurate and up to date — you must make sure that your writing is factually correct. Remember that any error or ambiguity in a health or medical feature can kill!

- **Don't be alarmist** Messages given through newspapers and magazines can have a greater impact than those given through professional journals. Make sure your work is sensitive enough for someone to read who actually has the condition you are writing about. It may be easy to frighten someone with a serious disease who has no knowledge of its implications. This is not to say that writing about serious conditions should be avoided.

- **Do not miss deadlines** Time is crucial. Newspapers may have only a short time to prepare, whereas magazines plan features months in advance.

- **Your work will not be peer reviewed** Unlike academic and professional journals, magazines and newspapers have no peer review system. An editor may seek further opinion, but this will be done informally. Your writing therefore has to please mainly the editor. If your article is rejected it may simply be returned with a rejection slip and no explanation. This is in contrast to a peer-reviewed journal, from which you should receive a reasoned explanation of a rejection because it has gone through a formal review system.

- **You may not see proofs** Few magazines will send you proofs, so you may not always see any changes made to your article. Editors may consider sending out proofs time-consuming and not worth the effort and delay to save missing a couple of typographical errors.

- **Study your market** Magazines and newspapers rarely produce instructions for authors. You will have to study publications you want to write for, work out what gets published and why.

## Generating ideas

Before writing any feature or article you must have something to say. This means generating ideas. Be aware that an idea for an article is more specific than deciding on a subject to write about. For example, 'The health risks of air travel' is a subject, whereas 'How to reduce your risk of DVT on a long-haul flight' is an idea, which may also be an acceptable title (depending on the magazine). Similarly, 'Pharmacists in the UK' is a subject, whereas 'Why should you ask your pharmacist for advice?' is an idea for an article. Coeliac disease is too vague for an article, but 'What to watch out for in restaurants if you have coeliac disease' is more specific.

People who work as staff writers on magazines or newspapers are surrounded by ideas, which have often built up around the publication. They can also share ideas informally or in an editorial meeting. Press releases and other literature appear daily; there is also the opportunity to attend press briefings and meetings. All of these may help to generate ideas for features. However, if you are a freelance or occasional writer, you will have to generate your own ideas — at least until you are known well enough by editors for them to commission you with their requirements. Some writers have no difficulty generating ideas: their problem may be having too many rather than too few.

If you are stuck for ideas, consider the following suggestions for inspiration:

- **Personal experience** These can form a good basis for health articles and features. You could write about an illness you or a member of your family has experienced; how you found the strength to cope with a disability or a frightening diagnosis; or how you coped with an operation or the side effects of a medicine. Such articles can provide an interesting insight, particularly when written by health professionals in light of their knowledge of evidence-based practice. For example, medical evidence suggests no role for complementary therapy in the cure of cancer, but you may have a personal experience of a benefit gained by using such a therapy that you could write about.
- **Professional experience** Interesting patient case scenarios could be adapted to use in an article. Perhaps a person has said something particularly illuminating about their disease or treatment that other people would find interesting and helpful. Also ask yourself what questions are

commonly asked by your clients? What are their common health concerns and misunderstandings? These, too, could form the basis for an article.

---

▶ Remember to respect patient confidentiality. Change all names and any personal details, or get permission from the patient to use their details.

---

- **Talking with people and listening to conversations** Become aware of people's health concerns. Observe the people round you. Keep your eyes and ears open. Carry a notebook to jot things down before you forget them.
- **Radio and television** Documentaries, phone-in programmes and chat shows can be a good source of ideas. Scan radio and TV listings for programmes on health issues. In the UK, the *Radio Times* is a good reference to scan. Most listings can also be found online (such as *www.bbc.co.uk/whatson* and *www.itv.com/listings*).
- **Printed material** Many ideas for writing come from reading: books, magazines, newspapers, professional journals, publicity material, personal and classified advertisements.
- **Magazines and newspapers** These are particularly useful sources if you are writing for them — current articles may suggest ideas for future articles, particularly if there is a hot topic getting a lot of coverage. Newspapers and magazines can also be useful models of particular types of article, such as a 'how-to' or 'self-help' feature, celebrity interviews, or a health politics feature.

---

▶ Look at a range of articles, not just those that interest you. What are the current topics of interest? What are the common approaches? Could you be more imaginative?

---

- **The internet** This can provide a fertile ground for ideas:
  - ○ Join newsgroups in your area of interest.
  - ○ Request contents pages of medical journals.
  - ○ Look at global news services that provide health news (e.g. the BBC, Eurekalert, Newswise and Reuters).

---

▶ If you are a bona fide journalist you can sometimes obtain a password for internet news sites that give you access to embargoed news. To get one of these you usually have to provide evidence that you are a journalist. The evidence required is usually a couple of recently published (usually within the last 6 months) articles with your name cited as the author. You must always respect embargoes, but they can be a useful source of ideas for stories and features.

---

Check question and answer sections on health sites to shed light and provide ideas about on current health concerns.

(For information about writing for the internet, see Chapter 21.)

- **Local and national concerns** Many national health issues can be used as the basis for articles of local interest. For example, concern about poor hydration in children at a national level can be made interesting at a local level if a child's behaviour in school appears to have improved through ready access to fluid. In contrast, a local concern can generate national interest when it is found to affect the lives of individuals with diverse backgrounds and geographical locations.

---

**The 'ideas folder'**

- Develop an 'interesting ideas' folder. Your filing system does not have to be elaborate, but should offer a means of saving interesting articles in clearly identified files or envelopes that you can find quickly.
- As you collect articles or write down ideas that appear in newspapers, magazines and radio programmes, add them to their subject folder and review them regularly.
- Consider carrying a notebook for jotting down ideas as they occur.

---

## Finding a market

When you have chosen an idea that seems to have potential, you need to decide whether it has marketable qualities. You may think it is a good idea, but will an editor want it? This is a hard question, particularly for an inexperienced writer. First and foremost, you need to have a clear theme and angle. Then you need to decide whether there is likely to be a market for the idea, and then how to access that market. This is when market research becomes crucial.

Because few magazines and newspapers produce guidelines for potential authors, there is no substitute for regular reading of publications you want to target. Subscribe to some and look through as many others as you can. You can also find out about the content, aims and readership of newspapers and magazines in the UK by consulting one of the following: *Willings Press Guide, The Writers' & Artists' Yearbook; The Writers' Handbook*. These guides also indicate which newspapers and magazines will consider freelance contributions. Some publications either use in-house staff or only commission articles from journalists they already know. Target those publications that say they will consider external contributors.

Take note of how different publications cover topics. Some useful questions to ask are:

- What topics are they interested in?
- Do their articles have a particular slant? (For example, some health magazines focus mainly on complementary therapies, whereas others favour more traditional therapies.)
- How do they approach topics? (For example, an illness might be covered from a personal perspective, or may be presented in factual terms in a detached and clinical manner.)
- What aspects of the topic have been covered in recent issues?
- Do their articles generally contain lots of facts and figures, for example on the incidence of a disease and its growth during recent years?
- Does it focus on issues such as how patients with the disease and their families cope?
- What is the tone and language favoured?

Keep an eye on ideas and trends — and remember these can change quickly.

Consider your own ideas and decide what sort of article you could write to fit one or more magazines or newspapers. Your articles should be closely tailored to fit a particular market: ignore this and you run the risk of getting many rejection slips.

## Understanding your reader

When selecting a publication to approach, you need to understand the needs and concerns of your target audience. Some good ways to do this are:

- Read previously published articles.
- Study the letters pages:
  - What are the main interests expressed?
  - Are there any letters about health?
- Study the advertisements:
  - What types of product are advertised?
  - What type of person do they appeal to?

Consideration of these points will help you to identify the age range, interests and social and educational level of the readers.

## Approaching editors

When you have worked out your idea for an article, done your market research and decided on one or more publications you would like to target, the next stage is to sell the idea to an editor. Opinions vary as to whether you should contact more than one editor at a time. Some would say that this is inadvisable. Certainly when you are starting out it is probably best to contact only one magazine or newspaper at a time, so start with the one at the top of your list. As you gain experience you may want to send the same ideas to various non-competing publications, perhaps in different areas of the UK, or different countries. However, make sure that you have ideas for adapting your article should you get a number of acceptances.

Make your initial approach in writing and address your letter to the appropriate editor. Obtain his or her name from one of the guides above, or you may be able to find it in an issue of the publication. You could also obtain it from the publication's switchboard or the editor's personal assistant. In general, do not phone editors with ideas until they know you and your work has been published.

### Submitting the article

Another question is whether to write the whole piece or send a preliminary letter containing a synopsis of the proposed article. Most editors prefer the latter approach, and few will read unsolicited manuscripts. However, if you are starting out, sending in an exceptionally good and original article, which is well researched, well written, well attuned to the readership and with a fresh, distinctive voice can result in success. Some editors are reluctant to respond to query letters from beginners because of past experience that the author delivers something unsatisfactory, or does not deliver at all. So if you can demonstrate talent, the editor may make room for your article.

### The query letter

The main function of a query letter is to sell an idea. It should look business-like, typed on headed paper with your name, address, telephone number and email address. Don't write a letter until you have done some preliminary research into your topic and have something to say. On the other hand, do not spend too long doing research before sending your letter, because you may find your idea has lost currency. Find out how far in advance the publication works. Some magazines may work 3 months in advance. Again, consider whether your idea will still be current by then.

Your query letter should be concise and include the following details:

- **Introduction about yourself** Include a brief paragraph on your qualifications and expertise for writing your proposed piece, including any writing experience. You must show you have the ability to do the work. Remember, you are selling yourself as well as your idea. A full curriculum vitae is not generally appreciated, but if you do send one, highlight the most relevant sections. Many editors also like to see hard copy of published work if you have any. If you have no samples to send, it may be a good idea to include a written introduction for your piece.
- **Your idea** This must be good, fresh, timely and important. Your job is to whet the editor's appetite. Include a provisional title, a brief summary of the content, its proposed length, and a description of any illustrations you may be able to provide.
- **Why your idea will suit the publication and interest the readers** You must show you have studied the publication. Make a conscious effort to fit your query letter to the target magazine without losing your individual tone. Do not waste words by saying how wonderful the publication is, or, worse still, how bad you think it is.
- **Any unique selling points** For example, any exclusive material or contacts you have, and why you are uniquely qualified to write the article.

### Example of a query letter to a newspaper or magazine editor

The Steppes
12 Peppercorn Drive
Rushley
ZX1 3YV

Mary Roberts
Editor
Healthy Child Magazine
21–25 Merton Street,
Southbourne
QA53 5JK

Dear Mary Roberts
I am a practising pharmacist and lecturer in pharmacy. I have enclosed an outline of an article on asthma in young children. It will be approximately 1500 words in length.

I feel this practical article will fit in with your magazine's approach to childcare. It provides advice on how to cope with acute asthma attacks in children and how inhalers can be managed at school. It includes two case studies.

I have previously had articles published in *The Parenting Magazine* and *The Rushley Gazette* and I enclose two samples. My four-year-old daughter suffers from asthma.

I enclose a stamped addressed envelope for your reply and look forward to hearing from you.

Yours sincerely
Signature
Name (title/qualifications)
Position

## The reply

Don't forget to include a self-addressed envelope for a reply, otherwise you may not get one. It may be weeks before you hear anything, but resist the temptation to call the editorial department in less than a month.

You will generally get one of three responses:

- **Acceptance** You may get an acceptance and the go-ahead to write your article. However, this is rare unless you are experienced and well known to the editor.
- **Interest** You may get interest, but with suggestions for revising your proposal. If editors are genuinely interested they will often make suggestions about the content and angle and the sort of things they would like to see. If you receive this type of response treat it positively. If you do your best to meet these requirements, you stand a better chance of being published.
- **Rejection** You may get a straight rejection. Try not to be too disheartened by this. Try to find out why you have had a negative response. It may not be the fault of your proposal — it might simply not be what the editor is looking for right now. If you think your idea is good, submit it to another publication. Before doing that, however, take account of any comments made by the first editor and consider doing some more market research.

(For further information about getting published, see Chapter 22.)

## Organising writing projects

### Make careful notes

If you get an acceptance of an idea or a commission to write an article, particularly if these come by telephone, write down the instructions very carefully. Make a careful note of the deadline. If there is anything you are unsure about — length, style, content and so on — check it with the editor at this point.

### Keep a diary

Consider keeping a desk diary in which you record all telephone conversations about writing assignments at the time you receive the call. Record the deadline twice in your diary — once on the day you get the deadline, and again on the day of the deadline itself. Use your diary also to make notes of appointments to speak to people about your writing projects. You might also want to keep a wall planner or an electronic diary in which you highlight any deadlines for articles, meetings to attend, interviews to conduct. But if you decide to keep more than one form of diary, be sure to transfer information across to all of them.

### Keep separate files

Start a file for each new assignment, using a different colour for each one. In them keep any letters and perhaps hard copies of emails from editors regarding the article. Add to the file any information, websites, references, possible contacts for interviews and notes you have made already. If you are feeling enthusiastic at this point, make more notes, questions to ask interviewees, perhaps even the structure of your article. You might also feel like writing a draft at this point if it is a subject you know a lot about.

## Research content

### Sources of information

Researching for your article is much the same as it is for any piece of writing. You can draw on any of the following resources:

- **Your own experience — personal and professional** This is unique and therefore helps to bring a fresh angle to your writing. Your article may be based entirely on personal experience (for example a personal journey through an illness). However, make sure you present personal experience in a way that is valuable to readers. Do not use it as an opportunity for personal therapy and self-promotion.
- **Experience of others** You may obtain this informally from family and friends, or you may decide to interview one or more experts (see below for interviewing).
- **Visits to relevant places (e.g. hospitals, clinics, GP surgeries, pharmacies, pharmaceutical companies)** Your article will be livelier if you have actually visited the places you are writing about, rather than just speaking to someone on the telephone. Make notes of everything you see, hear and, perhaps, smell, taste and touch. Take photographs too. It may be easier for you to recall detail from a photograph rather than notes.
- **Libraries** Despite the advent of the internet, it can be beneficial — even necessary — to visit a library. Some of the big libraries, including the British Library, have online databases with an enormous amount of information.
- **The internet** Many writers begin their research on the internet, but beware of using it as the only source. It is easy to miss relevant information, and your article may end up being superficial. The internet is a very useful source of information, but entries that are free of charge may just be abstracts or summaries — it may be best to buy entire papers, which you can also do online. The internet is not only a useful source of information for the factual content of your article, you can also use it to search for names and contact details of people who might be able to offer you personal expert quotes for use in your article. It is a good idea to learn how to use a search engine effectively.

## Organising your research

Be systematic in your information-collecting and note-taking. This is easier if you develop an outline for your feature before you start. If your article is based entirely on information from other written sources, divide the information you collect into the subjects of the sections identified in your outline.

Do the same for your written notes you have accumulated — using a tear-off pad rather than a notebook will make this easier. However, it may be more practical to extract information from interview notes as you go, rather than physically separating out the information.

## Interviewing experts

Most features can be enhanced by the inclusion of quotes or an interview with a carefully chosen person. Individual opinion can really bring a feature to life and is a useful way of making the oldest of ideas fresh and interesting. Although it may be easier to research your feature entirely from written information, editors of many publications — not just magazines and newspapers — expect to see quotes. Having access to a key contact for an interview can also help to improve your chances of having an idea accepted by an editor. Sometimes an entire article can be built around an interview with one person.

### Sources of experts

If you are new to feature writing you may not have many contacts to start with, but you will soon become adept at gathering them — keep a book for this purpose. Begin by making a note of likely names in the magazines and newspapers you read. Sources of names of experts may be:

- professional and academic journals (these publish papers by experts in their fields)
- trade magazines
- health news on the internet
- medical conference websites.

Attend health and medical conferences to get to know the experts, and listen for any interesting angles they have or new research they have conducted. Join newsgroups and mailing lists for topics in which you are interested. These will keep you in touch with new developments, and their press releases may offer you interviews with various experts. Many organisations have a public relations department or a press officer who may be able to put you in touch with a suitable contact. If you are commissioned to write a feature the editor may suggest experts to interview, often because they want to include a specific viewpoint.

### Contacting the expert

Before contacting an expert, decide what the aim of the interview is. This will help you to choose appropriate individuals as well as ask the right questions. When you have chosen your interviewee(s), read up as much as you can about them — their interests, views and expertise — if such information is available. You can then approach them with confidence.

## Preparing for the interview

Prepare your questions carefully. Never interview someone without good preparation because this wastes time. Research your topic thoroughly as well as the person you plan to talk to. Do not ask an expert something you should have found out already. The point of the interview is not to fill in gaps in your knowledge but to gain opinions your readers will be interested in.

### Constructing the questions

- Make your questions specific and be prepared to rephrase them on the spot if you don't get a clear answer.
- Avoid vague questions such as 'Do you enjoy being a doctor?': 'What do you most enjoy about being a doctor and what do you most dislike about being a doctor?' is better.
- Ask open-ended questions. Instead of 'Do you agree with the Government's policy on school meals', try 'What do you think of the view that the Government's policy on school meals is likely to alienate parents and teachers?' Discussion is more likely to arise from the second question.
- Try to avoid leading questions, such as 'You think that omega-3 fats improve dyslexia, don't you?' — these may generate noncommittal answers and you may not get any further on those points.

Arrange your questions in the order in which you want to ask them. This may not be the order in which you want to write them up. Ask them in an order that will help the conversation flow while minimising any sense of threat for the interviewee. Consider slipping in potentially contentious questions straight after friendly questions, and vice-versa. Try to sense the mood of your interviewee. If he or she is impatient, reduce the number of questions to those that are really important.

## The interview

### Approaching the interviewee

When you have prepared your questions approach your interviewee. It is best to do this by telephone rather than letter. In many cases this will mean speaking to a personal assistant or secretary in the first instance. If you have been commissioned by a well-known publication this can help you to get an interview, so mention it in the phone call. Depending on your article, you may want to interview the person face to face or by telephone. If your article is based on one key interview, face to face is best. If the material you want to cover is complex, correspondence by email or letter can help to clarify issues after a telephone interview.

Never presume that the person will be free to speak to you when you call. If the expert answers the phone, explain what you would like and ask whether he or she is free to speak now or should you phone back. Explain how long you think the interview will take, and if necessary make an appointment to call again.

### Recording the interview

Decide beforehand how you will record the interview — with a notebook or a tape recorder. A short interview is usually best recorded in a notebook, but if you are going to include quotes in your article, use the words actually spoken. If you paraphrase part or all of an interview, make sure you do so accurately, conveying the intention of the interviewee. A tape recorder can be useful for a longer interview, especially one that is potentially contentious. The editor may feel happier knowing there is access to the full original interview. However, a tape-recorded interview can take a long time to listen to and to transcribe.

### Keeping control of the interview

The interview should be controlled as much as possible by you, not the interviewee. People who are used to being interviewed are often adept at controlling them and saying what they want to say in spite of all your preparation. Experience will help you to deal with this, but always try to get the person back to answering your questions. A well-orchestrated interview should elicit some interesting responses, some of which come during unguarded moments. Take particular note of these, as they can help your story enormously.

### Writing it up

Before writing up an interview, study the way other magazines do it. It is a skill in its own right and not simply a matter of transcribing, editing and submitting it to the editor. Quotes must be used judiciously and woven into the story, interspersed between background material and comment. Convey to the reader why your interviewee is worth listening to.

- Pick out quotes with a common thread that move your storyline forward.
- Pick out a strong quote to start the feature and a strong quote to finish it.

Opinions vary as to whether you should show a copy of what you have written to your interviewee. Many experts appreciate this and some will specifically ask to see what you have written — they may want to ensure that they are not misquoted.

## Writing your article

An article consists of a title (and perhaps a subtitle — sometimes referred to as the 'strapline'), an introduction, a main body and an ending. Quotes, anecdotes and photographs should be used to illustrate the text.

As you begin to write, think of the structure as an inverted pyramid (see Figure 10.1). In other words, the most important information must come first. The introduction must follow on from the title and subtitle, grabbing the reader's attention. This can often be difficult for medical and science writers, who may be used to putting the most important information in the conclusion at the end. For magazines and newspapers this is not appropriate. Basically, you have at most a headline and an introductory paragraph to sell yourself to your readers. They will not look at the last paragraph to see what the article is about. The inverted pyramid structure is often considered useful only for 'news'-type pieces, but it is useful to keep it in mind for all articles, including features, particularly when writing for magazines and newspapers.

### Title

Always think of a title, even though an editor will probably rewrite it. Having a provisional title helps you to focus your article and give it direction.

A title must grab the reader's attention and intrigue, amuse, or demand a response.

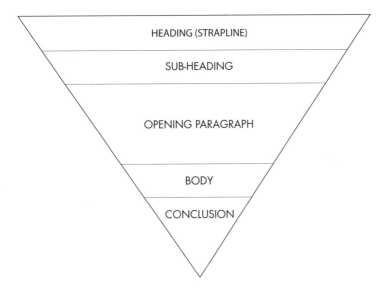

**Figure 10.1**    Inverted pyramid approach to writing an article.

Some titles, no matter how attention-grabbing, need a subtitle to explain them, particularly if they are likely to be misunderstood. Thus, a book entitled *Bloody Foreigners* has the subtitle *The story of immigration to Britain*. An article with the title 'A spoonful of sugar' could have a subtitle 'Why people with diabetes need not avoid sugar'.

---

**Creative titles**

Examples of titles and subtitles that could be attractive to magazines and newspapers include:

- 'What you should know about coughs' *rather than* 'Useful information about coughs'
- 'When your eyes itch and your nose streams' *rather than* 'The problem of hay fever'
- 'Dialling for dinner? A look at which takeaways deliver the least fat' *rather than* 'The fat content of takeaways'
- 'Are you tanorexic?' *rather than* 'The dangers of excessive sunbed use'
- 'How big is yours? Why portion sizes can make you fat' *rather than* 'Links between portion sizes and obesity'

- 'Know your body. How your monthly cycle affects your diet' *rather than* 'Hormones and dieting'
- 'Come up smiling! How to bounce back from the blues' *rather than* 'How to cope with emotional setbacks'
- 'Boost your immunity now. Your winning winter wellbeing plan' *rather than* 'How to help your immune system this winter'

## The introduction

Your introduction should be brief, give a taster of the topic to come, and persuade the reader to keep reading. The author's angle on the subject should also be conveyed to the reader in the introduction.

When writing your introduction, think of your readers, perhaps half-asleep on an early-morning train, or exhausted at the end of a working day. How will you wake them and their curiosity and entice them into the article? How will you make the introduction compelling enough to make them want to go back and read the rest if they have to break off to do something else?

Several techniques can be used, including starting with a quote — perhaps from someone you have interviewed — an anecdote, a shocking statement, or perhaps some striking facts and figures. Make sure that your introduction reveals your topic and the angle you will be taking on it.

## The body of the article

The main body of the article contains the bulk of the information. The main theme must be threaded throughout your article to create a unified whole, and all the material you use must be related to it. Be ruthless about removing anything that is not relevant. Your article must be coherent — that is, your material must be arranged logically and linked skilfully.

Newspapers and magazines do not have a lot of space because of the financial need to leave space for adverts. This means every paragraph of your article must contribute to the main theme, and the paragraphs must be ordered according to the importance of the information — the most important at the beginning and the least important at the end.

➤  The reader should be able to get the gist of your article just by reading the first sentence of every paragraph, so make sure the topic of each is in its first sentence.

## The climax and the ending

The climax of the article should satisfy or stir the emotions or thought, leaving the reader with a lingering feeling. This will help make the article memorable, particularly if it has also said something important. The introduction and the end of a feature should function as a partnership: a joint effort that shows the reader where you are going and where you have arrived in examining the topic. An effective ending gives the reader a sense of completeness and reinforces the writer's intention stated in the introduction. If the feature suggests a question, the article should answer that question and the ending should point to the answer or solution.

## Format, length and style

Remember you are writing for a lay audience. Break up your information into manageable chunks with plenty of headings. Write your headings from the outline you prepared before starting, then fit your content around them. Headings provide a framework and a focus for you the writer, and make the article easy to digest for the reader. They act as signposts for a change in topic and help the reader find specific information.

Put summary information in boxes and use plenty of bullet points where necessary. Your editor may break up your material even further, taking quotes from it and putting them in boxes and side bars.

**Creative text boxes**

Boxes of text or bullet points often appear in magazine articles. Do not overuse them, but consider the following headings for such sections:
- When giving information:
  - Did you know?
  - It's a fact

- When giving advice:
  - Top tips
  - Helpful hints
  - Three golden rules
  - Dos and don'ts
  - Four ways to help
- When challenging misconceptions:
  - Fact or fiction?
  - True or false?
  - Beliefs and myths
- When encouraging action:
  - You need help if
  - Get help if
  - Warning signs
  - Call a doctor if
  - Ask your pharmacist if

It is essential to stick to the length you have been given — be sure not to exceed it. Plan in advance how many words you will give to each section. If you exceed this, edit your work by removing anything that does not support your main theme, no matter how interesting or well written.

Magazine and newspaper articles are usually written in an easy-to-read style. This means short, simple sentences written in the active rather than the passive voice. Think carefully about your choice of words, particularly medical terminology. Readers are becoming increasingly informed about health and more familiar with medical jargon. Don't be patronising, using phrases such as, 'something we pharmacists call pharmacokinetics'. If you think the reader will not understand the term and you need to include it, explain it clearly and simply.

Beware of writing in a fine, fluent, pompous or grandiose style, creating sentences that wash over the reader but say nothing. Your article should flow and read well, but it must convey information, explanation and opinion. Your readers should gain more knowledge, understanding and insight as a result of reading your article.

### Finishing your article

When you have finished writing you are ready to edit, revise and create the finished article. Never submit a first draft to an editor — this is the best way to get a rejection. Print out your article and re-read it several times. Even if you are an experienced writer, leave your piece at least overnight before reading it. Sentences that seemed to be particularly good at the time you wrote them may, on re-reading, not fit your theme at all. Be ruthless and delete them.

Try reading your article aloud and listen to the flow of the sentences and paragraphs. Any awkward word order, rambling sentences or jarring transitions will be obvious. If you have to read any sentences twice, examine them carefully — they may need rewriting.

Consider asking a layperson to read your draft and comment. Ask for an honest opinion as to whether the article is clear, readable and understandable.

Newspapers often have short deadlines so you will not have time to create several drafts. This is where the upside-down pyramid structure helps you to organise your thoughts and write and edit quickly. Magazines usually have longer deadlines, which gives you the opportunity to polish your writing until it is irresistible.

**When writing, reviewing and editing your own work ask yourself:**

- Are the content and length of your article the same as you agreed with the editor?
- Is the organisation logical?
- Is the article consistent in theme and tone?
- Does the writing contain strong verbs and precise words?
- Are there too many adjectives and adverbs?
- Is the writing free of clichés and other well-worn phrases?
- Do the headline and introduction grab the reader's attention?
- Do the headline and introduction connect with the rest of the article?
- Do all the quotations add to the story, or are they there for padding?
- Are all quotations properly attributed?
- Does the first sentence of each paragraph summarise the content of that paragraph?
- Could the reader get the gist of the article from reading the headline, introduction, first sentence of each paragraph and ending?
- Do the ideas and the writing flow?
- Does your article read beautifully but say nothing?
- Does the ending complete the story?

Be brutal in answering these questions and make the necessary changes. Finally, when you are happy with your article, submit it in the format requested by the editor. Most editors accept electronic submissions, which should usually be in Microsoft Word or a similar format.

---

### In summary

- Selling copies is an overriding concern for magazines and newspapers. This means slanting your feature to the readership.
- Remember that readers are more important than writers.
- Messages given through magazines and newspapers can have a greater impact than those in professional journals. Be accurate and up-to-date, but not alarmist.
- Make sure you have something to say and say it. Avoid writing flowing text that says nothing.
- Research your newspapers and magazines. What are the aims of the publication? Who are the target readers? What is the style and general approach? How do they cover health and medicine?
- Target specific publications that have a content, approach and style you are comfortable with.
- Approach the editor by name using a preliminary letter giving brief details about yourself, your idea, a synopsis, and why you are the person to write the article.
- Agree content, word length and deadlines with the editor and stick to them.
- Write your article using the inverted pyramid structure.
- Make sure your headline and introduction grab the reader's attention and are connected to the rest of the article.
- Break up your article into manageable chunks using plenty of headings and boxes to give key points.
- Remember that your readers may have a limited knowledge of the topic. Be careful not only about the type of language you use but also the type and amount of information you give.

---

## Training resources

**National Council for the Training of Journalists (NCTJ)**
Latton Bush Centre
Southern Way
Harlow
Essex CM18 7BL
Tel: 01279 430009
*www.nctj.com*

The NCTJ is the main body concerned with the training of newspaper journalists. It offers distance learning courses and accredits colleges, universities and company training centres to run courses based on its own syllabuses. The website provides details of colleges and universities offering degrees and other courses in journalism.

### Medical Journalists' Association (MJA)
*www.mja-uk.org*
The MJA exists to support its membership, which comprises over 350 of the UK's leading medical and health journalists. It promotes and runs events of interest to medical journalists.

### Tim Albert Training
*www.timalbert.co.uk*
Tim Albert specialises in workshops for medical journalists, and offers courses on writing for magazines and newspapers.

## Further reading

Hennessy B (1997) *Writing Feature Articles. A Practical Guide to Methods and Markets*, 3rd edn. Oxford, UK: Focal Press.
Sova D (1998) *How to Write Articles for Newspapers and Magazines*. New Jersey, USA: Thomson Peterson.

# 11

## Writing press releases

*Pamela Mason*

Are you:

- setting up in a new business
- launching a new product
- planning an event you want to publicise
- publishing new research findings of your department
- receiving negative press about your company or product?

If any of these apply, writing and distributing a press release may be a key step in improving your publicity strategy.

## What is a press release?

Press releases (also known as media releases or news releases) are the basic written communication tool for those wanting to get a message across to the media. They contain a short, succinct message and should generally be no longer than one side — two at most — of double-spaced A4 paper.

Press releases are crucial to effective public relations. Although they are not a substitute for creating and maintaining good relationships with media contacts, press releases are a key method of spreading your organisation's news and making announcements.

## Function of a press release

The primary aim of issuing a press release is to get media coverage. It is not advertising. A press release provides information targeted at someone you hope will promote your news. Used in this way, a press release is potentially worth much more than an advertisement because it is much more likely to be noticed by the readers of the publication in which it is placed. If you want to advertise your product or an event directly, you should pay to do this through a publication's usual advertising channels.

The press release must therefore be sufficiently interesting to people outside your organisation to get them to use and promote its content. This means it must inform and grab the attention of the reader — who will usually be a journalist. All press releases should convey information that is newsworthy and timely, and which will clearly interest the media. If your press releases are boring — and sent too frequently — they will lose their impact and will usually be quickly discarded.

## How a press release is used

A press release can be used in two main ways. The journalist may decide to:

- use the information as it stands for a news item or article
- give the story greater prominence by commissioning or writing a feature to investigate the subject further, perhaps by interviewing the individuals mentioned in the press release.

### The 'hook'

A press release is most likely to be used in the latter way if it is based on a 'hook'. In other words, it provides enough information to create irresistible interest but is cleverly designed to leave out certain information. This technique may be useful to encourage a journalist to pick up the phone and ask for an interview or more information, or perhaps attend an event or briefing.

Say that your organisation promotes fish consumption. Recent media attention has focused on the risks of mercury and other possible toxins in fish, which has led to public concern about eating it; this will be an obvious concern for your organisation. You are made aware of a meta-analysis due to be published in a significant medical journal next month. This concludes that if British people reduce their fish intake there may be serious public health consequences, such as an increased risk of heart attack and stroke.

You decide to invite the authors of the meta-analysis to speak at a briefing for journalists. The 'hook' is the current public and media concern about the risks of fish consumption. However, you do not want to let journalists know from the outset that the briefing will be positive about fish (though knowing your organisation, they will expect this). So you might begin your press release with a heading such as 'Eat more salmon or less?' This suggests that there is no foregone conclusion and that there is information to be gained from attending the briefing.

## Intended audience

For press releases, the audience is usually journalists. Though you may not be a journalist yourself, you must get into their mindset: What will interest them? Use language and terminology they are comfortable and familiar with. Avoid extravagant language using highly technical medical terminology — remember that the journalists may not have a medical background. Also avoid using unsubstantiated claims to attract attention (for example 'Guaranteed to cure a cold within 24 hours'). Always be able to provide the evidence to back up your facts if required.

Journalists are busy people whose phones are constantly ringing and who receive new batches of information by post or email before they have processed the last lot. Your press release will therefore only maintain its impact if it is clear about what you are offering and why it is newsworthy. Just because a story seems interesting to you does not mean it will be to a reporter. Whereas your press release represents a major event in the life of your organisation, it may be just one of many that a journalist receives in a day.

Remember that the main aims of a journal or newspaper are to sell more copies and get higher ratings. This is therefore also the mission of journalists who work for them. Journalists may also be looking for promotion or a rise in salary, or to win an award for a good story. Informing the readers, though important, is not necessarily a high priority.

To achieve their aims, journalists need a newsworthy story. A newsworthy story is one that is new, significant, relevant and unique. Say you are planning a press release about a new generic 'me-too' medicine — this in itself is hardly newsworthy. If the product is significantly cheaper than its competitors, interest may be increased. If, however, your product is packaged using a new design to reduce the risk of dispensing errors — and if dispensing errors have been in the news recently — newsworthiness increases. If your product packaging is the first on the market to address this issue, and you have a study showing it works, your story is now new, significant, relevant and unique — a pharmaceutical journalist is likely to look at your press release.

If you have a particularly interesting story or piece of news, it may be better to target this at one type of media, or even offer an 'exclusive' to one journalist. Say your company makes vitamins. You have done a piece of research looking into the main groups of people who use vitamins and why. Your findings may be of limited interest to mainstream journalists, but a more attention-grabbing approach may be to turn it into a quiz for people to find out what type of 'vitamin user' they are. You may know one journalist who works for a magazine that publishes quizzes of this type. Offer your quiz idea as an 'exclusive' to that journalist and you may get some positive copy for your company.

Information presented to journalists which is sympathetic to the readers or listeners they write for is more likely to be used than one sent to every journalist you know. Alternatively, you may consider rewriting the same story for a number of different audiences. This could be more effective than a 'one size fits all' approach. Tell those you target that the information is intended for them, giving them a reason to continue reading it.

## Timing

The time to issue a press release is when you have something topical and newsworthy to say. All releases need a strong 'hook' or angle that will appeal to editors and give the story a good chance of gaining media coverage. Remember to keep up with current affairs for events into which you can hook.

> ➤ Greater impact and coverage may be achieved if you coordinate your press releases with significant national events, seasons of the year, health promotion events, issues of current media interest or charity events.

For example, if your organisation is involved in promoting public health among older people and National Osteoporosis Week is coming up in a couple of weeks' time, you could send out a press release detailing some new research showing that weightbearing physical activity can reduce the risk of fracture. Or perhaps a member of the royal family is due to have a special birthday in the height of the summer — this could be the hook if your company has developed a new product for sunburn. Another hook may be if you have conducted some medical research in a country that is currently in the news.

When delivering a press release, it is important to ensure your timing is appropriate for your target audience as well as your organisation. If your organisation is launching a new product or organising an event, do not wait until the day before it to send out a press release: send it early enough for the editor to decide whether the story will be interesting for their readers and when it could be used. The editor may also need time to check your facts and sources, or simply to rewrite parts of your press release to conform to the style and format of the publication. However, do not send press releases so early that — despite their appeal — they get buried on the editor's desk.

## Structure

### The 'inverted pyramid' approach

To increase the chance of having your press release used, it is important to present it in the professional structure that editors and journalists are used to. When you write your press release, think of an inverted pyramid (see Figure 10.1 on page 171). In other words, the most important information must come first. This can be difficult for medical writers who are used to writing research papers, where the most important information is revealed in the conclusions. This approach is not appropriate for a press release, where you need to get your main message across in the first sentence.

### The headline

Begin with a concise and compelling headline. This will usually be in the form of an incomplete sentence or a question that clearly encapsulates the main ideas in the press release and grabs the reader's attention. Using the example above, imagine how a journalist would react to the headline 'Eat more salmon or less?' compared with 'The risks and benefits of fish consumption'. Although the latter encapsulates the event as effectively as the first, it would most likely result in a yawn from the journalist and the press release being consigned to the waste basket.

### Subheadings

If necessary, use a subheading (also sometimes called the strapline) to include supporting details. In the above example, you might add 'Government urges people not to overreact on fish'. Never use the past tense in headlines or subheadings because it will make your announcement sound like old news.

## The first paragraph

The first paragraph sets the stage for your story and should encapsulate all the main facts. The first sentence should be the most powerful, as it will make or break your press release. Never start with a negative sentence. The combination of your headline, subheading, first sentence and first paragraph must grab the reader's attention and draw them into your story.

## The body

Subsequent paragraphs should provide supporting information in descending order of importance, putting the most newsworthy and exciting aspects first. These paragraphs should answer the following questions:

- **Who?** Who is launching the new product or event? Who will be presenting the new clinical research?
- **What?** What is the product or event you are launching?
- **When?** When (date and time) will the product or event be launched?
- **Where?** Where (address and postcode) will the event take place? Consider supplying a web link to a map of the location.
- **Why or how?** Why the event is happening and why people should be interested.

### Quotes

You may want to include a comment from a senior person in your organisation (for example a manager or lead researcher) or from an external expert, which journalists can use as a quote to support their story. Avoid using over-hyped and padded or meaningless quotes from company staff because these will come across as biased. Make sure you get permission for any quotes you use.

### Statistics

Statistics can be a useful way to make a point and add weight to an argument. Quoting the source of the statistics and specific findings would carry even more weight. For example, 'Department of Health statistics released last week show the number of deaths from breast cancer has reduced by 3 per cent over the last 5 years.'

### Release date

You should include the date you are sending the press release and also the release date: this tells the editor the general time frame when you want the information released, and should be typed in bold or capitals. Most press releases would simply say something like 'Release immediately', 'Release on March 18' or 'Embargoed until April 12'.

### The end

At the end of the press release, tell the journalist what to do next. Make their job easy. For example, you might mention the possibility of an interview or a photo opportunity.

You should also include a 'Notes to Editors' paragraph. This should provide background information on your organisation, when it was launched, its main areas of activity and any special achievements. This will enhance the credibility of your press release.

Finally, give the name, address and telephone/fax number of your appointed contact person. This should appear at the bottom of the press release so that journalists can get in touch if they want further information. In addition, make sure you include the name, address and telephone number of your organisation as the source of the release.

### Style

- **Make your press releases brief and to the point.** Be as detailed as you need to in as few words as possible. Make each word count — simple, concise sentences are preferable to long, protracted ones.
- **Avoid overuse of adjectives and flowery language.** Although you want to generate interest, cut hyperbole and avoid claims such as 'our service is absolutely unique' or 'the world's number one painkiller' unless you can back this up with published research.
- **Stick to logical and substantiated claims.** Avoid puffing up your press release with phrases such as 'our amazing new product' or 'this will be the best event this side of Christmas'. Don't use industry jargon and buzzwords such as 'cost-effective', 'cutting-edge', 'revolutionary' or 'one-stop-shop solution'. Such phrases are meaningless and tend to annoy journalists.
- **Grammar, spelling and punctuation must be correct.** Remember that journalists are wordsmiths and will probably be irritated by spelling mistakes and poor grammar. Badly written press releases stand a good chance of being consigned to the bin.
- **Avoid acronyms or abbreviations.** If you need to use them, spell them out in the first instance and then use the abbreviated versions afterwards.

- **Present the press release objectively and write in the third person.** For example, use 'he/she', 'they' or 'it' rather than 'I', 'we' or 'us'. Remember that a company is always singular, so it is 'it' not 'they'.

## Format

A press release should be typed on an A4 sheet of paper, double-spaced with wide margins. White paper is most commonly used, and if you have a logo, use it. Avoid fancy fonts. Stick to size 10 or 12 of a plain font such as Arial or Courier.

Press releases are increasingly sent in electronic format, but it is best to contact potential recipients to make sure they will accept them. Do not send your press release as an attachment because recipients may think it contains a virus and delete it. Include it in the main body of the email in plain text format. Remove italics and bold letters as, depending on the recipient's software, these may appear as illegible graphics.

## Checking

When your press release is ready, read it carefully yourself and also get a colleague to read it. Check all facts, dates, names, spelling and grammar. Ask yourself:

- Is it informative and easy to read?
- Do the headline and strapline grab your attention and make you want to find out more?
- Will it be understood by a journalist with perhaps limited medical knowledge?

## Sending it out

When you are satisfied that your press release covers all the above, you are ready to send it. Many newspapers, journals and magazines accept press releases via fax or email. If you post your press release, consider folding it with the copy side out, so that as soon as editors open the letter they see who it is from and what it is about.

## Monitoring

Keep an eye open for how and whether your press release is used. This is the best possible feedback. If your press releases are used, this should bring benefits to the organisation. If they are not, it may mean that they are too weak in style and content — aim to improve next time.

---

**Checklist for writing press releases**

Ask yourself:

- ☑ Do you have a newsworthy story?
- ☑ Why is the press release being written, and what do you want to achieve?
- ☑ Who is the audience, and how will they relate to the release?
- ☑ What do you want recipients to do with the press release?
- ☑ Follow the standard press release format: headline, opening paragraph, body text and closing paragraph.
- ☑ Follow the inverted pyramid structure, putting the most important information first.
- ☑ Make sure your headline and opening paragraph grab attention and include all salient facts.
- ☑ Make sure the press release answers the 'who, what, when, where, why and how' questions.
- ☑ Keep it punchy and don't use unnecessary adjectives and flowery language.
- ☑ Be factual and objective. Do not embellish, and refrain from using over-hyped quotes that may come across as being biased.
- ☑ Proofread your press release. Ensure that it is grammatically correct and does not contain spelling mistakes or factual errors.
- ☑ Make sure all sources and statistics are quoted and referenced correctly.
- ☑ Send your press release at the most opportune time — for both your organisation and the media.

# 12

## Advertisements

*Genevieve Meier*

### Principles of good advertising

We are subject to advertising messages at almost, if not every, moment of the day in every imaginable form. Our daily decisions are both consciously and subconsciously based on our perceived idea of the product we are using at the time, our car, the cereal we eat, the toothbrush we use. Another important part of making a decision, especially an expensive one, is our apparent perception of the company selling the product. Because of this, companies create a brand and guard it jealously because it is their identity and their guarantee of continued loyalty from their audience. It is about 'trust'. The importance of association between company and audience should never be underestimated.

However, the consumer is for the most part naïve to these facts and generally sees advertising as a nuisance. Advertising makes us aware of choices and allows us to purchase a product or service in preference to another. This requires us to take action, a difficult task in itself, human nature being what it is. By visually stimulating us, inviting us to become engaged, identifying with us or making us aware of our lack, the advertisers capture our attention for a mere few seconds and create a thought. This thought then needs to be reinforced over and over, either within the advertisement or later in repeat advertisements, using preferably as many types of media as possible to generate an action.

When does advertising move from being a nuisance to something we see as interesting, if not essential? What is it about a particular campaign that makes a consumer ultimately choose one product over another? These questions are very difficult to answer because there are a multitude of factors at play.

Companies spend huge amounts of money and resources on advertising for two fundamental reasons: revenue and brand building. Revenue is the short-term objective. The long-term objective is to gain customers and ultimately to keep them. This is done by creatively communicating trust through brand values. They are the essential keys to maintaining success. By persuading their audience that they share their values, a company ensures that it has lifelong customers.

In life there are various things that we want to optimise and preserve; these include youth, happiness, time, family, togetherness and life itself. Then there are taboos, which we attempt to ignore and avoid, including getting older, sickness, pain, failure and death. Astute companies incorporate and adopt these into their values and actively make us aware that they hold them dear, sometimes deliberately and sometimes by association. They can achieve this by associating themselves with a lifestyle, success, freedom, security or youthfulness.

Is Coca Cola selling a drink or are they selling sunshine and smiles, which magically appear when you drink their product? We automatically associate Volvo with 'the safest car on the road', and only cool, good-looking people wear Levi's. Endorsement is an easy one. Of course, the actor who plays James Bond doesn't necessarily choose to drive an Aston Martin — he is handsomely paid to do so — but to the consumer Aston Martin = James Bond and everything that goes with it. However, it need not be a celebrity that endorses a product: it could be an emotion such as humour, or tears — a classic is the use of children and animals — creating an association because we now feel something as well as seeing something we like. This additional use of the senses augments the effectiveness and the impact of the advertisement, and hence the chance that the consumer will remember the 'feeling' they had and ultimately buy the product.

In medical advertising, associations need to be approached with caution. Where possible, medical advertising should seek to achieve this ideal of trust. Dealing with illness and death is difficult: these are painful issues, which the consumer approaches with trepidation. The benefits of taking a medicine are also unfortunately inextricably linked to the likelihood of an associated disadvantage (side effect), and this is one of the hurdles that medical advertisers need to address. However, we need to grow and maintain trust, and this may be best achieved by creatively demonstrating accuracy and balance at every interaction. We need to remember that a company is more than just the products it sells (the ideals it embraces are very much a part of the product too). Most pharmaceutical companies already have a set of established values or company culture, and it is the function of the writer to incorporate this into the advertisement appropriately.

The framework of values and associations is of no consequence until it is made clear to the consumer at the most opportune time. The issue here is to choose the most appropriate channel and timing, which are as important as what is being conveyed. For example, an advertising campaign carried in a women's weekly magazine costing £1 and also broadcast on daytime television will probably suit a target audience of stay-at-home mothers, rather than high-powered businesswomen.

Furthermore, the fact that text for an advertisement (also known as copy) works in one format does not guarantee that it will work in another. Some degree of change needs to be made to suit the chosen medium, to make every contact with the target audience effective. A comprehensive knowledge of how a particular medium can benefit a campaign is important: it should not be used just because it is available, or because a competitor is using it. In this age, choices of media are endless. It is therefore beneficial for a writer to keep abreast and aware of current campaigns, market research and media planning. The following provides the keys to make the most impact with a campaign.

## Advertising drugs

The majority of the public unfortunately has a negative perception of the pharmaceutical industry, partly thanks to misleading and one-sided tabloid press reporting. To maintain credibility, it is therefore essential for the industry to explain its actions and maintain transparency.

Given the nature of the product, advertising drugs is not a simple matter. As with all advertising, there are rules and regulations. However, in drug advertising there are also additional stringent regulations. A medical writer involved in developing advertisements will benefit from understanding and applying the legislation that governs the advertising of drugs in the country where they are practising. More importantly, a good grasp of the codes of practice of the various statutory bodies will enable a writer to stay within those regulations.

The codes of practice provide a clear working approach to the laws and regulations that govern the advertising of medicines in the UK (see also Chapter 19). Knowing the legislation is essential, but the codes of practice make it simpler and easier to address. The codes of practice not only interpret the law, they also tend to be more rigorous and go beyond the constraints of the laws they reflect.

### Legal considerations

Advertising is a fundamental element of our consumer society, enabling us to make informed decisions based on the choices available. Advertising medicines is permissible, but highly regulated. It should be of a certain standard, and not exaggerated, misleading or offensive, and so additional legislation is in place to ensure that all medicine advertising is responsible and clearly states the benefits and risks of products in a balanced fashion.

The first obstacle to overcome is being able to recognise a medicine. This sounds easy, but there are many products on the borderline between medicinal products and food supplements, cosmetic or medical devices. Interestingly, homoeopathic medicines are not classed as true medicinal products but still have special provisions with regard to advertising. Since October 2005, traditional herbal medicinal products have been classified as medicines in the UK and therefore subject to medicines advertising legislation. For the purposes of this chapter, we will assume that products being advertised have been correctly licensed as medicines and that all legislation mentioned applies.

The advertising of all medicines in the UK is regulated by both European and UK legislation. The European legislation is contained in Title VIII European Directive 2001/83/EC (the Codified Directive). It is implemented in the UK by the Medicines (Advertising) Regulations 1994 (the Advertising Regulations) and the Medicines (Monitoring of Advertising) Regulations 1994 (the Monitoring Regulations). These are the statutory mandate of the Medicines and Healthcare Products Regulatory Agency (MHRA), which acts to protect the public by promoting the safe use of medicines and ensuring that advertising meets the legal requirements. In 1999 the MHRA introduced its Blue Guide (subsequently updated) to assist in the interpretation of, compliance with and understanding of regulations.

European law permits medicine advertising to be self-regulated. The MHRA in its statutory role supports the system of self-regulation employed in the UK. There are several such regulatory bodies, a brief mention of them and their respective codes follows. Later in the chapter, how to use each one with regard to audience and chosen media, where appropriate, will be addressed.

## Prescription Medicines Code of Practice Authority (PMCPA)

This code applies to the promotion of prescription-only medicines to healthcare professional and administrative staff.

The PMCPA was established in 1993 by the Association of the British Pharmaceutical Industry (ABPI) — the trade association of pharmaceutical manufacturers in the UK. The code of practice for the pharmaceutical industry is operated independently of the association itself.

The ABPI code of practice was drawn up in consultation with the British Medical Association, the Royal Pharmaceutical Society of Great Britain and the Medicines and Healthcare Product Regulatory Agency of the Department of Health. It is the intention of the ABPI that its members abide by the code in both spirit and letter. In the UK, virtually all pharmaceutical companies (including non-members) have accepted the code.

## Proprietary Association of Great Britain (PAGB)

The PAGB is responsible for administering the PAGB Medicines Advertising Codes. These are concerned with the advertising of OTC (over-the-counter) products both to the public and to persons qualified to prescribe.

The PAGB is the national trade association representing manufacturers of OTC medicines and food supplements. The codes are drawn up in consultation with the MHRA, the Office of Communications (OFCOM), Adverting Standards Authority (ASA), Committees of Advertising Practice (CAP), Broadcast Advertising Clearance Centre (BACC) and the Radio Advertising Clearance Centre (RACC).

## Office of Communications (OFCOM)

OFCOM in its statutory capacity endeavours to ensure the standards are maintained in the content of programmes and broadcast advertising in the UK. It is ultimately responsible in law for broadcast advertising and has clear procedures to monitor the effectiveness of self-regulation to ensure that the interests of consumers are properly protected. OFCOM is the independent regulator and competition authority for the UK communications industries, with responsibilities across television, radio, telecommunications and wireless communications services. In line with its responsibilities stated in the Communications Act 2003 and the Broadcasting Act 1996, OFCOM has formulated the code for television and radio, covering standards in programmes, sponsorship, fairness and privacy. The Broadcasting Code replaces previous codes set by the previous broadcasting regulators (the Independent Television Commission for commercial television, the Radio Authority for commercial radio, and the Broadcasting Standards Commission) on matters relating to taste, decency, fairness and privacy. This code came into force on 25 July 2005, its main objective being to protect children and to ensure that adults are given the information they need to make informed choices.

## Advertising Standards Authority (ASA)

The Advertising Standards Authority is the independent body set up by the advertising industry to maintain and uphold the advertising codes, in doing so protecting consumers and creating a level playing field for advertisers.

Since November 2004, OFCOM has contracted out the day-to-day regulation of broadcast advertising content to the Advertising Standards Authority. For 40 years before this the ASA regulated non-broadcast advertising (such as press, cinema, posters). However, it has now assumed responsibility for television and radio advertising under a new co-regulatory system with OFCOM, covering all advertising standards and consumer complaints.

As a result of these changes, three new bodies have been created within the structure of the ASA with specific responsibility for broadcast advertising:

*   The Advertising Standard Authority (Broadcast) ASA(B), which is responsible for handling complaints.
*   The Broadcast Committee of Advertising Practice (BCAP), responsible for setting, reviewing and revising standards codes for broadcast advertising.
*   The Broadcast Advertising Standards Board of Finance (BASBOF), responsible for funding the new system.

The ASA(B) and BCAP have inherited OFCOM's television and radio advertising codes. These will be reviewed and maintained by BCAP, and any changes must be consulted on and approved by OFCOM. The ASA, through the Committee of Advertising Practice (CAP), is responsible for administering the British Code of Advertising, Sales Promotion and Direct Marketing Code (BCAP). CAP itself is divided into a further two divisions, CAP (Broadcast) and CAP (Non-broadcast). CAP (Broadcast) is responsible for the TV and radio advertising codes, and CAP (Non-broadcast) is responsible for the codes for non-broadcast advertisements, sales promotions and direct marketing.

## Vetting of advertisements

Several regulatory bodies require advertisements to be submitted to them for vetting against their codes of practice. In addition, those that are to be broadcast via television or radio need to be submitted to the appropriate clearance centres.

## MHRA

The MHRA will now vet advertisements for any newly licensed medicines before they are advertised. Pre-vetting is also required where a product is reclassified, such as from prescription-only medicine (POM) to pharmacy medicine (P), and where previous advertising has breached the regulations. The period of vetting will normally be 3–6 months, but could take longer should any problems be identified. Under previous arrangements the MHRA only vetted advertisements for new medicines on the basis of a risk assessment. The decision to pre-vet promotional material for all new active substances is in line with the recommendations laid down in the Health Select Committee's Report *The Influence of the Pharmaceutical Industry* (2005).

Promotional material submitted for vetting to the MHRA should indicate the target audience (public, or person qualified to prescribe or supply medicines) and include references in support of claims made in the promotional material. All material should have already undergone a full set of internal quality control and compliance checks before submission to the MHRA. Normally 5 working days should be allowed for assessment, but where substantial data are submitted the MHRA will give an estimate of the time necessary to complete the assessment if a delay is unavoidable. The company may be asked to advise the MHRA of the form of the advertisement, the intended audience, and the intended date and duration of issue for each piece of copy submitted. (See also Chapter 18 on how to write a marketing authorisation.)

## Proprietary Association of Great Britain (PAGB)

Pre-vetting and approval prior to issue is only a prerequisite for advertising material directed at consumers. There is no re-publication approval of advertising aimed at persons qualified to prescribe and supply.

## Broadcast Advertising Clearance Centre (BACC)

The BACC pre-vets all television advertisements at the preproduction script stage and then again at pre-transmission of the finished advertisement. Pre-vetting is by applying the Television Advertising Standards Code (BCAP). Most broadcasters will not permit transmission without a certificate of clearance by the BACC.

## Applying the law

All forms of advertising for licensed medicine are subject to various legal requirements, including medicines supplied on prescription, OTC preparations, general sale items, generic and branded products, and homoeopathic remedies.

The law defines an advertisement as the spoken or written word having the intention to promote the prescription, supply or sale of drugs by healthcare professionals, or to encourage their use by the general public. Generally, in some form or other, a product claim is stated or alluded to. It is important to remember that the definition of an advertisement is not limited to a particular medium. Advertising can also include articles in journals, magazines and newspapers, posters and notices on display, photographs, film, broadcast material, video recordings, electronic transmissions, and material posted on the internet.

The two basic principles that govern the advertising of medicines in the UK and Europe are:

- only products that are correctly licensed as a medicine can make claims.
- no prescription-only medication can be advertised directly to the public.

For this reason, advertisements directly promoting prescription-only medication will not appear on television, in the newspaper or in main-stream magazines. These products can only be directed at healthcare professionals in medical journals or at medical conferences.

## Minimum requirements

### Product licence

Only fully licensed medicines may be advertised. The MHRA offers advice if it is not clear whether a product should be licensed as a medicine. With regard to unlicensed products it is permissible to provide factual information only to key budgetary decision makers and public advisory bodies, and only where it is thought to significantly affect future planning.

### Approved Summary of Product Characteristics

Statements in the advertisement must comply with the particulars listed in the Summary of Product Characteristics. These need not be identical, but should never contradict. Only promotion of those therapeutic indications that are listed in the approved Summary of Product Characteristics is permitted. An advertisement cannot promote use by a patient group not indicated in the summary.

## Balance

An advertisement must encourage the rational use of the product by representing it objectively and without exaggerating its properties. An advertisement should be objective, and should therefore make reference to any significant limitations, not unduly minimise side effects, or be inconsistent with the Summary of Product Characteristics.

## Accuracy

The advertisement should reflect accurate, up-to-date, verifiable claims and data. Any statement that cannot be supported by the Summary of Product Characteristics should be substantiated. Reference citations should be provided and presented in a faithful and balanced manner, avoiding 'cherry-picking' and the use of obscure data.

## Complete information

Every advertisement should be sufficiently complete to enable the recipients to form their own opinion of the therapeutic value of the product. It is not acceptable to use 'teaser' advertising with the intention of gaining attention for something that is to come, or that will be available at a later date, without providing any actual information.

## Misleading information

No advertisement should be misleading, either in word or in overall impression. This also applies to images that appear in any advertisement.

## Industry reputation

An advertisement should not bring the industry into disrepute.

## Advertising OTC products

Advertisements that are directed at patients and those qualified to prescribe must comply with the minimum requirements described above, as well as some additional prerequisites. A useful tool here is the PAGB Medicines Advertising Codes. The principles of these codes reflect the law and go beyond the legal requirements in an attempt to maintain high standards, ensuring responsible promotion of self-medication products. The aim is to encourage and educate the public and professionals in the safe, effective use of medicines.

The codes provide the primary methods that control the advertising of OTC medicines and food supplements. The PAGB operates a pre-vetting approval system, and all advertising aimed at the public must be submitted to the PAGB for approval prior to the first occasion on which the public will see the advertisement. Those advertisements that are fully compliant will have a stamp of approval. This process does not detract from the responsibility of the member company to ensure that all applicable legal requirements are met and upheld.

> ➤ The primary consideration when preparing an advertisement is that the overall impression gained, whether by careful study, brief overview or partial reading, must be carefully constructed.

Only those products available from a pharmacy without a prescription (P) and those on the general sale list (GSL) can be advertised to the public. However, there are some exceptions to this: government vaccine campaigns are permitted, but products that claim to treat cancer, some psychotropic products, and those used in abortion, may not be advertised to the public.

## Advertising to the public

As advertising covers a multitude of media it is important to remember that most, if not all, of them are subject to legislation. If there is uncertainty it is worth referring to section 3.2.1 of the PAGB consumer code for further information.

**Essentials for public advertising**

- Product name
- Indication (information on correct use)
- Active ingredient (if product has only one)
- Invitation to read the leaflet/label

An advertisement should:

- be clearly definable from editorial material
- use plain language that is easily understood, being neither confusing nor misleading
- not suggest that health would be adversely affected if the product were not used, or create unjustified anxiety about a condition
- not encourage unnecessary use of medicine
- never discourage consumers from seeking medical advice or purport to offer diagnosis
- not contain details or testimonials that could lead to incorrect self-diagnosis
- not imply that 'licensed for use' is equivalent to an endorsement
- only mention establishments that genuinely exist
- not offer a 'money-back guarantee', samples or voucher redemptions
- not imply that a product is recommended or used by a particular health professional or scientist
- not use personal recommendations by celebrities to directly or indirectly encourage use
- only include testimonials that are less than 3 years old, are genuine views, and which comply with all aspects of the code
- not be directed principally or exclusively at children, or show children using or in reach of medicines without adult supervision.

## Claims made in an advertisement

- Most homoeopathic medicines are unlicensed therefore only those that have undergone the full licensing procedure are allowed to make claims in advertisements. Whereas the unlicensed homoeopathic medicines can only state what is found on the label.
- Advertisements cannot suggest in any way that results are guaranteed.
- Claims should not mislead as to the true nature of the medicine or indication.
- Claims must be supported by comprehensive evidence, especially if they comment on speed of action, absorption, dissolution or other pharmacokinetic properties.
- Claims must not be improper, alarming or misleading with regard to recovery, or visuals used to depict physical changes.
- Advertisements can only state that a product is 'new' for up to 1 year from the time a product is made available for purchase.
- Statements about 'uniqueness' must be based on significant differences from anything else on the market.

- Advertisements should not suggest that the active ingredient is unknown, or that the product is anything other than a medicine.
- Advertisements can state that a product is herbal, provided all the active ingredients are plants or plant extracts.
- Advertisements can use the word 'natural' to describe a product provided that all components occur naturally, or to describe only those elements that are naturally occurring.
- Advertisements cannot suggest that safety or efficacy is due to the product being 'natural'.
- Advertisements cannot suggest enhancement of normal good health, or claim to be side-effect-free.
- Advertisements for homoeopathic products cannot claim any action or health-improving effects: they can only list what is on the product label.
- The word 'safe' cannot be used without qualification.
- Advertisements cannot suggest that a product is or has been available on prescription, but can claim that a product's active ingredient, formulation or preparation has been prescribed by a health professional, if there is appropriate evidence.

### Use of comparisons in an advertisement:

- must be fair, balanced and verifiable
- may never, in any way, unjustly discredit a competitor or treatment
- cannot mention brand names of other products without permission
- cannot be based on the lack of an ingredient found in a competitor product
- should not be hanging comparisons (each comparison must be qualified: for example 'product $y$ is better than product $x$ in the treatment of hypertension')
- must not suggest that efficacy is better than or equivalent to that of another identifiable product
- can use top parity provided this is supported by direct comparative data, and only until another product proves superior.

### Advertising to professionals

Advertising to professionals is regulated by the PAGB with the aid of its Professional Code. Pre-vetting is not required, and the PAGB exercises a post-event complaints procedure. However, there is an advisory service available.

Advertisements covered by the Professional Code are aimed at persons qualified to prescribe or supply medicines, with the aim of affecting sales and/or recommendations to the public. The term 'advertising' is meant to imply and encompass print media, electronic, audio, audio-visual, any gift, hospitality or sponsorship at meetings/events, samples, and activities of representatives (refer to section 4.2.2. of the PAGB Professional Code). Furthermore, the Code stipulates that there be a process in place to ensure compliance, and that a signatory of senior status within the company be nominated who will be responsible for ensuring that advertising undertaken by the company is produced in line with the Code, in both letter and spirit.

The items covered by the Code are broad and the following is intended as a guide rather than a comprehensive assessment.

Items are excluded if:

- the medicine is not mentioned by name
- it names the product but only makes claims found in a genuine pack shot
- it names the product but only mentions new labelling, adverse events or price.

(For further details refer to section 4.3 of the PAGB Professional Code.)

**Professional advertisement essentials**

- The seven minimum requirements mentioned earlier in this chapter apply.
- Use of 'safe' must be qualified.
- Information on side effects must reflect evidence.
- A product can not claim to be side-effect free.
- All claims must be fair and verifiable.
- Images (tables, artwork, photographs) must give a true and fair view; those taken from other publications must be accurately reproduced.
- Claims about speed of action and the like must be supported and in line with the Summary of Product Characteristics.
- Use of 'new' can only be used for the first year after launch.
- No reference is made to the MHRA or other regulators.
- Studies used to make claims must be fully referenced.
- Comparisons are permissible but must comply with the Code.
- Uniqueness must be based on significant differences from anything already on the market.
- Only testimonials that are the genuine views of the author and which comply with all aspects of the Code may be used.
- A product can only be 'herbal' if all the active ingredients are plants or plant extracts.
- A product can only be called 'natural' if all its components occur naturally, or the word used to describe only those elements that are naturally occurring.
- A product cannot suggest safety or efficacy is due to its 'natural' nature.

## Essential information for professional advertisements

All advertising to professionals must contain certain essential information, according to the size of the advertisement, and whether it is bound in a dated publication, a loose insert or a detail aid.

In the case of audiovisual material or interactive data systems, the essential information can be either incorporated into the material or provided as an additional document. For audio (sound only) material it must be provided as a document. Promotional aids that feature only the product name and company name do not require this information. Most importantly, wherever required, the information must be prominent and clearly legible.

### Essential information for items over A5 (420 cm²) (unless a promotional aid or dummy pack)

- Active ingredients must be listed immediately adjacent to the most prominent use of the product name. They should either occupy the same amount of space as the name, or use a font size in which the lower-case letter 'a' measures at least 2 mm in height. (This equates to point size of 10 for the majority of fonts.)
- Product licence number
- Name and address of the licence holder, or the part of the licence holder's business responsible for the supply of the product
- Supply classification: P or GSL
- Product indication(s)
- A concise statement describing side effects, precautions and contraindications related to the indication(s)
- Statement about dosage, dosage frequency and, only if not obvious, method of use
- Any warning required as part of the advertising conditions of the Marketing Authorisation
- Cost (excluding VAT) of a specified pack size, specified quantity or recommended daily dose. It should be clear whether the quoted price refers to trade or retail (both are acceptable)
- Date essential information was drawn up or revised

### Essential information for items under A5 (420 cm²) and part of a bound publication

- Active ingredients listed immediately adjacent to the most prominent use of the product name. These should either use the same amount of space as the name, or use a font size in which the lower-case letter 'a' measures at least 2 mm in height. (This equates to a point size of 10 for the majority of fonts.)

- Supply classification: P or GSL
- Product indication(s)
- Any warning required as part of the advertising conditions of the Marketing Authorisation
- Statement that *'further information is available from'* followed by the name and address of the licence holder or the part of the licence holder's business responsible for the supply

## Loose inserts and detail aids:

- must comply with the essential information requirements based on the page size
- must be accurate, up to date, verifiable
- must be sufficiently complete for the recipient to be able to form an opinion of the therapeutic value of the product
- must state the date the information was last drawn up or revised.

## Sponsorship

In order to strengthen a brand or increase product recognition, companies may choose the route of sponsorship. This is when a product or company associates itself with an event (conferences and the like), programme or organisation. For example, a company producing a cardiac drug might wish to associate itself with the British Heart Foundation, which will be reflected on the leaflet the BHF publicises. Similarly, a company producing a children's cough syrup might choose to sponsor a child-related programme on television. The sponsor will therefore take on some of the costs of the event or advertising, but in so doing will indirectly promote itself.

A brand of medicine can be linked to a sponsorship campaign as long as it is classified for over-the-counter sale.

## Advertising of prescription medicines

There is much debate about whether medicines should be advertised at all. Some believe that the amount of funding invested by pharmaceutical companies in their advertising campaigns would be better spent elsewhere. Others understand the economic need for competition and awareness created by advertising. All agree that advertising should be regulated.

The PMCPA (ABPI Code of Practice) is concerned with regulating the promotion of medicines to UK health professionals and the information supplied with prescription-only medicines. The Code is the fundamental reference used in the pharmaceutical industry. It goes beyond the law to provide detailed guidance for ABPI members, who must adhere to the Code both in letter and in spirit.

The ABPI was formed in 1930 and represents more than 80 member companies that research, develop, manufacture and supply more than 80 per cent of the medicines prescribed though the National Health Service.

When examining the functions of the ABPI it will become clearer how they relate to advertising and why almost all highly esteemed pharmaceutical companies in the UK are members and hence subscribe to the Code. The main function of the ABPI is to represent the pharmaceutical industry in such a way that consumers can be assured that they are receiving the best available medicines. First and foremost, the ABPI functions to safeguard the interests of the patient and to promote health through the effective use of medicines. The association has other major objectives, but we will focus on how the ABPI, with the aid of its Code of Practice, is able to promote the industry, protect the patient and reassure health professionals, ensuring that the promotion of medicines is carried out in a responsible, ethical and professional manner.

Pharmaceutical companies go to enormous lengths to ensure that their marketing campaigns comply with ABPI standards. Most have 'copy approval' working practices if not standard operating procedures (SOPs) (see also Chapter 17) to do this. The code requires that two signatories of senior status (CEO or MD) within a company be nominated to certify all final work for publication and take full responsibility for promotion activities undertaken by a company. One of the two nominees must be a registered medical practitioner or a dentist (if the product is for dental use only), and the Code now also allows a practising UK-registered pharmacist, working under the direction of a registered medical practitioner, to certify certain promotional material. A complaint or a breach of the Code is a serious matter, and therefore it is crucial as a medical copywriter that you understand and apply the Code. The ABPI exercises a 'name and shame' policy as its most powerful sanction, the ultimate being expulsion from the Association. This has never happened, but many question whether it is a sufficient sanction for breaching the Code.

The Code is far more comprehensive than the legislative requirements for the advertising of medicines. It has also been recently extensively reviewed, and these reviews came into effect on 1 January 2006. The primary reasons for review were to:

- increase awareness of patient safety by reminding prescribers to report adverse events on all promotions
- apply further restrictions on the amount of advertising in journals and sent to customers
- suspend circulation of material if the information is under appeal
- report more serious cases in the press.

The Code incorporates the principles set out in:

- The International Federation of Pharmaceutical Manufacturers Associations' (IFPMA) Code of Pharmaceutical Marketing Practices
- The European Federation of Pharmaceutical Industries and Associations' (EFPIA) European Code of Practice for the Promotion of Medicines
- The European Directive on the Advertising of Medicinal Products for Human Use (92/28/EEC) (now consolidated as Articles 86–100 of Directive 2001/83/EC)
- The World Health Organization's ethical criteria for medicinal drug promotion.

The following need to be considered in light of the ABPI Code when advertising prescription medicines.

## What is considered promotion?

Promotion is any of the following:

- journal and direct mail advertising
- detail aids carried by sales representatives
- information provided to the general public, either directly or indirectly
- exhibitions, audio cassettes, films, recordings, tapes, video recordings, soundtracks, radio, television, the internet, electronic media, interactive data systems and the like
- any point-of-sale material, booklet, leaflet or other material supplied separately from the product that makes a claim.

## What is not considered an advertisement (as long as no product claims are included)?

- A disease awareness campaign
- Correspondence
- Announcements
- Reference material

- Labels and leaflets
- Price lists and trade catalogues

## Which audience can be addressed?

- Prescribers
- Pharmacy staff
- Suppliers under patient Group Directions
- General sale suppliers

## Size matters

As for OTC medicines, minimum requirements in an advertisement depend on the size of the advertisement. An advertisement is classified as either abbreviated (smaller than A5, with some other provisions as mentioned below) or full (larger than A5).

## Abbreviated advertisements

An abbreviated advertisement, which requires less detail than a full advert, must be no larger than A5 and may only appear in a professional publication. A loose insert cannot be regarded as an abbreviated advertisement, regardless of its size. Abbreviated medicines advertisements are not permitted in audiovisual, interactive or internet material (including internet journals). The minimum requirements for abbreviated advertisements appear later in this section.

**Minimum requirements for a full advertisement**

- The seven minimum requirements discussed on page 194 apply.
- Clear and legible prescribing information (size of letter 'x' no less than 1 mm in height, no more than 100 characters per line, including spaces) must be included in all promotions except promotional aids featuring only product name or company name, and abbreviated advertisements.
- Prescribing information essentials:
  - Name of medicine
  - List of active ingredients
  - Indication(s)
  - Dosage, method of use and route of administration if necessary

- List common and serious adverse events, precautions, contraindications referenced in the SPC, and also include a recommendation to consult the SPC for the complete information
- Any warning required as part of the advertising conditions of the Marketing Authorisation
- Cost (excl. VAT) of a specified pack size, specified quantity or recommended daily dose (not required in journals circulated outside the UK, and in audiovisual or associated material)
- Product classification (POM)
- Name and address of the product licence holder, or the part of the product licence holder's business responsible for the supply of the product
- Date prescribing information was drawn up or last revised
- Promotional aids that feature only the product name and company name do not require any essential information

- Product name and active ingredients listed immediately adjacent to the most prominent use of the product name. The active ingredients should either use the same amount of space as the name, or use a font size in which the lower-case letter 'x' measures at least 2 mm in height.
- In a journal, if the prescribing information is overleaf this must be stated on the advert at the beginning or end, on the outer edge in type size (lower-case 'x' no smaller than 2 mm)
- In a journal, if the pages of a two-page advertisement do not face each other, the advert must not be misleading if read in isolation
- In a journal, a loose insert can be only be a single sheet printed on both sides but cannot be larger than the pages of the journal
- In a journal, a product can only be advertised on two pages per issue
- Printed promotions of more than four pages must clearly state the location of the prescribing information
- In the case of audiovisual material or interactive data systems, the prescribing information can be part of the material or provided as an additional document made available to all persons who are shown or sent the material, but must be provided as a document for audio (sound only) material
- Date item was drawn up or revised, except where part of a dated professional publication
- Promotions on the internet or in an electronic journal must have a clear prominent statement on where to find prescribing information, and a direct link if part of an electronic journal
- All promotional material (except promotional aids) must include, in a text size larger than the prescribing information and in a prominent location, 'information about adverse reporting can be found at www.yellowcard.gov.uk' or similar, and 'Adverse events should also be reported to [company name, telephone number and department]'

**Minimum requirements for an abbreviated advertisement**

- Product name
- Active ingredient(s)
- Indication
- Statement to consult SPC before prescribing
- Product classification (POM)
- Any warning required as part of the advertising conditions of the Marketing Authorisation
- Name and address of the product licence holder, or the part of the licence holder's business responsible for the supply of the product
- Statement that further information is available on request from licence holder or SPC
- Product name and active ingredients listed immediately adjacent to the most prominent use of the product name. The active ingredients should either use the same amount of space as the name, or use a font size in which the lower case letter 'x' measures at least 2 mm in height
- In a prominent location 'information about adverse reporting can be found at www.yellowcard.gov.uk' or similar and 'Adverse events should also be reported to [company name]'
- Statement in line with the SPC giving reason why product is recommended for indication(s)

## Content, claims, comparisons and quotations for all advertisements for prescription-only medicines

- The advertisement should reflect accurate, up-to-date, verifiable claims and comparisons. Any statements in the advertisement that cannot be supported by the Summary of Product Characteristics should be substantiated. The quoted reference citation should be provided and presented in a faithful and balanced manner, avoiding 'cherry-picking' and the use of obscure data.
- Every advertisement should be sufficiently complete to enable the recipients to form their own opinion of the therapeutic value of the product.
- Tables and graphs must give a true, fair and balanced view, conform to the Code, and must be faithfully reproduced and fully referenced.
- Use of the word 'safe' must be as a qualification: it must not suggest that the product is side-effect or dependence free.
- Superlatives must be limited to facts, and claims of special merits or properties must be substantiated.
- The use of 'new' is only permissible to describe a product or indication for up to 12 months from the time it is made available.

- Use of comparisons must not be disparaging but rather fair, balanced and verifiable.
- Must make no reference, unless required as part of its product licence, to a regulatory agency.
- Reproduced official documents need permission in writing from the appropriate body.
- Postcards, envelopes and mailings must not contain information that might be construed as advertising to the public.
- Telephone, text messaging and email cannot be used without the prior permission of the recipient.
- Material relating to medicine or the use of it which is sponsored by a pharmaceutical company must make this fact prominently clear.
- Advertising must be not be disguised and must be clearly distinguishable from editorial material.
- Quotations must reflect the meaning and the current views of the author, be referenced and faithfully reproduced, and modified only to comply with the Code if necessary.
- Quotations from public broadcasts or conferences must have permission from the speaker.

The above information can be found in detail in the PMCPA. This should be consulted and fully understood before attempting to write an advertisement that includes all the necessary items and which complies with the Code in both letter and spirit.

## Images in advertising

The purpose of advertising is to create — to create change, thought and emotion. Images may be present to support the text, or the text can be there to support the images. Reliant on visuals as we are, it is hard to separate the two. However, the marriage of text and images is a powerful tool to support the ultimate message of the advertisement.

## A thousand words

We need not know how to read to be subject to the persuasions of advertising, because through our knowledge of life we create associations with visual elements in order to help us make decisions. For example, a toddler given a box of sweets, who likes what he has tasted, might create an association with the images on the box. Next time he sees the same box in the store, he may ask his parent to buy it for him, even though he cannot read: his actions are a demonstration of the effects of images and associations.

People have always used images to communicate. We have the innate ability to decipher images, knowing that they can provide more information than is visible to the naked eye. Images influence belief and behaviour by association. When you think of a skull and crossbones, you think of pirates, toxic material, danger, death and fear, all thanks to a simple image. From this exercise we can see that images have the power both to inform and to misinform. Even if we are unaware of the context in which the image has been used, we are still able to generate feeling and thoughts, and the meaning taken by one person might be different from that taken by another. Images thus add another layer to language, with meanings and dimensions far beyond what words can convey. Advertisers are more than aware of the impact images have on the human psyche, and because of this we are bombarded with images from a multitude of visual media.

When choosing a particular image, we must be clear about what message we wish to convey with that image. Images that reflect the strategy of an advertisement will achieve more than if they have been selected just because they are good images in themselves. In our demanding and sophisticated market images that demonstrate benefit and which are novel will attract attention.

An interesting article in the *British Medical Journal*[1] concerning the use of images in medical journals provides good examples of medical advertising campaigns that use images in a powerful way, indicating how much can be denoted by associations between the images and the text. Anyone reading these advertisements will agree that thought and insight can generate a whole new undercurrent and an appreciation of the impact images offer. Scott[1] believes that by using strong imagery to underpin the mythical associations between the product being advertised and the condition it treats, advertisers unleash their most powerful weapon, so that the professionals the advertisements are aimed at may not be fully aware of the impact of these images. His statement that: 'In law and science, words are precise and accountable, justified by evidence. In advertising, the image is ambiguous and unaccountable. It makes its "killing" (an aggressive metaphor for selling) softly' is apt and sums up the understated power of speaking without words.

## Legal requirements

Images used in the promotions of medicines must conform to certain requirements. First and foremost they should not exaggerate any claim, either directly or indirectly. Second, images must be tasteful and decent, and not offensive; in this respect it is unacceptable to display naked or partially naked people to attract attention, or to use sexual imagery for that same purpose. Third, no advertisement should mislead in its over-all impression — this also applies to the use of images. Last, images of people in advertisements should not show someone younger than the minimum age, or not within the patient group the medicine is licensed for. (This is irrespective of the true age of the model, but rather their age as perceived by the audience.)

## Global versus international advertising

All advertising must comply with the laws of each country in which it is broadcast, displayed or used. It is not difficult to use an advertisement produced to UK standards within Europe, because UK legislation is based on European Directives. An important matter to consider here is the internet, where anything is available for viewing by the global community.

The United States and New Zealand are the only two countries in which direct-to-consumer advertising of prescription-only medicine is permitted. Television advertisements in the US can now mention both brand and disease, provided that the 'major' risks of the drug and other sources of information, such as websites, magazines and toll-free numbers, are also given. In the UK, pharmaceutical compa-nies can use disease awareness campaigns to create public interest, as long as no drugs are mentioned or drug claims made; if any products are mentioned, all available therapies must be presented in a fair and balanced manner, and it must be clear which company is sponsoring the campaign.

### Advertising in international journals (Taken from the PMCPA, which differs from the MHRA Blue Guide)

- Journals produced (even if they are not distributed) in the UK are subject to UK legislation if they are circulated to a UK audience (consider stating that the advertisement is in respect to a UK licence).
- Journals produced in the UK but only for overseas distribution must follow local requirements and/or the International Federation of Pharmaceutical Manufacturers and Associations' (IFMA) Code of Pharmaceutical Marketing Practices.

## Promotional material

Any UK company preparing an item to be used in another country must ensure that the material complies with both countries' regulations. If there is uncertainty about an issue between the relative codes, the more stringent regulation applies.

In order to be able to promote indications not licensed in the UK, where the product holds a licence for that indication in another country, at a UK meeting, the meeting must be truly international and have a significant international audience. The material should be relevant, proportionate to the purpose of the meeting, and should clearly and prominently indicate that the product or indication is unlicensed in the UK.

## Internet

Material posted on UK websites and/or aimed at a UK audience is subject to UK medicines advertising legislation. As with other media, the promotion of prescription-only medicines to the UK public on the internet is prohibited. However, it is permissible to advertise prescription-only medicines on websites whose nature and content are directed at health professionals. For websites that provide information for both consumers and health professionals the target markets should be separated and clearly identified.

Where companies include links from their UK website to sites that serve other countries, it should be clear to UK users that they have chosen to access material aimed at users from other countries. The UK site should have all the minimum basic information about the company's products, such as the prescribing information and Summary of Product Characteristics. A statement on each page of the website making clear the intended audience is also suggested by the Code of Practice.

## Advertising on internet journals

Journals which are published or posted on the internet and directed expressly at persons qualified to prescribe or supply medicines, and the advertising contained within that journal, should comply with respective regulations of the Code. Each page of an advertisement for a prescription-only medicine (POM) should be clearly labelled as intended for health professionals.

## Radio and television advertising

The advertising standards for both television and radio encompass the medicines advertising laws. There seems to be much overlap with the PAGB Code described earlier, the main reason for which is to ensure that non-PAGB members also comply with the law. Both Codes reflect the same law, with only a few subtle differences. For this reason, here I will concentrate on the additional requirements of the Advertising Standards Codes.

OFCOM ensures that the content of programmes and advertising on television and radio meets the appropriate standards. OFCOM can insist that an advertisement be removed or amended. It can also impose broadcast restrictions on the timing of an advertisement, particularly when children might be watching.

### Television

All advertisements must be sent for pre-vetting by the Broadcast Advertising Clearance Centre (BACC) and PAGB (if a member company). No broadcaster will air an advertisement without a clearance certificate from the BACC. The BACC sends medicine advertisements to a medical panel for advice.

**Requirements for medicine advertisements on television**

- An advertisement can only direct the viewer to seek advice on medicines or health matters from a health professional regulated by a statutory/recognised professional body (list of recognised bodies available from ASA and BCAP).
- An advertisement cannot offer to treat or diagnose remotely (e.g. by phone, post, internet, e-mail, fax).
- Use of the word 'tonic' in medicine advertising is not permitted unless authorised by the product licence.
- Products for the treatment of alcohol and substance misuse or dependence cannot be advertised, with the exception of products to aid smoking cessation.
- Smoking cessation advertisements must make clear that the product is no more than an aid and that willpower is crucial.
- Adverts must not suggest that smoking is safer while the habit is being reduced.
- Advertisements for homoeopathic products can make no claims or mention an ailment.

- Invitations to read the label should read: 'Always read the label' or 'Always read the leaflet'.
- No advertisement can suggest that a medicine is a foodstuff, cosmetic or other consumer product.
- Medicine advertisements cannot offer to donate money to charity.
- A product cannot claim to be side-effect free, but can refer to the likely absence of a specific side effect (i.e. 'unlikely to cause weight gain').
- No medicines may be advertised to anyone under the age of 16.
- No product can claim to relieve tension, but relief of a 'tension headache' is permitted because this is a recognised medical condition.

## Radio

Radio advertisements must also be vetted before they are broadcast. The body responsible for this is the Radio Advertising Clearance Centre (RACC). The RACC is authorised by OFCOM, the commercial radio regulator. PAGB member companies are required to submit advertisements to both the PAGB and the RACC for approval. The requirements assessed by the BACC are much the same as those stipulated in the PAGB. The points highlighted here are just some extra items that the BACC mentions.

### Requirements for medicine advertisements on radio

- All radio advertisements must use the words 'Always read the label' or 'Always read the leaflet'.
- An advertisement cannot offer to treat or diagnose remotely (e.g. by phone, post, internet, e-mail, fax).
- An advisement can offer additional advice and information remotely by a health professional service recognised by the ASA and BCAP, including the provision of brochures and leaflets.
- Recommendations and testimonial by celebrities or medical charities, patients' groups and medical professionals are not permitted.
- The words 'help' or 'relieve' should be used to state claims and not imply cure.
- Use of the word 'tonic' in medicine advertising is not permitted unless authorised by the product licence.
- A product cannot claim to be side-effect free, but can refer to the likely absence of a specific side effect (e.g. 'unlikely to cause weight gain').
- No advertisement for medicine can target anyone under the age of 16.

- No product can claim to relieve tension; relief of a 'tension headache' is permitted because this is a recognised medical condition.
- Sales promotions, offers and samples are not allowed in medicines advertising.
- Jingles cannot be used in the promotion of medicines.

## Useful resources

The Advertising Unit
Medicines and Healthcare Products Regulatory Agency
*www.mhra.gov.uk*
(MHRA Blue Guide and advice available on the website)

Proprietary Association of Great Britain (PAGB)
Tel. 020 7242 8331
*www.pagb.co.uk*

Association of the British Pharmaceutical Industry (ABPI)
Tel. 020 7930 3477
*www.abpi.org.uk*

Prescription Medicines Code of Practice Authority (PMCPA)
Tel. 020 7930 9677
*www.pmcpa.org.uk*

OFCOM Contact Centre
Tel 020 7981 3040
*www.ofcom.org.uk*

Advertising Standards Authority (ASA)
Tel. 020 7492 2222
*www.asa.org.uk*

Committee of Advertising Practice and Broadcast (BCAP)
Committee of Advertising Practice (CAP)
Tel. 020 7492 2222
*www.cap.org.uk*

CAP Copy Advice
Tel. 020 7492 2100
E-mail: *copyadvice@cap.org.uk*

Broadcast Advertising Clearance Centre (BACC)
Tel. 020 7633 2935
*www.bacc.org.uk*

**Radio Advertising Clearance Centre (RACC)**
Tel. 020 7306 2620
*www.racc.co.uk*

# Reference

1.  Scott T, Stanford N, Thompson DR (2004) Killing me softly: myth in pharmaceutical advertising. *BMJ* 329: 1484–1487.

# Section Four

Medical writing in education

# 13

# Writing examination and assessment papers

*Lilian M Azzopardi, Anthony Serracino-Inglott,*
*Maurice Zarb-Adami*

Recent decades have witnessed major changes in medical and pharmaceutical technology and innovation. Patients' receptiveness and participation in their own healthcare have also evolved considerably. This has led to changes in educational requirements. The development of the curriculum and medical education must prepare graduates for the needs of today, as well as providing the necessary skills for continuous lifelong learning.

The requirements of quality assurance in professional healthcare services and within the pharmaceutical industry are well established, and quality assurance in education is an accepted practice. In education, quality assurance aims to demonstrate that the educational programme is preparing the graduate for contemporary needs and that they have acquired the necessary skills. This scenario emphasises the need to develop examination papers and assessment documents that will evaluate the student. Such evaluation should not only look at the student's ability to recall knowledge acquired, but also at their ability to apply that knowledge to practice, whether this relates directly to patient care or not.

Quality in education is important. Assessment strategies and curriculum development are used to assure that the education programme is accomplishing its intended objectives. This chapter provides an overview of the issues concerning the development of assessment strategies for medical education. This includes the principles and characteristics involved in the preparation of appraisal schemes, and approaches and methods that could be adopted to prepare the documents.

Assessment in medical education programmes is essential. Examinations are known to induce stress in those sitting them, and sometimes also in those who set them. There is also the possibility that they might not give an accurate evaluation of those examined. They may produce elation (which may be unwarranted) in those candidates who are successful and despair in those who are not. However, they are necessary to assess candidates' knowledge of facts and academic abilities, and they are less subject to bias than any other means of assessment available.

There is variability in both assessment practices and assessment-related terms. The glossary below explains the terms used in this chapter.

**Glossary**

**Assessment**: a systematic process involving the collection, review and interpretation of information to aid student learning and development and/or to certify competence
**Assessment document**: tools used in the assessment process which include examinations and other assessment activities
**Candidate competence**: the candidate's ability to perform in an assessment
**Certification**: qualifying examinations
**Diagnostic assessment**: early assessment of candidates' knowledge in a course programme
**Evaluation**: judgement made about a candidate's mark which measures the extent of learning by comparing the mark obtained with a standard or with the marks of other candidates
**Examination**: an assessment process prepared by an institution to certify candidates' performances
**Formative assessment**: assessment conducted during course of instruction
**Measurement**: the process of gathering objective information about candidate's performance
**Reliability**: an index of the extent to which the data resulting from the measurement instrument (examination/test paper) can vary due to external factors, such as bias of the assessors
**Self-assessment**: candidates assess themselves during a course programme to identify their learning needs
**Summative assessment**: assessment conducted after instruction is completed
**Test**: assessment process carried out to evaluate candidates' performances
**Validity**: a measure of how well the instrument measures what it is supposed to measure

## Preparation

When you are preparing examination papers and assessment documents it is necessary to plan their structure to ensure that each serves the objectives of the examination or test.

## Defining objectives

Examination papers and assessment documents should be developed within an educational programme structure with the objective of measuring candidates' learning and ability. The objectives of the examination or test should be outlined at the planning stage, well before you begin to write the questions for it.

Objectives may include:

- recruitment of candidates from a group (a selective process)
- grading and classification of candidates based on performance
- confirmation that candidates have acquired a standard level of knowledge (certification) and ability (skill)
- assessing candidates' knowledge within a continuous assessment programme.

## Duration of the assessment

Examination papers or assessment documents must be practical and feasible within the environment where the assessment is undertaken. They must take into consideration the time and costs involved and the ability of the candidates attempting the assessment. Therefore, you should prepare the questions in such a way that the candidates have enough time to complete all the sections of the paper. The number of questions they should be expected to address will depend on the expected depth of their knowledge of the topic.

---

➤ Word questions in a way that enables them to be answered within the allotted time.

---

Where the candidate is given just a few minutes to answer a question, you could use the words 'briefly' or 'in summary' as a guide, or give keywords. This will highlight the issues they should focus on and the amount of time they should spend on the question.

> **Example 1. Extract from a test for third-year pharmacy students where the approximate time to be dedicated to the question is 12 minutes**
> Giving examples, write briefly on the use of atypical antipsychotics in schizophrenia using the following keywords as a guide to the content of your answer: efficacy, side effects, patient advice and monitoring, cautions, and contraindications.

## Type of assessment

The type of assessment should take its objectives into consideration. This will depend on whether a comprehensive approach to a broad subject area is required, or rather an assessment of knowledge on a specific topic. When the assessment is intended as an ancillary test to assess candidates' knowledge of an individual topic, for example management of disorders of the gastrointestinal tract, the questions need to be very specific. On the other hand, when the assessment aims to evaluate comprehensive knowledge in an area such as the management of minor ailments, the document should touch on different issues and not be specific to a particular area: for example, questions should not only address ailments related to nausea.

> ➤ For a comprehensive assessment, include a range of interrelated subjects such as pharmacological issues, pharmacotherapy and clinical skills.

## Target audience

The target audience of the assessment needs to be defined before the assessment is set. The terminology used should be accessible and able to be understood by your audience. For example, if the audience is first-year undergraduates the terminology should be simpler than that used for third-year students. When the target audience is final-year undergraduates or clinical practitioners, then the terminology should reflect a higher standard.

Example 2. Extract from a test on diuretics for first-year pharmacy students (5 marks allocated)

1.   Give *one* example of each of the following stating trade name and active ingredient:
     a.   loop diuretic
     b.   thiazide diuretic.
2.   Compare the two products considering indications, mode of action, and side effects.
3.   What product is used with loop and thiazide diuretics to reduce the occurrence of unwanted effects, and how is this achieved?

Example 3. Extract from a test on diuretics for third-year pharmacy students (5 marks allocated)

1.   When is a diuretic required in congestive heart failure?

2.    Give *two* examples of diuretics that may be used in heart failure.
3.    For each example, state trade name, active ingredient, dose and side effects to be expected.

## Scoring and measuring candidates' performances

Assigning marks for the different questions of the examination or test paper is important, as it reveals the relative significance of each item. Therefore, easier questions should be assigned fewer marks than the more difficult ones. This system also gives candidates a guide to the amount of material they should provide for each question. If the scoring system gives all questions the same number of marks (for example multiple-choice questions), the questions should as far as possible have the same level of difficulty.

▶ Plan the scoring system to reflect the level of answer expected. This will help you maintain consistency when marking.

The scoring system should be based on the objectives of the assessment. If it is intended for a qualifying process or as a competitive evaluation, the scoring system is of great significance. In such cases, marks should be assigned for specific aspects rather than assigned in bulk. This will give you better control over the marking outcome and will result in a much fairer measurement of candidates' performances.

▶ Scatter the marks across a number of separate related questions, rather than allocate them all to one question that addresses all the issues (especially with case-based questions).

Example 4. Extract from an examination for fourth-year pharmacy students. A total of 20 marks have been allocated, and these have been divided between short response questions

- BD is a 55-year-old woman who has been diagnosed with breast cancer. She is receiving chemotherapy cycles of cyclophosphamide, methotrexate and fluorouracil.
  - Explain the rationale of using cytotoxic chemotherapy and of using combination regimens.                               (2 marks)
  - Explain the term chemotherapy cycles.                        (1 mark)
  - What are the options for the route of administration for the above drugs and what is their mode of action?       (4 marks)

- ○ What is the emetic potential for the drugs used? Describe therapeutic options for preventing nausea and vomiting.

  (3 marks)

- ○ What advice should be given to the patient regarding bone marrow suppression?                                          (3 marks)

- ○ Which drug could be used to counteract neutropenia that may occur? Describe monitoring requirements, precautions and side effects when this drug is used.                              (4 marks)

- ○ Describe pharmacist interventions in a cancer chemotherapy day-care setting.                                               (3 marks)

**Preparation checklist**

☑ Define objectives
☑ Establish duration of assessment process
☑ Draw up a scoring system

## Document layout

An examination paper can be compared to a work of art: it must be sculpted and painted into a pleasing format. The layout of the paper should make the candidate feel relaxed. Their efforts should be dedicated to tackling the problems presented, and not to deciphering the questions. Well-prepared candidates should consider the assessment as a positive experience and not as an exercise in trickery. It should not be seen as a weapon intended to stress, threaten, or create tension. Candidates should emerge from a test without feeling unduly exhausted, and certainly the majority should have their confidence enhanced rather than destroyed.

The candidate should be drawn comfortably into the assessment process. Start with questions that contain familiar elements. The paper can then progress to other questions that rely more on the intelligence of the candidate. The layout should be stimulating, imaginative and interesting.

### Typesetting

Typesetting is of the utmost importance. Italics or handwritten script may not be as effective as other fonts: using bold text for emphasis will serve the same function and will be certainly clearer to the candidate.

The typesetting of the paper is often left until the last minute, sometimes to someone who has no knowledge of the text. The text must be prepared in sufficient time so that amendments can be made to the typeset paper if necessary, and not just to proofread for technical or typographical errors. This is easier said than done. It is even more important to take care when setting test papers for the international market, as those taking the tests may come from very diverse linguistic and cultural backgrounds — the format of the document must enable it to be fully accessible.

**Layout checklist**

- ☑ Make the administration of the tests user-friendly
- ☑ Ensure instructions are clear
- ☑ Give examples to clarify what is being asked
- ☑ Keep the layout uncluttered
- ☑ Allow plenty of space for handwritten answers

## Task division

The questions on a topic such as a case study must be divided into tasks: each question should have five or six tasks, but none should have more than ten. The text should be divided into paragraphs with a maximum of 240 words each.

Preferably, each question should not take longer than 15 minutes to answer. In medical-related questions the tasks should be brief and varied, and should also reflect, as far as possible, the types of tasks normally carried out in real case scenarios. Such questions correspond more with reality and make the objectives of the test easier to achieve.

Few of us would take tests just for fun. However, making a test more light-hearted is acceptable today, even for serious and higher-standard assessments and examinations (such as in surgery or oncology). Even in this type of examination a touch of humour (especially in a diagram setting) and a feeling of a game challenge (for example in a calculation, epidemiology or statistical setting) is also encouraged. Although you should not overload the test with material that creates continual time-watching and pressure, the candidate should be occupied throughout and the occupation should be interesting and not just a race against time.

The choice of language should also reflect today's ways of communication. Gone are the days where medical personnel had to use archaic language, poorly legible handwriting, mysterious measuring units (such as minims) and the apothecary's ounce, or long Greek or Latin names. There is no need to use language other than that used during ward rounds, in the *British National Formulary* and in the *Physician's Desk Reference*. When wording questions try to use common subjects, daily nomenclature, drugs, medical devices, and as few abbreviations as possible so as to relate to the candidate's own experience and culture and to allow for differences in the particular settings. This is especially appropriate where candidates come from different backgrounds.

The use of fiction and whether it has a place in the examination setting is often discussed. For example, should an assessment deal with a fantasy patient with a blood pressure of 480/290 and still alive? Should the concept of visiting aliens be used to ensure that the test is original and not a regurgitation of material? This would appear to be a fair way of assessment, as it is far from any example that candidates will have met in their familiar surroundings. This concept may have a place in formative assessments, which are conducted during the course of instruction and are used as a learning exercise. Nevertheless, we are of the opinion that there is definitely no room for such fantasy in summative examinations. The advantages of using topics and language associated with daily practice are said to outweigh the disadvantages that such criteria may present.

## Using computers for assessment

Until recently computer-based testing has been used mainly for formative assessment, such as giving students feedback on their performance during the course. It is now also used for summative examinations, such as state board examinations for the purpose of registration. Computers can be used to design assessment papers that include drawings and even multimedia. The principles of good layout that apply to printed scripts must still be taken into consideration, however do not let the creative possibilities offered by computer software go beyond a feasible and practical layout.

Using computers for assessment allows for an interactive scenario to be used whereby, for example, the results of laboratory investigations are presented to introduce the next question. However, interactive media should not be used unless they enhance the outcome of the assessment.

➤ Be sure to set the document in such a way as to achieve its objectives without testing the candidate's computer skills.

## Writing the questions

For any assessment process the measurement instrument must be:

- practical
- feasible
- reliable
- valid.

These attributes give confidence in the data generated by the process and hence in any judgements based on the candidates' results. In the medical field, such judgements might include performance in undergraduate education, certification in an undergraduate degree such as medicine or pharmacy, postgraduate certification in a speciality such as medicine, clinical pharmacy, surgery, or revalidation for practice (renewal of licence).

### Reliability and validity

Reliability is a measure of the reproducibility of the data generated by the assessment. It is also an index of the extent to which the data resulting from the measurement instrument (examination paper) is dependent on the assessors and/or environmental factors. If the measurement instrument is reliable, a candidate should obtain the same results if the test is re-taken in similar circumstances. Various factors can influence the reliability of an examination, e.g. inconsistency in the assessors, interpretation of language used in the questions, and the presentation and layout of the paper.

Reliability can be measured using different statistical methods, such as inter-rater or test–retest reliability, and then calculating internal consistency. Examination questions should be prepared in such a way as to provide consistent and reproducible results, using simple terms to avoid ambiguity, which might lead to different interpretations. A good marking scheme should also be constructed to reduce inconsistencies in marking.

Validity is a measure of how well the instrument measures what it is supposed to measure. In education, validity refers to:

- appropriateness of the results
- meaningfulness of the results
- whether the assessment produces useful, specific and appropriate decisions.

An assessment document may be reliable, but it may not be valid because it does not measure what was intended. For example, a practice-oriented examination for first-year undergraduates may be reliable in that it yields similar results within a cohort of students; however, if the candidates' performance is heavily dependent on knowledge of the terminology used, rather than of the different classes of drugs (as stipulated in the module objectives), then the validity of the assessment is highly questionable.

It is not always feasible in an educational setting to undertake statistical validity tests for assessment processes. Therefore, when writing questions, assessors should bear in mind the concept of validity in terms of a meaningful and appropriate process.

➤ Ensure validity by adhering to the objectives of the assessment process when writing questions. Have the questions reviewed by a colleague who was not involved in writing them.

To balance errors that may arise, more than one assessment method may be used, for example a written assessment combined with a practical one, or a written assessment at the end of a course combined with the results of continuous assessment of clinical or experimental practice. This method of collecting results is referred to as triangulation.

## Types of questions

Different types of questions can be used in examination papers and assessment documents. Each type has its advantages and disadvantages in terms of the writing process, the assessment process and the scoring process.

### Created response questions

In created response questions candidates are required to compose an answer and the questions vary in terms of the flexibility they offer. Candidates may be required to give a brief answer of a few words or sentences (restricted response), or they may be expected to write a multiple-page essay (extended response).

It is quite easy for assessors to prepare created response questions, as they require less time to word. A characteristic of such questions is that they provide an opportunity for the candidates to demonstrate their writing skills as well as their skills in organising knowledge and concepts. Hence the assessors are in a position to assess candidates' ability in report writing and communication of knowledge. There is also the advantage that when candidates do not know their material it is more difficult for them to guess successfully.

Although easy to prepare, created response questions are time-consuming to score, especially if the expected response is an essay. Therefore, such questions are not indicated when the assessment requires very careful or mathematically calculated scoring (such as in qualifying examinations), or when prompt and detailed feedback to the candidates is required. In fact, the difficulty of scoring reliability in this type of question is a major disadvantage. Several issues may interfere with the scoring, such as the legibility of the candidate's handwriting, their grammar, writing style, and the length of the essay. How candidates are penalised for spelling mistakes in technical terms (such as disease states, diagnostic markers, or generic and proprietary names of medicines) may also interfere with scoring reliability. Reliability may be enhanced by establishing certain marking criteria before the marking process begins.

> Prepare a model answer and then develop a scoring system based on the issues that feature in it. The original question will need modifying if the marks cannot be easily allocated to the model answer.

**Example 5. Extract from an examination for fourth-year pharmacy students, including a model answer and a marking scheme**

*Question:* Which drug could be used to counteract the neutropenia that may occur with cancer chemotherapy? Describe monitoring requirements, precautions necessary and common side effects when this drug is used.                                          (4 marks)

*Model answer and marking scheme:*

Drug: Filgrastim                                                          (0.5 marks)

Monitoring: temperature, complete blood count, cardiac function                                         (0.5 marks each, 1.5 marks total)

Precaution: do not use within 24 hours of cytotoxic
chemotherapy                                              (1 mark)
Side effects: bone pain, fever          (0.5 marks each, 1 mark total)

Created response questions limit the amount of material that can be covered by the assessment, as time must be allowed for the candidate to write the required text.

---

➤    Created response questions are most useful in formative assessments. It is best to avoid them in comprehensive certifying assessments.

---

### Selected response questions

In selected response questions, candidates are required to select the most appropriate answer or to answer the question with a single word (e.g. true or false) or a short phrase. Carefully written selected response questions can be used to classify candidates in a similar way as created response questions. However, selected response items can be more difficult and time-consuming to write. Sometimes you will need to re-write questions a number of times before the correct style is achieved.

Selected response questions need to be clear, intelligible and unambiguous, as the candidate does not have the opportunity to express any different possibilities. Having the questions reviewed by colleagues provides an external control, eliminates problem questions and reduces invalid questions.

If you wish to present a highly cognitive assessment in order to classify candidates, then the questions should be simple and clear but address a higher order of knowledge. This could be achieved by presenting questions that require the candidate to carry out thinking and/or mathematical skills, which requires a more comprehensive knowledge base.

An advantage of selected response questions is that they are very much less subject to assessors' scoring bias, so that the reliability and robustness of the assessment process are greater than can be achieved with created response questions. Tests and examinations based on selected response questions also take less time to mark. Another advantage is that because candidates take less time to complete each question, more material can be covered within the same timeframe.

Rather than measuring candidates' abilities in report writing and communication as do created response questions, selected response questions measure their knowledge of the material and their skills in applying that knowledge.

The term 'multiple choice' is often used to refer to selected response questions. Table 13.1 presents a range of various formats that can be used for these questions.

**Table 13.1**   Different possibilities for selected response questions

| Description | Example | Characteristics |
| --- | --- | --- |
| Stem and alternative responses to select correct answer* | *Select the correct answer* Common side effects of salbutamol include all EXCEPT:<br>A   fine tremor<br>B   tachycardia<br>C   headache<br>D   constipation<br>E   muscle cramps | Difficult to prepare a number of realistic but wrong alternative responses; may be used in the initial part of a test or examination which is based on selected response questions as a warming-up exercise. |
| Matching items* | A   furosemide<br>B   spironolactone<br>C   bendroflumethiazide<br>*Select from A to C, which one of the above is a potassium-sparing diuretic* | Useful to assess ability of candidates to identify relationships. May be used to assess knowledge of abbreviations and drug characteristics. |
| Stem and multiple correct answers* | *Decide which response(s) is (are) correct. Then choose the answer between A to E according to the key provided (e.g. if 1, 2 and 3 are correct — A; if 1 and 2 only are correct — B)* Clinical features of hyperthyroidism include:<br>1   palpitations<br>2   tremor<br>3   weight gain | Useful to assess candidates' grasp of knowledge in depth, difficult for candidates to guess the answer. |
| True or false | *Indicate whether True or False* | Very easy to prepare, but memorisation and |

(continued)

**Table 13.1** *Continued*

| Description | Example | Characteristics |
|---|---|---|
| | a) By increasing the gastric pH, proton pump inhibitors may promote haemostasis in upper gastrointestinal bleeding.<br><br>b) Both omeprazole and ranitidine should be used with caution in hepatic impairment. | guessing by the candidates may compromise reliability and robustness of the assessment process. |
| Combined statements with true or false* | *Decide whether first statement is true or false. Decide whether second statement is true or false. Then choose answer from A to E based on key provided (e.g. A if both statements are correct and the second statement is a correct explanation of the first, B if both statements are correct but the second statement is not a correct explanation of the first, C if first statement is true but the second is false, D if first statement is false but the second is true, E if both statements are false)* Tardive dyskinesia is a chronic movement disorder characterised by uncontrolled facial movements. Tardive dyskinesia is associated with the use of trifluoperazine. | Easy to prepare, good to identify candidates' skills in understanding and applying the knowledge to address the questions, difficult for the candidates to guess the answer. |

*Examples taken from Azzopardi LM (ed) (2003) *MCQs in Pharmacy Practice*. London: Pharmaceutical Press.

> Remember:

- to ensure the reliability of the assessment process to achieve consistent and reproducible results
- to ensure the validity of the assessment process to produce meaningful results
- to use selected response questions to minimise scoring bias
- that created response questions allow candidates' reporting skills to be scored.

---

**In summary**

- Always identify the objectives of the assessment and start planning the writing of assessment documents in advance.
- Before you start writing the questions, prepare a plan of the assessment procedure (duration, type of assessment, scoring system).
- Give particular attention to the layout of the assessment document.
- When writing the questions, prepare a model answer and establish a scoring plan; doing this at this stage will avoid problems during the marking of the scripts.
- Give the questions to a colleague, who will be able to add an external perception to them.
- Write questions that are simple and clear, to avoid ambiguity both in interpretation of the question and in the answer the candidate provides.

## Useful contacts

American Journal of Pharmaceutical Education (online)
*www.ajpe.org*

American Association of Colleges of Pharmacy (AACP)
www.aacp.org

European Association of Faculties of Pharmacy (EAFP)
*www.eafponline.org*

Royal Pharmaceutical Society of Great Britain
*www.rpsgb.org.uk*

British Medical Association
*www.bma.org.uk*

232 Writing examination and assessment papers

## Further reading

Abate MA, Stamatakis MK, Haggett RR (2003) Excellence in curriculum development and assessment. *Am J Pharm Educ* 67: 1–22.

Anderson HM (2005) Preface: A methodological series on assessment. *Am J Pharm Educ* 69: 81–83.

Azzopardi LM (ed) (2003) *MCQs in Pharmacy Practice*. London: Pharmaceutical Press.

Bearne E (2002) *Differentiation and Diversity in the Primary School*. London: Routledge-Falmer.

Bird E, Anderson H, Anaya G, Moore DL (2005) Beginning an assessment project: A case study using data audit and content analysis. *Am J Pharm Educ* 69: 356–369.

Cantillon P, Irish B, Sales D (2004) Using computers for assessment in medicine. *BMJ* 329: 606–609.

Cohen L, Manion L, Morrison K (2004) *A Guide to Teaching Practice*. London: Routledge-Falmer.

Cruickshank DR, Bainer DL, Metcalf KK (1999) *The Act of Teaching*. New York, USA: McGraw-Hill College.

McKinley RK, Fraser RC, Baker R (2001) Model for directly assessing and improving clinical competence and performance in revalidation of clinicians. *BMJ* 322: 712–715.

Mifsud C, Mallia G (eds) (2000) *Ways and Measures: Teaching and Assessing Young Learners of English as a Foreign Language*. Malta: World Academic.

# 14

## Presentation materials

*Matthew Shaw*

'*It was a great presentation! They gave out all the handouts at the start, so I could read my book while the presenter was droning on . . .*'

Have you ever been in this position or felt that way? We can't promise to turn you into a star at conferences or any other presentation events, but if this phrase sounds familiar, then this chapter may be helpful! Throughout, we have categorised presentations according to their scale. There are the large-scale shows, including slide shows, overhead projectors and PowerPoint. Then there's the mid-scale approach — flipcharts, whiteboards, chalkboards and the like. Finally, there's the small scale — the handouts. This chapter focuses on the common resources and approaches used in selecting and preparing presentations. We will give you an insight into these and review their use in practice. We will also give personal viewpoints on what to avoid.

When selecting which type of presentation to prepare, the following should be considered:

- benefits and limitations
- cost
- ease of use
- ease of maintenance.

The three approaches can be pulled together: a large-scale presentation can be used to set the scene, then the mid-scale can be used to gather information or support feedback, and finally the distribution of handouts can underpin content, key messages, and provide references or resources.

### The large-scale presentation

A number of formats are used for large-scale presentations, including the following:

- slides
- overhead projection, using acetates
- powerPoint
- films
- video technology.

The use of films or video technology is not covered here, but you may find that many of the points raised are relevant to both these methods. When choosing which method to use there are some key questions to consider (see Box 14.1).

---

**Box 14.1**    Questions to consider

- What type of presentation do I want to give?
- What do I have available?
- What equipment does the venue have?
- What am I comfortable using?
- What is my budget?
- What is the timescale?
- What is the purpose?

---

### What type of presentation do I want to give?

One of the main things to remember is that it is *your* presentation. This may sound obvious, but if you are not comfortable with the approach you take, you are not likely to perform well.

### What do I have available?

It is of course important to remember the software, stationery, technical assistance, etc. that you have to hand, and the availability of such at the venue.

### What equipment does the venue have available?

In general only larger centres will have a slide projector, although most venues will offer an overhead projector. Increasingly data projectors (for PowerPoint) are being provided. However, with both types the quality is hugely variable. If you choose to take your own projector along, does the venue offer sufficient power points, or an extension cable to keep your computer up and running?

➤ Remember your responsibility under Health and Safety legislation. If you need lots of cables, you must ensure that they are covered. Options include both cable cover mats and brightly coloured carpet tape.

## What am I comfortable using?

Don't get carried away with what everyone else is using. If you know how to use a particular method, stick with it. If you do need to use a different approach, practise it well beforehand, as regardless of the quality of the content, you will be judged on the proficiency of your delivery.

## What is my budget?

Whichever method you decide to use, there will be financial implications — what budget do you have? If you give yourself longer to get things ready, does that bring the cost down? Will that then affect the currency and timeliness of the content?

For each approach we indicate how much it is likely to cost. Budgets should often be linked to currency of content as well as final materials. For example, a topic that requires frequent updates will affect the cost of the method chosen. If it is to be used on one occasion only, is it worth the investment in money and time?

## What is the timescale?

If you have been called in to give a presentation at short notice, you may be restricted as to the options available. Consider what is realistically possible in the timeframe. Planning well in advance will ensure your production time is optimised. If you have been given plenty of notice, there is little excuse for not planning well in advance!

## What is the purpose?

In all of these considerations you should constantly remind yourself of the purpose of your presentation. Don't allow your messages to be taken over by the presentation itself. Films, flashing lights, walking text or gory images may be useful — but is that what you want your audience to remember? They are likely to be receiving this information for the first time, so keep it simple, clear, and focused on the key points you wish to make.

The following compares the main forms of presentation media.

## Slides and projectors

### Benefits

- Compact
- Durable
- Excellent for picture detailing
- Useful for medical library images
- Useful where paper distribution is not practical or possible for copyright reasons
- Allows you to create pre-timed recorded presentations, when the machine is set to display the slides in a timed sequence
- Allows use of your own photographs (if you use slide film)

### Limitations

- Needs professional production to develop slides
- Needs more storage space than electronic formats
- Machinery may break down
- Requires skill and knowledge to operate machinery
- Deterioration or dust may be visible during the presentation
- Slides can get stuck in the machine, which disrupts presentation
- You may need your own carousel

---

➤ Try to ensure that technical support will be available at the venue to ensure the smooth operation of projection equipment.

---

In our opinion slides are not really a modern option. They are often associated with university lectures and their use nowadays is quite dated. However, they can still be used with skill to enhance the style, humour and panache of a presentation.

### Cost considerations

The initial production costs of slides are higher than for either PowerPoint or overhead projectors (OHPs). However, if the content is durable — for example pictures of wounds, human organs, etc. — this may lead to longer-term savings.

As fewer venues use slides regularly, the cost of using them is likely to increase.

Many postgraduate medical centres offer a slide projection facility, and this is likely to remain a viable option in these situations, but hotels, for example, will probably not have this as an option — can you borrow a reliable projector? If not, you may need to invest in your own system.

As slide projections have a habit of breaking down it is always worth investing in a projection support assistant, both to get a presentation up and running again and to take the flak for anything that goes wrong! It is very difficult to maintain rapport with your audience once you start trying to mend the projector yourself.

### Maintenance

Slides can be tricky to maintain. If you have a slide film in your camera you can take pictures to your heart's content, but you then have to try to find somewhere to get them developed, which can be difficult.

## Overhead projectors and acetates

### Benefits

- Versatile, flexible
- Majority of venues have a projector
- Can use colour or black and white
- Little IT or projector experience needed
- Easy to flick back and forth
- Easy to skip images in order to manage time
- Good to have as an additional backup to other formats
- Reproduction of presentation easy
- Handwriting possible — but spelling and legibility must be checked manually
- Useful for recording feedback and key points for small group presentations
- Versatile — images can be hand drawn or produced using high-tech printing technology
- One of the few methods that really allow the flexibility of amending live, by drawing or writing on them to make a point or gain audience buy-in

## Limitations

- Not fashionable
- A projector in poor condition can affect the quality of projection
- Focusing the projected image can be difficult
- Colours and scratches can be hard to rectify
- Physical damage to projectors is often ignored by venue personnel
- Less durable than slides: fade, brittle, dirt, creasing, curve at edges
- Requires ability to present and use the equipment at the same time

---

▶ Invest in some spare bulbs to take to the venue.

---

▶ Remember, there are different types of acetate for handwriting, inkjet, photo and laser, so be sure to purchase the correct ones.

---

Our personal opinion is that OHPs can be the easiest option because of their ease of use and their forgiving nature. Although we use PowerPoint to prepare the OHPs and are more than happy to use the data projector, we always print off OHPs as a second backup.

OHPs allow you to maintain total control of the content of your presentation. Who has not seen a presenter realise how little time they have left and suddenly skip through half a dozen PowerPoint slides to get back on track? You simply pick up a slide from lower down the pile — no-one needs to know what you have missed out (unless you put it on the handouts of course!).

## Cost considerations

Perhaps the most cost-effective method of presentation available, OHPs are cheap and easy to print, reproduce and store.

Older OHP acetates are likely to harden, curl and crack, and so may need to be replaced, but regular quality checks will ensure that you notice this before your audience does.

## Maintenance

OHPs are generally replaced quickly and easily. Whether they are old, the content needs to be changed, or you scrawled all over it last time to make a point, it takes little time to print a new acetate.

**PowerPoint**

*Benefits*

- Easy to change and update
- Very professional look if used effectively
- Allows video, sound clips and live web links
- Wide range of colours, templates and backgrounds
- Can spell-check content
- Corporate imaging (such as logos) very easy to include
- Watermarks possible
- Can use to print backup OHPs
- Can cut-and-paste and mix-and-match presentations
- Easy to file electronically
- Version numbering easy
- Mobility of presenter allowed by roving mouse devices
- Easy to maintain and keep current
- Easy to take to the venue on a computer disk

*Disadvantages*

- Projector quality can vary
- Delay between presenters in switching and opening files
- Harder to skip slides than with OHPs
- Need to have computer skills
- Some screens and magnification of projector limited
- Easy to get carried away with animation gimmicks just for the sake of it
- Different software versions may affect your presentation
- Consider version of programme and your file — but pack-and-go possible (the pack-and-go facility on PowerPoint allows you to save your presentation in a format that will work on any version of PowerPoint — useful if you don't know how old the version is at your venue)

Venues are increasingly investing in decent data projection facilities. If you can practise using PowerPoint, reduce your reliance on slide content and stand clear of the centre of the screen, where you inadvertently set up your computer, then this is the method of choice.

---

➤ If animation is included in a PowerPoint presentation, the images used will overlay each other on the handouts. Make sure that your handouts are printed before you create the animation.

---

*Cost considerations*

With most IT solutions it can become more challenging to identify what costs are associated with the final presentation. For example, many people will use PowerPoint to prepare and print the OHPs, so perhaps the set-up costs for the computer package should not be included only in this section.

Once the hardware and software are in place, PowerPoint has very low running costs.

Many presenters would benefit from training in using PowerPoint, so that they look a little less surprised when words start tumbling across the screen because their admin assistant knew a bit more than they did! Therefore, training may be a cost to consider.

The key cost with PowerPoint is the frequency of release of new versions. Although these tend to support the older versions for a couple of years, eventually the pace of change means you need to update your software to cope with the destination computer.

*Maintenance*

PowerPoint is the fastest and simplest of all. We have changed a presentation in the minutes before we were due to give a presentation because of items arising in the news or the arrival of conflicting evidence. As long as you are familiar with the version at the venue, you will benefit from the advantages of this option.

---

➤ Hiring equipment can be much more expensive than you realise. Check this out, particularly if you have not booked the venue yourself and the equipment costs are going to be your responsibility.

---

---

➤ Whatever you choose, make sure you have tried the equipment out well before you are due to make your presentation.

---

## Medium-scale presentation methods to engage your audience

### Flipcharts, whiteboards, chalkboards

All of these methods offer the same flexibility with regard to making a live record of what your audience says. Flipcharts offers an extra advantage in that you can tear off the comments and record them later.

If you are planning to use any of these approaches as part of your presentation, then it is always worth carrying your own supplies with you. Don't rely on the venue to provide suitable marker pens: you may end up with red and green to write with, and most of the people sitting two or more rows back will not be able to read a thing!

Carry a selection of dry-wipe pens (for whiteboards), flipchart markers, and white chalk for chalkboards. Check that they work well before you start to use them — just draw a quick line with each as you set the room up. We recommend that you use chisel-tip pens, as these tend to be the most forgiving option if your handwriting is less than legible.

Other options to engage your audience include the use of Post-it notes: consider giving a Post-it pad and a pen to each participant and letting them write their own answers to questions on pre-prepared flipcharts. You may find yourself surprised at how much more you find out.

*Use in presentations*

The key use of the mid-scale presentation tool is to gain participant comment and feedback. It demonstrates to your audience that you are listening to them, as you write down exactly what they say. It is tempting to improve on their comments, or to ignore comments that you don't like, but this is likely to alienate the majority of the group. This method also offers the potential to make a specific point and to interact with your participants (for example to create a graph, or to build up a picture stepwise). You may find, though, that many participants are so busy copying down what you are doing that they forget to listen to you.

## Small-scale presentation methods for the take-home message

### Handouts

Handouts are probably the most durable and hence the most important element of your presentation. It is surprising, therefore, how many presenters simply give out a copy of what was on the slides.

To work effectively, handouts should:

* remind participants of what your presentation covered
* be clear and easy to read
* facilitate note-taking

- support your presentation
- stand alone if necessary.

Consider using them as a complete resource for your presentation. Rather than putting illegible graphs, tables or references on the main screen, include these only on your handouts. You can choose the font size and the amount of space allocated to each point — you don't have to go with 'six slides to a page' for everything.

Why not include a summary of your presentation as an introduction to the handouts? This will reinforce your message, the way you intend. Take care if your visuals contain animations, as these will overlay each other and the text.

---

**In summary**

- Select the large-scale presentation method that works for you.
- Use the mid-scale presentation methods to show that you are working with your audience and building rapport.
- Design handouts that continue your presentation and carry your message away after you finish talking.

---

## Putting the presentation together

This section looks at how the presentation comes together and considers how the presenter gets their message across to the audience. This information comes from our experience as presenters and a great deal of the honest feedback we have received.

The basic rules for the good presenter are:

- Know your message.
- Know your audience.
- Meet your time parameters.

### Know your message

> 'That was a fantastic presentation. He had great slides, amusing anecdotes and finished in time for us to grab a coffee. I don't know what he was on about though . . .'

Have you ever laughed your way through a presentation and been completely convinced that it was one of the best of a conference or learning event, but had no real idea what its purpose was?

The style and approach you use in your presentation are important, and gaining rapport with the audience increases the chances of them listening to you and believing you, but it is no use if they don't know what you are trying to tell them.

As you are putting the presentation together, ask yourself what your key messages are. For most presentations, it is worth restricting yourself to one key message for each 20 minutes of talk time. It is also worth finding a way to break up your presentation into 20-minute blocks.

## Content flagging

Make use of techniques such as 'content flagging' to prepare people to listen. For example:

- Start by telling people what you are going to tell them.
- Begin each section by repeating what that section will cover.
- End each section by summarising what you have said.
- At the end of the presentation, summarise your summaries.

Being clear about your main message increases the chance that the audience will listen and remember what you told them.

## Know your audience

The key here is to remember that although you are giving the presentation, you are not the one receiving it. The presentation should meet the needs of those who are listening to it and those who are seeing it.

You must bear in mind the nature and make-up of your audience. Pitching the presentation at too basic a level may insult your audience; pitching it too high may affect what your audience thinks you are saying. Including too much personal comment or insight may result in the audience judging you as a person, rather than your presentation.

Whichever pitch you choose, the risk is that the audience will stop listening to what you say, or will read your notes in advance. Others may start to discuss a variety of issues with others in the room, and some may even go to sleep. This will disturb the focus of those who are interested in what you are presenting. Getting your pitch right will increase the proportion of those present who hear and understand your message.

> The job of the presenter is to talk. The job of the audience is to listen. The trick is to get both to finish at the same time.

## Meet your time parameters

Most events will have a published timetable for presentations, and the time allocated to you may include time for questions. Your audience will expect you to start on time and to finish on time. Even if you are late starting — for whatever reason — it is still your fault if you run over your allotted time!

The course providers will expect you to deliver their objective, which includes supporting the smooth running of the day as well as presenting your topic within a set period of time.

As discussed earlier, the use of OHP acetates allows you to leave out elements of the presentation to save time. This is less easy with the other methods, but you can reduce the amount of talking per slide, or skip through them without comment.

When preparing your presentation, plan for time shortages by asking yourself which parts you could reduce coverage of, or where you could suggest additional reading attached to points on the handouts.

## The presentation itself

*So then the presenter said 'I know that you won't be able to read this on the slide' — so why put it up there?*

We assume that the presenter wants the audience to be able to see the words or pictures on the screen clearly. Working on this basis, it is worth remembering that no matter what font size you use, your presentation will be affected by many factors at the event itself, including the magnification of the projector, where people sit, and how far the screen is from the audience.

### Background, themes, fonts and content

To make sure that your audience can read your presentation, we suggest the following as a guide:

- **Font colour** — black or dark blue
- **Background** — yellow, white or cream

- **Lines on slide** — not more than eight. Aim for five
- **Words on line** — not more than eight. Aim for five

## Graphs

With medical presentations there is often the need to show graphs, for example to indicate results or epidemiology, including the reference from which the graph was taken. There may be a need to show flowcharts to describe how a process is followed, or for a chemical structure to be displayed. Each of these makes it hard to follow the rule of thumb. There are ways around this, but all require just a little more work on the part of the presenter.

If you need to show graphs, then why not show the graph on one slide and the reference on a subsequent one — or provide handouts for this purpose. Make it clear from the title or subtitle that one slide is a continuation of the other.

Make sure that any graphs are clear from a distance. Avoid the use of pale colours such as yellow or green for line graphs — people at the back will not be able to see them. Also, make sure that titles and subtitles are relevant to the message on the slide, and be clear about the reason a slide has been used.

 Only use underlining or bold to stress key points.
Remember that UPPERCASE is SHOUTING!

## Photographs

If you are including photographs, for example for clinical conditions, be clear about their purpose, either by stating it on the slide or by discussing it in your presentation. It is important to link all the material into your presentation in some way. When including photographs (in PowerPoint, for example), remember to use the highest resolution possible, as the quality will be reduced when they are magnified.

## Pointing devices

Our personal preference is not to use car aerials, laser pointers and other such tools. As participants we are generally more fascinated by watching the presenter fiddle with them than in seeing what they are pointing at! They also show up any nerves on the part of the presenter by magnifying the tremor in their hands. They do have a place when it is necessary to point out a particular lesion, anomaly or result on the screen, but when this has been achieved, put them down and leave them alone.

## Tables

Many medical presentations make wide use of tables. Tables are great in written documents, offering a way to summarise key points or highlight issues, but if you can't read them, don't use them. As your presentation allows you total flexibility with regard to what the audience sees and when, there is often little need to use tables: presenting the individual findings can have much more impact. Depending on the message you are giving, consider presenting the table one line at a time, or just the section of the table you are covering. Provide the audience with the full reference and put a full copy of the table on the handouts.

## Diagrams

If you are including diagrams, start by showing the whole thing, then highlight and expand the area you wish to talk about. Use blow-up images. If your skills are up to it, PowerPoint will allow you to make a section of an image fly out and expand automatically.

## Cartoons

Cartoons are a great way of breaking the ice and encouraging your audience to relax. They can also help you to build rapport. Be cautious, though, as cartoons may contain discriminatory content and you will then create rather than remove barriers.

## Clip Art

Clip Art is increasingly used to provide a visual shorthand of an intended message — for example to show that a statement is worth thinking about, or to demonstrate reaching a peak. There may, however, be copyright issues associated with the use of Clip Art. Certain pictures also suffer from a degree of overuse, and participants may spend more time trying to recognise where the artwork came from than listening to the presentation.

## Flowcharts

Flowcharts are often best shown first in full, then with each step magnified on a separate slide. Use of the overall chart will allow a return to recurrent themes and permit the audience to see the temporal relationship between the separate elements.

## Presenting to people with visual impairment

There is an obligation under the Disability Discrimination Act 1995 to meet the needs of those with disabilities, and you must consider this when putting your presentation together. In general, this means you need to actively remove the barriers to access experienced by disabled people in your target audience.

As a simple test, put yourself in the position of a friend or colleague with, say, a visual impairment:

- Can you read the screen clearly and easily?
- Is the letter size big enough to read?

Also, think hard about the handouts you are giving out. If someone can't read the screen, can they read your handouts? The Royal Institute for the Blind issues guidance on making printed information more accessible for those with visual impairment ('See it Right', published by the Royal Institute for the Blind, is available from *www.rnib.org.uk/seeitright*).

# 15

## Writing a thesis

*Steven Kayne*

Because of the diversity of subjects studied there is no one format that governs the production of a thesis or dissertation. However, some cross-discipline commonality can be identified. In this chapter general guidance is offered on how to approach the production of a thesis. With assistance from a supervisor you should be able to modify the information to satisfy your own requirements.

### What is a thesis?

The term 'thesis' (from the Greek for 'position') is an intellectual pro-position. A thesis statement is the statement that begins a formal essay or argument and may take the form of a hypothesis, a question, or an account of a problem. Strictly speaking, a 'dissertation' presents the author's research and findings in support of the thesis, but in practice both terms are widely used to describe the document submitted in support of a canditure for a higher qualification.

In the UK the term is usually associated with a PhD (doctoral) or Master's degree, whereas 'dissertation' is the more common term for research projects required for other postgraduate qualifications. In the US the reverse is often true. In this chapter the term 'thesis' will be used exclusively, but may also be taken to refer to a dissertation.

There are different expectations for doctoral and Master's theses. These lie in the significance and level of the problem and the research undertaken:

- A doctoral thesis necessarily requires a substantial and innovative contribution to knowledge.
- The contribution to knowledge of a Master's thesis is more likely to be an incremental improvement in an area of knowledge, or the application of known techniques in a new area.

In undergraduate programmes, limited research activities and the resulting report are usually referred to as a 'research project', whereas 'assignment' is a synonym for homework.

## Aims and objectives of a thesis

In order to satisfy the examiners, a thesis for a higher degree must achieve the following:

- A worthwhile and previously unaddressed problem or question is clearly identified.
- A worthwhile contribution to knowledge is made by solving the problem or answering the question.
- The solution is derived from robust research accompanied by arguments presented in an organised and coherent manner.

The candidate's objectives should be:

- to demonstrate original critical thinking and an understanding of research techniques, as well as reporting experimental data.
- to locate and use statements of critical thinking and analysis in the literature as fact, and refer the reader to the primary source for further clarification rather than just repeating the details.
- to concentrate on principles and state clearly the lessons learned from the research that has been undertaken.
- to support every statement either by a reference to published scientific literature or by original work.

The completed text must be capable of withstanding the scrutiny of experts, some of whom will have been working in the area of study (but perhaps not on the exact topic of the thesis) for many years.

## Preliminary work

Before starting work on a thesis there are some important preliminary tasks to complete.

### Read the regulations

It is a good idea to get some idea of what is involved by reading a typical set of thesis regulations. When you start writing, you will need to consult the regulations carefully on several occasions to ensure that you produce a thesis that meets your institution's requirements. Many are posted on the internet. They may differ in the detail from one institution to another (or even between faculties and departments), but the basic content is similar. Glancing at one or more finished theses is also useful, provided this volume of work does not intimidate you.

### Obtain finance

Think about finance at an early stage. Make some enquiries about how your fees and living expenses are going to be funded. If you need to take on casual work to generate funds this could restrict the time that you have available to study. The university may offer you a grant, and perhaps some teaching duties.

### Choose a topic

Students rarely know exactly what they want to do when they first consider carrying out research. Often they have some vague notion, but have little in the way of a concrete plan. With any research it is necessary to collect background information on the subject so that you can choose a topic about which you are curious and which interests you: bear in mind you are going to be living with it for at least 3 years.

The area of study must be manageable and at the same time provide enough scope for meaningful research. Make some notes on key words that describe your topic and see how they interlink to give an indication of the potential breadth and depth of your work. It will also establish the wider context within which your project fits. This will be useful in choosing where you are going to study, and during negotiations with a supervisor. For example, if you were interested in diabetes there would be an obvious choice to work in type 1 or type 2 diabetes. To this topic could be added diseases associated with diabetes. Each of these could perhaps be further split into drug therapy and lifestyle management.

### Obtain a place to study

For the sake of continuity it is often best to seek a place at your current university, but if this is not possible and you are strongly committed to a particular area of research, look around for a university that matches your interest. If you have no particular preference, choose a topic in which a target university already has an interest, and where there will be colleagues to assist you when you get stuck. You are more likely to get a place to study for a PhD if you are contributing to an established research programme. Discuss your ideas with one or more prospective supervisors.

## The role of the supervisor

Your research will be overseen by one or more members of the academic staff acting as supervisors. The supervisor has many important roles in the production of a thesis, so try to establish an early rapport with him or her. He or she should:

- encourage and motivate you
- give guidance on research methodology
- advise on the structure of your thesis and the writing-up process
- tell you when you are ready to submit your thesis to the examiners
- possibly even act as one of your examiners.

The writing of a thesis should involve an efficient working partnership between student and supervisor, each respecting the other's position. If your preferred supervisor is unable to take on any new research students there is little you can do about this and you will need to seek someone else.

## Problems that can arise

It is well to be aware of problems that can arise while the thesis is being produced, so that the symptoms can be identified and rectified as quickly as possible. Any one may contribute to severe difficulties during the writing stage; collectively they spell disaster. These difficulties may include the following:

- inadequate awareness of what is to be achieved in writing a thesis
- methodological difficulties experienced during the research phase, making the thesis statement incapable of resolution
- inadequate supervision arising from a laxity in control and support from the supervisor, or an unwillingness of the student to respond positively to guidance and criticism
- poor planning, resulting in a loss of focus and a 'butterfly approach' — flitting from one task to another without concentrating in depth on any, although this may happen at the start of the project, as time goes on the planning process assumes even greater significance
- poor time management due partly or wholly to personal problems not directly associated with the research.

## Research proposal

When an informal agreement on the field of study has been reached with the supervisor and department head, candidates in PhD programmes are generally required to present a research proposal. This will be of great use in the initial stages of planning the thesis. It normally runs to a maximum of about 2500 words, with 15–20 references, and broadly follows the following format:

- **Objectives** — justification for the research, highlighting its innovative nature and the perceived importance of the contribution to current knowledge.
- **Relation to existing work** — preliminary literature review and model of the theoretical basis of the research if appropriate. An indication of how the intended topic fits into the ongoing university research programme.
- **Background of the researcher** — brief details of any previous interest, for example a student project or published paper, or other experience of the topic.
- **Methodology** — a concise justification of the particular methods being advocated, including references. If any specialised equipment is necessary then costings should be included.
- **Timescale** — an indication of the various important targets that should be met during the study programme.

Following acceptance of the proposal the research element can be organised and work on the thesis begun.

## Getting started: things to consider

### Time management

*'It seems like hundreds of years and it also seems like no time at all.'*
Jerome John Garcia (1942–1995), American musician

Three years seems a long time when you start, but they will pass quickly. It is essential that a timetable for the research and writing stages should be drawn up. Table 15.1 provides an approximate guide to the pro rata times and emphasis that might be allocated in writing a thesis. You may well be writing more than one section concurrently. Research activities will continue during most of a typical 3-year PhD, and in addition there may be lectures to attend on research techniques. A modest time allowance for holidays should be included in your timetable. Be pragmatic about the time allocated to each task — try not to be too optimistic.

Make your own series of sub-goals for the thesis — small sections of work that you are confident of achieving — rather than trying to complete whole sections at one sitting. This means that even small

**Table 15.1** Approximate guidelines for writing a thesis

| Topic | % thesis | Approx Words | Approx time to produce (months) |
|---|---|---|---|
| Initial work; producing proposal | | | 1 |
| Introduction | 5 | 5000 | 4 |
| Literature review | 30 | 30 000 | 6 |
| Methodology | 25 | 25 000 | 5 |
| Data analysis | 20 | 20 000 | 4 |
| Conclusions; further work | 20 | 20 000 | 6 |
| | 100 | 100 000 | |
| Appendices | | | |
| Final production, production graphics, binding, etc. | | | 2 |

windows of opportunity can be used effectively rather than waiting for a substantial period of free time that might not materialise.

There are numerous systems to assist with time management. Figure 15.1 illustrates one such method that may be drawn out on a sheet of paper or constructed electronically. Items in each category may be written on adhesive notes, with different colours to represent different sections of your thesis and stuck in the appropriate box. As writing proceeds the notes can be moved around within each quarter or from box to box. If you are using a computer, a new version of the plan can be printed out weekly.

A crucial phase in the research process is the transition from analysis to synthesis, that is, from the collection and analysis of literature or data to the writing of the first draft.

You should establish a list of dates on which you will hand over the first and subsequent drafts of each chapter to your supervisor. If you merely aim to have the whole thing done by some date that may be months or even years away, you can easily fall into the trap of thinking — and worrying — about the writing, rather than actually getting down to it. Targets focus your attention. Beware of adopting the typical undergraduate practice of leaving coursework until the night before it is due for submission.

A thesis is a substantial piece of work and takes a considerable time to complete — much longer than you may think. You can turn

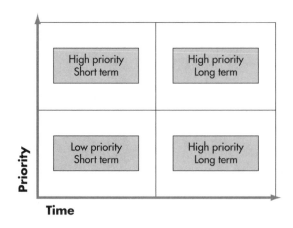

**Figure 15.1**  Example of a time management system.

your timetable into a chart with items that you can check off as you complete them. This is particularly useful towards the end of the thesis, when you will find there are quite a few loose ends. Start writing a first draft early, based on preliminary ideas that emerge during your literature search (see below).

Apart from this intellectual activity there are the production procedures to be considered. These include preparing graphics, spell-checking, formatting and binding, all of which seem to take an inordinate length of time. The university regulations will give an idea of the time involved in the submission process, and by working back it is possible to set the deadlines.

## The title

A working title for your thesis should emerge following discussions with your supervisor, but this may be revisited several times during the progress of your studies. The title should not be too long and should contain key words that indicate its content, so that when it is listed in the literature other workers may locate items of interest to them.

## Length of thesis

The length of a thesis varies greatly. In the 1950s and 1960s about 250–300 pages (70 000–100 000 words) was the norm, but now they tend to be much more comprehensive. Students carrying out research involving scientific experimentation, for example in pharmaceutical science, tend to produce rather shorter theses than those working in areas such as pharmacy practice, where it is not uncommon to see two volumes of perhaps 400 pages each at some universities.

The aim is to create a balance between quantity and quality. The actual number of pages depends on how many graphics and equations are included, and whether the regulations specify a particular format (see below).

## Style of writing

### Grammar

A thesis should be written in a formal style — more formal than this chapter — without the use of colloquialisms (e.g. 'loads of . . .'), undefined technical jargon and slang (even when certain words or phrases are widely used in spoken language). Words such as 'awesome', 'bad', 'fabulous', 'good' and 'nice' should be avoided. Hidden jokes, puns and exclamation marks are also inappropriate. In general it is better to use short simple phrases rather than long complicated sentences. 'At this point in time' uses up more words than 'now', but the number of words is not the only criterion by which theses are judged.

Ensure that all tenses and conjugations are correct. Remember that 'data' is the plural of 'datum', defined as being 'a known or assumed fact that is used as the basis for a theory, conclusion or inference'.

An important stylistic choice is between using the active voice and the passive voice. The active voice ('I measured the pH . . .' or 'Heat encouraged the reaction') is simpler, and it makes clear exactly what happened. The passive voice ('The pH was measured . . .' or 'The reaction was encouraged by heat') is more often used in books, journals and other published material and may be favoured by your supervisor. In this chapter both structures are used, but the first person has been avoided. (For more information on style, see Chapter 1.)

### Format

It is helpful to examine the use of headings, overall style, typeface and organisation in two or three completed theses on a similar topic, or from a similar institution. Use them as a guide for the preparation of your own work. Check the regulations of your institution carefully, as there are likely to be regulations governing the style and size of font that may be used and the margins required. Although both may be readily changed at a later stage, it is sensible to start using them from the beginning.

## Clarity

Good writing is essential, but it cannot compensate for a lack of ideas, or clearly explained concepts. In fact, a clear presentation may well expose weaknesses in your arguments. Each technical term and key word must be defined either by a reference to a previously published definition in the case of standard terms, or by a definition that appears before the term is used (in the case of a new term, or a standard term used in a novel way).

A page of standard abbreviations may be inserted in the preamble to your thesis (see below). Each term should be used in only one way throughout the dissertation. Readers find it confusing if an author keeps using alternative words to mean the same thing. Tables and graphics should be introduced to improve the clarity of the information, discussed in the text and clearly labelled.

## Plagiarism

Plagiarism is an attempt to pass off the ideas, research, theories or words of others as one's own. Copying an entire piece out of a book or buying a paper off the internet without citing the source is a serious academic offence and contravenes the whole spirit of originality embodied in a thesis. With the development of anti-plagiarism software (an online service is also available), it is now possible to identify the practice by detecting different word patterns. In some instances it is difficult to present long-established facts in an innovative way, but you should use your own words to précis these ideas rather than simply copy verbatim the words of others.

## Wordprocessing

A discipline for identifying different versions of your work, saving and backing up files regularly should be established at an early stage. It is a good idea to keep at least one backup at a location away from your workplace, just in case something untoward happens. Ensure that your spell-checker is set to the appropriate version of English.

Create a folder for each chapter, with separate files for text, graphics and references, for both security and convenience. It is easy to lose a sense of where you have placed material in a very long document. You can also put notes in these files, as well as text.

While writing one chapter, something relevant to another chapter may well come to mind. You can easily access the second file without disrupting the current session. You might also use a paper folder for each chapter, in which snippets of information, cuttings or papers can be filed.

If you prefer to work from hard copies of your text rather than on screen, consider using different-coloured paper to identify the versions.

It is often easier to draw up graphics or complicated tables altogether in one long session, rather than one at a time over several weeks or even months, when all the wordprocessing commands need to be re-learnt each time. In the interim, hand-drawn versions will suffice. A scan will obviate the necessity of struggling with unfamiliar graphics programs. Computer-drawn graphs do not always reach the required quality, and should be checked carefully for anomalies and errors.

## The writing process

### Producing an outline

The best way to start work on a thesis is to prepare an outline that will form the basis of an embryonic table of contents. If a research proposal was prepared (see above) it can be used to prompt your thoughts.

The outline should include each section and subsection, with a bullet point description of the contents of that section. The finished outline might run to three or four pages and should be reviewed carefully with your supervisor to determine whether:

- there is material not directly related to the thesis statement that needs to be deleted
- there are topics that need to be included or expanded.

Following this interaction you are likely to end up with notes scribbled all over the pages. It is then best to generate a revised copy of the outline to ensure that nothing is left out. This will form the basis of your table of contents (see below).

Once the outline is agreed, the most productive approach is to begin writing those parts of the thesis that interest you most and with which you are familiar. Items do not need to be written in chronological order.

➤ Generating text, even a small quantity, will give you the confidence to continue, so try and write something every time you sit down, even if it is just a set of notes.

At some point sections can be structured and any omissions identified.

**Establishing a structure**

There is no definitive model for structuring a thesis. In scientific theses it is possible to work within a generic framework. In non-scientific disciplines this is not possible: the structure varies widely and often has to be tailored to the requirements of the project.

Essentially the thesis comprises a number of standard pages, some of which are required by the regulations (often called 'the preamble'). The main body of text is split into chapters, sections and sub sections. In its *simplest* form, a thesis may comprise just three extremely long chapters:

• an introduction that includes all the supporting and explanatory material
• a chapter detailing the experimental work
• a final chapter for the conclusions.

Another model separates the various topics into a number of chapters, as shown in Figure 15.2. Within the main text the first four chapters may be grouped together as Part 1 (Introduction). Chapters 1 and 2 underpin the reasons for carrying out the research, and Chapters 3 and 4 show that a good problem or question has been chosen. Part 2 (Experimental work) comprises the next three chapters. Chapter 5 describes how the problem was solved, Chapter 6 highlights the main knowledge generated by the whole project, and Chapter 7 gives the conclusions and recommendations for extra work.

*Declaration*

Many universities require one or more declarations that the thesis represents a student's own work. The wording required will be specified in the regulations of the institution.

**Example of a declaration**

This thesis is the result of my own independent work/investigation, except where otherwise stated. Other sources are acknowledged by giving explicit references. This work has not previously been accepted in substance for any other degree and is not being concurrently submitted in candidature for another degree.

Preamble
- Declaration
- Title page
- Acknowledgements
- Table of contents
- List of abbreviations
- Abstract

Main text
- Chapter 1 Introduction
- Chapter 2 Thesis statement
- Chapter 3 Background information (optional)
- Chapter 4 Literature review
- Chapter 5 Materials and methods
- Chapter 6 Results and discussion
- Chapter 7 Conclusions
- References and bibliography
- Appendices

**Figure 15.2**  Skeleton outline for a thesis.

*Title page*

**Box 15.1**  The following is an example of a title page.

**Title of thesis**
A thesis presented by (name of student) in fulfilment of the requirements for the degree of Doctor of Philosophy of the University of [name]
**Name of Department or School**
**Month and year**

*Acknowledgments*

Most thesis authors acknowledge those who have contributed to their personal and academic development by providing guidance, support, advice, friendship, etc. Such people could include supervisors, the head of the department, family members and friends. If any of the work is collaborative, it should be made clear who contributed to which sections.

### *Table of contents*

The table of contents is usually developed from the outline described above. The introduction starts on page 1; the pages before this are usually given roman numerals. The chapter titles and up to two levels of sub-heading should be given as shown in Figure 15.3.

### *List of abbreviations/glossary of terms*

To ensure that there is no confusion about the meaning of abbreviations and key terms used in the text, an explanatory list may be given here.

### *Abstract (Summary)*

The abstract (approximately 500 words) should provide a synopsis of the thesis stating the nature and scope of the work undertaken and the contribution made to the knowledge of the subject treated. This part will be the most widely read and published, and is best written towards the end of the project. The abstract does not usually contain references, but if a reference is necessary its details may be included in the text. (For more information on abstracts, see page 65.)

### *Chapter 1 — Introduction*

This is a general overview of what the thesis is all about and serves to amplify the first few sentences of the abstract. The hypothesis, question

| | |
|---|---|
| 2. The determination of number-average micellar molecular weight by membrane osmometry | 8 |
| 2.1 Principles of osmosis | 8 |
| 2.2 Applications of membrane osmometry | 12 |
| 2.2.1 Difficulties in applying osmometry | 13 |
| 2.2.2 Procedures | 15 |
| 2.2.3 Limitations and sources of error | 20 |
| 2.3 Vapour pressure osmometry | 22 |
| 3. The determination of number-average micellar molecular weight by light scattering | 30 |

**Figure 15.3** Extract from a table of contents.

or problem statement should be summarised briefly (it will be covered in more detail in the next section), and some of the reasons given as to why it is a worthwhile project. Material from the research proposal may be used here.

## Chapter 2 — Thesis statement (hypothesis, research question or problem statement)

This section has three main parts:

1) a concise statement of the question the thesis tackles
2) justification (with direct reference to Chapter 3) that the question is previously unanswered
3) discussion of why it is worthwhile to answer this question.

## Chapter 3 — Background information

A brief section giving background information is included here if necessary, for example if your work spans more than one traditional field, and if your readers are unlikely to have the experience or sufficient background knowledge needed to follow your thesis.

## Chapter 4 — Literature review

A literature review surveys academic articles, books, dissertations and conference proceedings relevant to a particular issue, area of research, or theory. The literature review provides a description, summary and critical evaluation of each work. Full references to each piece of work that you cite must be given. Specifically, you should:

- Review published work that contributes to an understanding of the subject you are studying. The material may be divided into categories (e.g. work in support of a particular position, work that opposes it, and work that offers a different approach.
- Describe the relationship of previous work to your project, and demonstrate that your research is worth doing.
- Identify novel ways to interpret and critically assess previous research with regard to the methodological approach and the way in which the results have been interpreted.
- Identify any gaps in the current knowledge.
- Resolve conflicts among seemingly contradictory previous studies.
- Identify areas where similar work has been carried out to prevent duplication of effort and ensure the originality of your research.

This chapter should represent about one-third of your whole thesis.

**Locating material for a literature review**

Material can be obtained from university libraries, from other institutions, from the British Library (through the interlibrary loan system). You will probably have to have requests for loan materials countersigned by your supervisor.

Online searches may be carried out at journal sites (e.g. *British Medical Journal, Pharmaceutical Journal*) and databases (e.g. Medline, PubMed). Medline (*http://medline.cos.com*) is the US National Library of Medicine's bibliographic database covering the fields of medicine, nursing, dentistry, veterinary medicine, the healthcare system and the preclinical sciences. It provides access to abstracts of articles and citations from more than 4000 biomedical journals published worldwide. There are many organisations that offer access to this database, and all of these services offer different ways of searching Medline. The key Medline service is offered by the US National Library of Medicine itself, via its PubMed service (*www.ncbi.nlm.nih.gov/entrez/query.fcgi*).

ATHENS is an extremely valuable access management system for controlling secure access to web-based services in the education and health sectors. Full details on how to get started with ATHENS may be found at *www.athens.ac.uk*. The system provides users with a single sign-on to numerous web-based services throughout the UK and overseas, including journal sites that are normally subscription only. Your supervisor will be able to advise you on how to obtain the necessary user name and password.

*Chapter 5 — Methodology: materials and methods*

The factors underpinning your choice of methodology will have been fully explained in previous chapters, so here you report how you carried out the study. How much should you include?

The clue here is to decide how much information would be needed by another competent scientist, a specialist in the field, to repeat the study or experiment. Such a person will be familiar with most of the commonly used techniques. Your equipment and methodology only need to be described in detail if you have developed a new technique or extensively modified an existing one in some way. However, enough information needs to be given to convince the reader that your methodology was robust and that they can be confident in your results. Characterisation of any materials involved is important, and the source and any applicable standards or analytical details should be given. (For more information on scientific methods see page 68.)

## Chapter 6 — Results and discussion

In this part of the thesis you should record your results and show how they were relevant to answering the question or solving the problem you set for yourself. This means treating the results in an appropriate way and discussing them fully. Any limitations of your work should be mentioned, but do stay positive: only mention research problems that you experienced if they were part of the process to find a solution. You might mention trying out several methods involving subtle changes in methodology before finding one that worked, but you would not mention a series of experiments that had to be repeated because the suppliers had sent you the wrong materials.

## Chapter 7 — Conclusions

This part of the dissertation is sometimes best written after stepping away from your research for a short period, so that you can put it into perspective. The following sections are usually included in this chapter:

1) conclusions
2) summary of contribution
3) recommendations for further work.

All three sections should be concise statements and are often presented as a series of short numbered paragraphs, ordered from most to least important.

1) **Conclusions** — these should be the inferences you have drawn from your work.
2) **Summary of contributions** — here you list the contributions of new knowledge that your thesis makes. (There may be some overlap with the conclusions.)
3) **Recommendations for future work** — this section is included so that researchers reading your thesis in the future have the benefit of the ideas that you generated while you were carrying out the research. Ensure you make suggestions that emanate directly from your experiences over the time that you were carrying out your research. Do not merely repeat items that you were considering when you wrote your initial proposal. Although this will probably be the last section that you write, you should not rush it, for if it is lacking in content the

examiners may think you have not sufficiently considered the wider context within which your work fits, and focus on this area in the oral examination.

### References and bibliography

You should note the difference between a list of references and a bibliography. References should be cited throughout the text and collected together at the end of your thesis (or possibly at the end of each chapter).

### Appendices

Any material that is likely to impede the smooth development of your argument, because it is too detailed, should be included in one or more appendices. Examples include program listings, lengthy mathematical proofs and derivations, questionnaires, and accompanying documentation.

## Managing references

The management of references can be a challenge. Always check the regulations before you start on your literature review, because universities have their own variants of the two most widely used systems, Harvard and Vancouver. A complete guide to using these systems can be found in Chapter 3.

A decision on the referencing system should be made right at the start of work on the literature review, because trying to change later on will just involve extra time.

> Make sure you record the complete reference at the time of first access — finding it again may not be as easy as you might think.

Making sure you have a complete list of references is vital because it adds to the credibility of your work and allows others to follow up on your review. For web references be careful to cite only academic sites, and quote the date of access. If there is a protracted length of time between your first access and submission of the thesis, the addresses will need to be checked to ensure they are still live. If you are intending to use an abstract from Medline direct or through PubMed then you should state this after the reference. For example:

Smith JP (2006) Use of DMARDs in the treatment of rheumatoid arthritis. *NZ Medical Journal*; 43: 14–16 (PubMed).

▶ Examiners generally scan your list of references to ensure that you have found the most important works in the field and cited them accurately.

They are also likely to look for their own publications if they are working in the area you have chosen — it would be appropriate to cite these too. Reading your examiners' papers will give some indication of the questions they might ask at your oral examination (also known as a *'viva voce'* or simply a *'viva'*).

### Harvard (author/date) style

This system uses the author's name and date of publication in the body of the text. The list of references is arranged alphabetically by author at the end of the chapter or thesis. See page 55 for a guide to using the Harvard style of referencing.

### Vancouver (author/number) style

The Vancouver system differs from Harvard by using a numbered series to indicate references. They are listed at the end of the chapter or thesis in numerical order as they appear in the text. The main advantage of the Vancouver style is that the text reads more easily, and the numbers may be considered less obtrusive. See page 52 for a guide to using the Vancouver style of referencing.

Vancouver style is so named as it is based on the work of a group, first meeting in Vancouver in 1978, which became the International Committee of Medical Journal Editors (ICMJE). The style was developed by the US National Library of Medicine (NLM) and adopted by the ICMJE as part of their 'uniform requirements for manuscripts submitted to biomedical journals'. The NLM has an ICMJE page (*www.nlm.nih.gov/bsd/uniform_requirements.html*) that gives sample references for 41 different circumstances, and should be considered as the authoritative style.

Students sometimes find difficulty in managing the Vancouver system, especially when extra references are added to the text necessitating the renumbering of successive citations. All major wordprocessors have a scheme for inserting references and allow text to be copied and pasted easily while still maintaining the link. This may be useful, depending on the referencing system chosen.

## Final checks

In this frustrating but nonetheless important stage of writing your thesis you need to make the final checks before moving to completion. You need to ensure the following.

---

**Pre-binding checklist**

- ✓ Check that all the chapter and section headings are worded exactly as they appear in the table of contents.
- ✓ Check that the formatting has not changed and that the pages are numbered in the right order.
- ✓ Check that you have the right binding margins (check these with the binder).
- ✓ Check that all the graphics and tables are correct, in the right place, correctly labelled and introduced in the text.
- ✓ Check that references in the text have been correctly inserted.
- ✓ Check that the list of references is complete.
- ✓ Check that there are no obvious spelling mistakes or typographical errors — run a spell-check and re-read thoroughly.

---

### Binding your thesis

When all the checking is completed and your supervisor has given the green light, it is time for the final stage. There are usually several companies who will bind your thesis; the university might also offer a service and provides useful guidance online (e.g. *http://www.ncl.ac.uk/bindery/thesfaq.html*).

You only need to deposit one carefully checked printed copy of your manuscript with the binder. For a modest extra charge they will provide as many photocopies as you need. If you give the binders a disk or email your thesis, ensure that it is in a format that will not be corrupted during the printing process (e.g. PDF), particularly if a change of computing platform is involved.

The binders normally have copies of the regulations for each university and are aware of the very precise requirements for binding and titling. They will advise you on the inclusion of photographs or large fold-out items. Typically, universities require you to submit three copies of your dissertation. Most students get a further two or three copies for their own use.

There are two types of binding: soft and hard. The former may be sewn and glued with card covers, or comb bound; the latter will have stiff board covers and a card-covered spine (Figures 15.4–15.7). Some universities allow the initial submission for examination purposes to be soft bound; following the examination and incorporation of any amendments to the text, the final hard-bound copies may be submitted for depositing in the departmental and university libraries. Other universities require the initial submission to be hard bound.

You must bear the cost of binding yourself. At the time of writing this varied from around £30 per hard copy for a 4–5-day turnaround to around £45 for a 24-hour service. If you choose to have your thesis bound at a busy time of the year you might have to wait a little longer. Spine lettering and the first two lines of title text on the front cover are usually included in the price, but an extra charge will be added for each additional line on the front cover. Soft binding costs about £6 per copy for a 1-week turnaround.

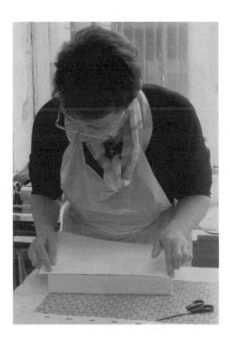

**Figure 15.4**  Hard covers for the final copy.

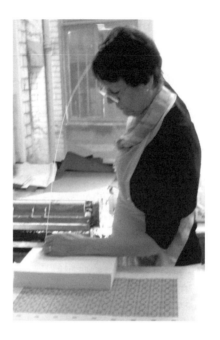

**Figure 15.5** Sewing the sections together.

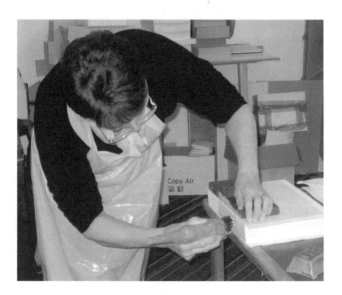

**Figure 15.6** Glueing the spine.

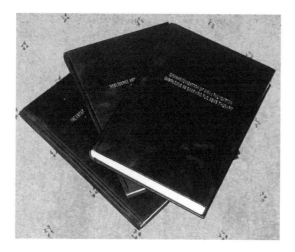

**Figure 15.7**    The final hard-bound copies.

## Submission — and beyond

Following a PhD submission you will be given a date for an oral examination, prior to which the examiners will have inspected your thesis. They
may point out some statements with which they do not agree, or some
small errors that need to be corrected. These matters need to be rectified
before your degree is awarded. If you submitted soft-bound copies you
can now reprint a final copy of the manuscript and have it hard bound.
If you submitted a hard-bound copy you will have to change the text
neatly with a pen or insert a page of errata. After successful completion
of the thesis it is time to enjoy the fruits of your labour – graduation and
the future opportunities associated with a higher degree.

## Further reading

MHRA (2004) *MHRA Style Guide. A Handbook for Authors, Editors and Writers
of Theses.* London: Modern Humanities Research Association.
Murray R (2002) *How to Write a Thesis.* Maidenhead, UK: Open University Press.
Turabian K (1996) *A Manual for Writers of Term Papers, Theses and Dissertations,*
6th edn. Chicago, IL: University of Chicago Press.

## Acknowledgement

The author wishes to thank A. Cameron Bookbinders, 73 Robertson
Street, Glasgow G2 8QD, for facilitating Figures 15.4 to 15.7.

# Section Five

Medical writing for
medical professionals

# 16

# Writing medicines information for healthcare professionals

*Angela Bussey*

Poor presentation of medicines information can result in loss of professional credibility and may lead to the recipient ignoring the advice or information given. More seriously, it could result in clinical error and patient harm. This chapter is to help you present reliable, relevant and robust information about medicines in a format suitable for health professionals. It cannot provide you with all of the tools or skills required to search and evaluate information, but it will provide you with guidance to help you improve your current practice. It will also help you consider how you can develop and use your core skills and knowledge to provide written medicines information, such as letters and bulletins to health professionals, in your particular field of practice.

If you are not a pharmacist, I recommend that you always involve a pharmacist in the development of any written information about medicines, both to draw on their expertise and to ensure clinical accuracy.

Some skills and competences used to provide information to patients and the public, such as gathering and interpreting data, are similar to those used to provide information to health professionals. However, the language and style used to present data to these groups are quite different (see Chapters 1 and 2).

## Practical issues of medicines information provision

To present medicines information effectively you will need:

- planning, prioritisation and time management
- to know your audience and your limits
- use of resources and search strategies
- accurate, up-to-date information from reputable evidence-based sources
- suitable skills and knowledge.

## Planning, prioritisation and time management

As the roles of healthcare professionals change or are created and services are redesigned, you will need to adapt in order to offer services that support these new roles and to manage increased public expectations. You may identify a knowledge gap in an individual or group; you may have recognised how you can add value to an existing service; or there may be new partners you want or need to work with locally and nationally. The fundamental principles of planning, prioritisation and time management apply to the provision of medicines information.

Consider the resources you will need (such as people, reference sources, information technology) and how you will search for and use the information gathered. Planning must also consider funding as well as staff recruitment and retention.

To deliver quality information you also need:

- suitable training and competencies
- standard search strategies
- checklists
- templates.

You will also need to plan how you will present the information and have a realistic timescale based on clinical urgency and current workload.

## Knowing your audience and your limits

In order to present information usefully you must know what your audience wants and needs, as well as their working practices. You may need to interpret statistical data and present it in a way that your audience will understand.

All pharmacists can become involved in providing information about medicines to health professionals or across the various healthcare sectors. With the changing role of pharmacists, the increasing use of electronic communication such as email or online publishing, and the ongoing rapid advances in therapeutics and medicine, it is useful to have the skill to present medicines information in a variety of formats.

There is also a need to be aware of the requirements of strategic organisations, other health professionals, patients and the public in order to develop services according to their needs.

United Kingdom Medicines Information (UKMI) pharmacists provide medicines information services for the National Health Service (NHS) in the UK. UKMI has a strategy and framework to oversee the development of UKMI services.[1]

Part of the skill of providing medicines information is being aware of your own limitations. This includes being able to recognise when a request for information is beyond your expertise, or that you do not have the requisite resources to find the information (see Table 16.1).

**Table 16.1** Examples demonstrating innovative provision of medicines information[2-5]

| Type of service | Types of written medicines information highlighted or with potential |
| --- | --- |
| A pharmacist-led information and advice service based in a voluntary sector drugs service[2] | Patient information<br>Review of forensic report on analysis of ecstasy tablets<br>Fact sheet on OTC medicines and false-positive results for urine screens |
| Assisting Aboriginal patients with medication management[3] | Local formulary development<br>Patient information<br>Medicines information training packages for health workers<br>Development of communication strategies about medicines, between pharmacists and community health workers |
| Supporting general practitioners to solve medicine-related problems[4] | Enquiry answering to support clinical problem solving for GPs. This could include supporting verbal answers in writing. It could also include the use of newsletters and bulletins |
| Setting up a medicines information service in Uganda[5] | Enquiry answering to support clinical problems for hospital staff and external health providers. This could include supporting verbal answers in writing. It could also include the use of newsletters and bulletins |

## Resources

Any information you produce should be accurate, up to date, from a reputable evidence-based source and referenced.

Information resources are classified as primary, secondary and tertiary. In practice, this classification will not affect your day-to-day searching, apart from the fact that, in answering an enquiry, you will often start with tertiary sources.

Many resources are now available via the internet, although you may need to purchase subscriptions to certain journals or to register for access to them.

Primary resources:

- contain original research (for example the *British Medical Journal*)
- are new original information, clinical trials, systematic reviews (for example the Cochrane database)
- require you to read and evaluate their contents.

Secondary resources:

- essentially abstract the primary sources (for example Medline, Pharmline)
- help you scan a large volume of original material
- locate primary sources that are relevant to your work.

Tertiary sources:

- are useful starting resources
- evaluate many resources to give a summary of the literature (for example the *British National Formulary* (BNF), Martindale)
- interpreting tertiary sources can introduce author bias and important detail may be missed in summarising research
- can become out of date quite quickly.

## Use of resources and search strategies

To ensure that you do not miss any important information sources, it is essential that you develop an organised and systematic search strategy.

You should have a clear strategy about how and when to use all of your resources. In this you need to include when to seek support or refer to medicines information services or other specialists.

A common enquiry strategy is to start by using a tertiary source (reference books such as the *British National Formulary* (BNF) or Martindale) to get a good overview of the subject and fill any gaps in your knowledge. This will help to put things into a historical and therapeutic perspective and may be all you require.

Search strategies change depending on your experience and knowledge of the various information sources, and you may adapt your strategy over time to suit the way you work. Any search is dependent on the complexity of the enquiry as well as the needs of the enquirer or audience.

### Suitable skills and knowledge

You need at least basic computer skills in order to retrieve, store and present information, including using the internet and databases. If you enhance your PC skills you will save much time and effort as well as improving your presentation of information. Knowledge also includes having access to the right resources, so your IT systems must be able to support your needs. The UKMI website provides information on minimum resource requirements.

## The role of different formats of medicines information

**Different types of medicines information:**

- enquiry answering
- frequently asked questions (FAQs)
- development of local services and decision-making
- news
- newsletters
- critical appraisals and drug reviews.

### Enquiry answering

How you respond to medicines information enquiries depends on several things, including the needs of the enquirer and the complexity and urgency of the enquiry.

If you receive an enquiry in writing, the enquirer will often expect a written reply. On other occasions you may wish to send a written answer to avoid misinterpretation, or because a large amount of information needs to be provided. Your reply should not only serve as an *aide mémoire* for the answer, but also give an evaluation of the information itself, to enable decision-making. If you give your own opinion on the information you should make it clear that you are doing so and provide further information to support it.

### Frequently asked questions (FAQs)

Some enquiries will arise more frequently than others. To save time and effort, it is useful to develop a list of frequently asked questions and answers. This will save time, avoid duplication of work and maintain the quality and consistency of the answers given. You could keep these on a database or share them with your service users via a website.

### Development of local services and decision-making

The provision of medicines information can be useful in many environments. Identify and work with key health providers and individuals to explore the needs of your health community, whether local or strategic, and consider the benefit of providing medicines information.

### News

Health professionals are bombarded with new information every day, and it can be difficult to keep up with developments — practitioners usually sift out the most useful information for their particular specialty.

The National electronic Library for Medicines (NeLM) produces medicines news summaries every day and covers ground-breaking clinical trials, new guidelines, regulatory and government information.

To help identify your role in the healthcare team you could consult with your colleagues and circulate selected news items relevant to their practice either regularly or periodically.

### Newsletter

A newsletter can pull together useful information, tailored to the needs of your audience. Table 16.2 illustrates types of newsletter and potential target audiences, using asthma as an example.

Figure 16.1 is an example of a health promotion newsletter, produced by a regional medicines information centre for health professionals involved in public health campaigns. This can be accessed electronically and would have URL links to the references to signpost the reader to the relevant resources.

## Spring Health Newsletter

Pollen Forecast for the UK *http://www.bbc.co.uk/weather/pollen/index.shtml*

| | |
|---|---|
| Effects of Treatments for Symptoms of Hay Fever Clinical Evidence: Jan 2003.<br><br>***Evidence-based evaluations of the effectiveness of oral and intranasal antihistamines, oral decongestants and various miscellaneous drugs, e.g. montelukast.*** | National Prescribing Centre Hay Fever Review MeReC Bulletin. Treatment of seasonal allergic rhinitis (hay fever) 1998; 9: 9–12.<br><br>Examines the choice of treatments available to patients and their effectiveness.<br><br>See also *Common Questions About Hay Fever* MeReC Bulletin March 2004. |
| Oral Antihistamines for Allergic Disorders<br><br>**Drug & Therapeutics Bulletin 2002; 40 (8): 59–62.**<br><br>First generation antihistamines may be suitable in patients where sedation not likely to be problematic. Chlorpheniramine is a reasonable choice in pregnancy. Second generation antihistamines are agents of choice for most patients. Cetirizine and fexofenadine considered preferable compared to terfenadine and mizolastine as latter can cause cardiac adverse effects. Acrivastine requires frequent dosing. Experience with levocetirizine and desloratidine is still limited. | Butterbur vs. Cetirizine for Treating Hay Fever<br><br>**Randomised controlled trials of butterbur and cetirizine for treating seasonal allergic rhinitis. Br Med J 2002; 324: 144–153.**<br><br>❏ ***After two weeks, the effects of butterbur and cetirizine were comparable in patients with hay fever.***<br>❏ ***Butterbur produced fewer sedating effects than cetirizine.***<br>❏ ***Butterbur could be considered when the sedating effects of antihistamines must be avoided.***<br><br>*Safety Concerns about Butterbur* News. Pharmaceutical Journal 2003; 268: 123–30.<br><br>Crude butterbur herb can be toxic, especially to the liver. |
| *Information for Patients* **BBC Health guide to hay fever and other allergic conditions.** | Management of Rhinitis: e-Guidelines [ENT section; registration required] The British Society for Allergy and Clinical Immunology, 2000. |
| RPSGB Practice Checklist **Pharmaceutical Journal Practice Checklist for OTC Treatment of Hay Fever. Produced in the Pharmaceutical Journal November 1997 (updated January 2001).**<br><br>Points to consider when selecting products for hay fever. | Management of Hay Fever **Management of Hay Fever in the Pharmacy. Pharmaceutical Journal 2003; 270: 443–445.**<br><br>General article about the causes, symptoms and management of hay fever in the pharmacy. |

**Figure 16.1** Example of a periodic and seasonal health promotion bulletin.[6]

**Table 16.2**  Types of newsletter and potential target audiences, using asthma as an example

| Newsletter content | Audience examples |
|---|---|
| Critical appraisal of a clinical trial of new asthma drug | Decision-makers such as pharmaceutical advisors, formulary management pharmacists, prescribers with a specialist interest in asthma/chronic lung disease |
| Abstracts of recent asthma articles | Prescribers with a specialist interest in asthma/chronic lung disease, including GPs, respiratory care nurses, clinical pharmacists for respiratory medicine |
| Medicines news, for example, details of the above article plus latest BTS guidelines, plus latest on a complementary therapy | Community pharmacists, GPs, respiratory care nurses, independent and supplementary prescribers |
| Health promotion campaign information, for example, stopping smoking | Community pharmacists/local surgeries/respiratory care nurses |

## Critical appraisals and drug reviews

Critical appraisals and drug reviews can be produced to anticipate the information needs of a particular audience and to support decision-making. They may be useful in providing valid evidence of clinical benefit and cost-effectiveness to purchasers of healthcare and to support prescribing practice.

Statistical analysis forms part of a critical appraisal and you need at least an understanding of basic statistical concepts before you can do this. Misinterpretation of data could lead to inappropriate patient care or harm. For further information about writing reviews see Chapter 5.

## Why, what and how to document enquiries

### Importance of documentation

The documentation, storage and retrieval of enquiries are important to ensure that the safeguards and standards necessary for effective clinical governance are met.

The components of clinical governance, such as risk management, audit and performance management, help to ensure continuous improvement to deliver high standards of care. For this reason, clinical governance is as important in the provision of medicines information as it is in any other area of health service provision.

## Risk management and quality assurance

Risk management in medicines information includes:

* having a clear definition of the scope of your service
* having robust procedures
* ensuring that the information provided is accurate, up to date and of high quality
* ensuring that working practices are safe and comply with legal and ethical requirements
* maintaining adequate and appropriate resources
* involving personnel who are appropriately qualified and trained.

You will find more about writing instructions and procedures in Chapter 17, and how to answer an enquiry in writing is dealt with later in this chapter.

As part of the clinical governance framework, quality assurance initiatives should be in place.[7] These include setting, reviewing and monitoring standards, audit, and user-satisfaction surveys. UK Medicines Information (UKMI) has a long history of quality assurance initiatives, including setting standards, peer review and external audit. Guidance documents on clinical governance and risk management have also been produced.[8]

Documentation of enquiries supports safe working practices and compliance with legal and ethical requirements. The enquirer may need to be reminded of the answer given; it saves work if the same question is asked again; is useful in case of complaint and in education and training; and is necessary for collating workload statistics. A record of enquiries also allows quality assurance measures such as audit to be introduced.

Error reporting and documentation are both vital to maintain and improve upon practice standards. Reporting adverse events/near misses while maintaining anonymity and a culture of 'fair blame' is a fundamental organisational requirement.[9]

The Clinical Governance Working Group of UKMI has developed an Incident Reporting in Medicines Information Scheme (IRMIS)[10] whereby data about incidents in UKMI practice are collected in a central database to determine trends and share learning. Although reporting of incidents must still be carried out to feed into local schemes, a separate MI database helps to reduce the likelihood of similar incidents occurring in other MI services, and informs training programmes, risk management strategies and national standards accordingly. Learning from IRMIS is shared with national agencies such as the National Patient Safety Agency (NPSA).

Recording enquiries also gives some training examples for new staff. Completed enquiries can be used to show 'how it is done', and recording illustrates the range of enquiries that are asked. You can also use completed enquiries as articles in bulletins or at training events. You can use them for your own continuing professional development too, as evidence of reflective learning and competencies.

### Repeat enquiries

Enquirers sometimes mislay original answers, or they may come back to you with new details concerning a completed enquiry and ask for new information. If someone else presents a similar enquiry at a later date, looking back at a previous enquiry can give you a head start.

If an enquirer complains that you gave an incorrect or misleading answer, or were slow to respond, you have documentation to show how you acted. This is also important in the event of any litigation.

### Workload statistics

Documenting enquiries enables you to provide workload statistics to demonstrate the value of your service and to support funding applications. Some commissioning bodies may make it a requirement of funding that such data be available.

### What should be documented?

In order to have a full audit trail of the enquiry and to be able to provide an answer of acceptable standard, you should record:

1) enquirer details
2) the urgency of the enquiry
3) the enquiry itself
4) all relevant background information
5) resources used and details

6)    the answer, or a summary of the answer
7)    time taken to answer the enquiry.

Figure 16.2 is an example of a medicines information enquiry form used by a regional medicines information centre.

**Document an enquiry if:**

it requires professional judgement
it demands an appreciable amount of time
it involves use of your specialist resources, especially if these are not available elsewhere
it could be the subject of a complaint.

Documenting enquiries takes time and effort, so you need to decide on limits for what you should and should not document. You could choose *not* to record the following because they do not need clinical input:

• requests for drug company/rep contact
• enquiries referred to another source without any input
• completion of questionnaires or surveys
• enquiries about stock held in the dispensary.

However, this will vary according to local needs and what you want to achieve with your service.

**Hints and tips when documenting an enquiry**

| Always record | Note |
| --- | --- |
| Full name of enquirer | Even if you know who they are — consider the need to refer back in future |
| Contact details of enquirer | Do not assume that you will not need to contact them. A full postal address is needed for all enquiries to enable follow-up if required, e.g. for survey purposes |
| Agree a mutually realistic timescale | Consider the clinical urgency and your current workload |
| State clearly why the enquiry is needed by a specific day/time | Someone else may take over the enquiry; also a useful workload statistic |

| | |
|---|---|
| Get a clear explanation of the question | Ensure that it is clear from the enquiry form that you have fully understood the question. Ensures quality assurance |
| All relevant background information, e.g. age of patient | It saves time and supports clinical accuracy. Ensures quality assurance |
| Names of people you speak to, e.g. in company medical information departments | Ensures quality assurance. Useful if you have to contact them again |
| Names of all resources used | Have you checked all the key texts required for that level of enquiry? Have you worked through the sources in a systematic fashion? Ensures quality assurance |
| Editions/dates of books, and name/ full address of websites used | Ensures quality assurance |
| Summary of Product Characteristics (SPC): specify the date accessed and date of revision of the text (e.g. Section 10 of SPC in electronic Medicines Compendium)[11] | Ensures quality assurance |
| Search terms used and dates searched | Ensures quality assurance |
| Summary of answer | Ensures quality assurance |

## Ways to document

Despite efforts to work towards the 'paperless office', many of us still either use paper systems or support electronic systems with paper documentation. It is useful to have knowledge of both.

A basic system assigns each enquiry a number according to the date, with an ongoing hard copy list of enquiries. Filing is by both numerical and date order. Alternatively, electronic databases are useful for quick retrieval of information as well as allowing several users to share information. You can also improve retrieval systems that use a database by assigning medicine or clinical categories.

There are standards and recommended periods for the storage and retrieval of information that should be adhered to and which may vary according to the organisation or country where you work. The UKMI standard for storage of medicines information enquiries is in

| LONDON & SOUTH EAST MEDICINES INFORMATION SERVICE | PAGE |
|---|---|
| ENQUIRY TITLE | Enquiry Number<br><br>Keywords |

| CALLER NAME | CALLER STATUS | DATE | DEADLINE |
|---|---|---|---|
| | | TIME | |

| CONTACT DETAILS | PATIENT NAME<br>AGE<br>WEIGHT<br>SEX<br>LOCATION |
|---|---|

| QUESTION: Pregnancy | Trimester | Renal Status | Hepatic Status |
|---|---|---|---|
| CHECK:    Cardiac Status | U And E's | Paediatric | Other Drugs |

QUESTION AND BACKGROUND

| Taken By | Answered By | Checked By | Enquirer Informed By | Date<br><br>Time |
|---|---|---|---|---|
| QA Check | Database Entry Date | Reason For Any Delay | Others Who Have Been Informed | Answered time YES/NO |

| STATUS ENQUIRER | ORIGIN | CATEGORY OF ENQUIRY | SOURCES USED |
|---|---|---|---|

| STATUS ENQUIRER | ORIGIN | CATEGORY OF ENQUIRY | SOURCES USED | |
|---|---|---|---|---|
| 01 Consultant | 01 Base Hospital | 01 Admin/dose | 01 Pharmline | 12 Press Index |
| 02 Reg | 02 Private Hosp | 02 Adverse effects | 02 Micromedex | 13 Specialist MIC |
| 03 SHO/HO | 03 Region/Trust | 03 Availability/supply | 03 IOWA | 14 PubMed |
| 04 GP | 04 Region HA/community | 04 Therapy choice | 04 TicTac | 15 Medline |
| 05 Hosp Pharm/Pre reg | 05 Outside region | 05 Pregnancy | 05 CSM | 16 Embase |
| 06 Pharm Tech | 06 BFG | 06 Breast feeding | 06 Cochrane | 17 Online other |
| 07 Comm Pharm | 07 PASA | 07 Identification | 07 ADIS R+D | 18 Internet |
| 08 Hosp nurse | 08 MOD | 08 Interaction | 08 UKMI new product evaluation | 19 Library |
| 09 Comm nurse | | 09 Pharmaceutical | 09 Industry | 20 MI resources |
| 10 Practice nurse/health visitor/midwife | Time taken | 10 P'cology P'kinetics | 10 RPSGB | (not 1–19 |
| 11 Dentist | Min | 11 Poisoning/toxicity | 11 Expert Opinion | 21 Other (specify) |
| 12 Dietician | (minimum 10) | 12 Press Index | | |
| 13 Patient | | 13 General Info | | |
| 14 Public | Directorate /MIC/HA | 14 Costing | | |
| 15 HA/Pharm Adviser | | 15 Find a reference | | |
| 16 PCT Pharm | Urgency of answer | | | |
| 17 Practice Pharm | 01 Immediate | | | |
| 18 Comm Services Pharm | 02 Same day | | | |
| 19 Student | < 1 week | | | |
| 20 Other (specify) | > 1 week | | | |

| ROUTE OF ENQUIRY | | ROUTE OF ANSWER |
|---|---|---|
| 01 | Phone | 01 |
| 02 | Person | 02 |
| 03 | Letter | 03 |
| 04 | Email | 04 |
| 05 | Fax | 05 |

| SOURCE USED | ANSWER |
|---|---|

SUMMARY

| PENDING – REASON | DATE | | INITIALS |
|---|---|---|---|
| 1 | SEARCH NOT COMPLETE | | |
| 2 | ENQUIRER NOT CONTACTABLE | | |
| 3 | WAITING FOR OUTSIDE INFO | | |
| 4 | WAITING FOR INFO FROM ENQUIRER | | |

**Figure 16.2** Example of an enquiry form from an NHS Regional Medicines Information Service.

line with current National Health Service Regulations.[12] This may be subject to change, however, so you should check for the latest updated information.

## Effective ways to communicate responses to enquiries

### Delivery of an impartial, evaluated, accurate and timely response

When dealing with a medicines information enquiry, your response must be impartial, evaluated, accurate and timely. In order to deliver this, you need to understand what the question is, who the enquirer is, and what their needs and expectations are. To begin gathering this information, you need to know:

- if it is a general enquiry, or about a specific patient
- the name of the enquirer
- the job or role of the enquirer and their specific interest in this enquiry
- the enquirer's contact details
- any deadlines for providing an answer.

This will provide you with the basic information, the enquirer's level of understanding of the subject, and will help you manage their expectations at an early stage. For example, they may want an answer the same day, but this may not be possible if the enquiry is more complex than they realise, or you do not have the resources to answer the enquiry within that timeframe.

Misunderstandings can occur because of poor communication, assumptions about what either party already knows, and if a question is misinterpreted. Misunderstandings can also occur if you do not provide sufficient information or background to support your answer.

If you do not gather enough information at the point of enquiry, you may not fully understand what the enquirer needs. For example, if you are asked for information on the side effects of a drug and provide a list, have you really answered the question? The question might actually relate to a particular symptom in a particular patient. Gathering all of the facts avoids these misunderstandings, and it is sometimes necessary to contact an enquirer for more information as you research your answer.

When you receive a written enquiry you still need to obtain this information, whether in writing or by phone.

## Supporting telephone answers by letter or email

As outlined in the introduction, the two main reasons for writing well are clarity and professionalism. It can therefore be useful to support any answer you provide over the telephone or in person with a written response. This allows you to provide a fully referenced, evidence-based response. On other occasions you may need to send a written answer by post or by email to avoid misinterpretation, or because a large amount of information needs to be provided.

Email is a useful tool as you can often provide electronic links to relevant references to support your answer. If full articles are required that cannot be accessed by the enquirer, you may have to photocopy the relevant information and provide a covering letter, bearing in mind any copyrights.

## How to write a response to an enquiry

If the enquiry is in writing, the enquirer will often expect a written reply. Whether by letter or email or telephone, acknowledge receipt immediately, provide the enquirer with an estimated timeframe for your reply, and agree a deadline.

## Writing a response to an enquiry

Whether the written correspondence is an email or a letter, you should:

- use a template
- provide your contact details
- write the enquirer's name, address and date at the top
- have a subject heading so that the recipient can see instantly what it is about
- answer the question!
- use an appropriately professional tone
- if there are limits on your answer, say what they are
- tailor the answer to the enquirer's needs
- answer within the enquirer's deadline
- anticipate further questions
- provide references.

## Presentation and content

A letter or email should also contain:

- a summary of the question(s) at the beginning
- arguments and facts presented in a logical order

- concise information. Avoid over-burdening the enquirer with details. Stick to the point
- headings and bullets to break your text down into readable chunks (this may not be necessary if the answer is very short)
- a summary of your answer in the final paragraph (again, this may not be necessary if the answer is very short)
- 'Yours sincerely' or 'Yours faithfully', as grammatically appropriate (you may wish to use a more familiar term, such as 'kind regards' or similar if you know the person well enough)
- your job title after your name
- your contact details
- any organisational logos and details as required.

Always check:

- that your answer is clear
- readability (see Chapter X for more information):
- select appropriate font style and size.
- use of correct grammar, punctuation and spelling
- sentences are not too long (aim for 15–20 words)
- overall presentation.

### Referral of inappropriate enquiries

When enquiries are inappropriate for you to answer, always acknowledge the request and then explain why you cannot (or will not) answer it, e.g. a third-party enquiry that breaches patient confidentiality. Refer the enquirer to a more appropriate resource if possible, e.g. a poisoning or overdose enquiry to a poisons information service.

---

**In summary — responding to an enquiry**

- provide an impartial, evaluated, accurate and timely response
- make sure you understand the enquiry
- make sure you understand the enquirer
- avoid misunderstandings
- presentation of written correspondence should reflect the professional standard of your answer
- refer inappropriate enquiries elsewhere.

# Producing a medicines information newsletter

## Content

There are no hard and fast rules about the content of a medicines information newsletter.

Points to consider are:

- the aims of the newsletter, for example advanced notice, to influence prescribing, or for signposting
- the audience: the group of health professionals you are targeting, their level of knowledge and interest, the locality
- the frequency and length: get a balance between the needs of the audience and your ability to stay in regular production.

Examples of newsletter content:

- abstracts of medicines news, e.g. ground-breaking clinical trials
- critical appraisals and reviews
- frequently asked questions
- important health service announcements relating to medicines
- new published guidelines
- new products
- product licence changes.

## Using abstracts

Abstracts provide a brief but comprehensive summary that is useful to include in a newsletter or news item. It should give the reader an overview without their having to read the full article.

*Hitting the Headlines* is a product of the National electronic Library for Health which discusses a topic that has hit the headlines in the UK media. It uses an abstract at the beginning of an article to describe a recent health story, then goes on to evaluate what the evidence is behind the headlines and provides further references and supporting information. It is a very good example of how an abstract provides the reader with an instant snapshot of the work and illustrates how evaluated information can be summarised effectively.

## Frequently asked questions

The purpose of a list of frequently asked questions (FAQs) is twofold: it may answer a common question or provide an answer to a difficult one.

Having standard answers saves time, avoids duplication of work, and can maintain the quality and consistency of answers given.

### Tips for writing a FAQ

- Present your arguments and facts in a logical order.
- Be concise.
- Provide qualifiers for the answer and references.
- Explain any limitations to your answer.
- If there is no answer, say so and explain why.
- Provide a review and expiry date.

---

**In summary — producing a medicines information newsletter**

- There are no rules about what to put in a newsletter.
- Use abstracts to present snippets of news.
- Frequently asked questions are useful both for enquiry-answering purposes and to deliver to an audience with a specific interest.
- Critical appraisals add value (see Chapter 5 on writing a review).

---

## Presenting a case for local formulary choice

Medicines information skills allow you to use your expertise to provide evaluated information for local decision-makers and commissioners, to support the development of local services and decision-making.

As well as evaluating clinical effectiveness, formulary management involves economic evaluation. As well as comparative costs, it could include any comparative cost implications for the local health economy.

You can also use a newsletter format to publicise changes or developments in formulary choice or policies and publications.

## Legal and ethical considerations

**Legal and ethical considerations**

- Dealing with any ethical dilemma requires an element of professional judgement, discretion and experience.
- Have a clear policy for dealing with enquiries relating to legal proceedings.
- Ensure you are working within your professional codes of ethics and the law.
- Be aware of how current legislation affects your practice.

## Enquiry answering and ethical dilemmas

It is not possible to plan for, or advise on, every conceivable ethical dilemma that you may encounter when answering medicines information enquiries. No guidance, however comprehensive, will cover every possible situation. Each problem encountered will be different and will require an element of professional judgement, discretion and experience.

### Dealing with ethical dilemmas

- You do not *have* to answer *every* question that you are asked.
- Always give yourself time to think before replying.
- It may be useful to consult with colleagues and/or managers before answering.
- There is no 'right' answer to most ethical dilemmas, but you should be able to justify what you do.
- Do not answer queries that are beyond your sphere of expertise or available resources.
- Research your answers thoroughly, and document carefully everything that you do.

## Enquiry answering for legal proceedings

Enquiries with legal overtones are like other enquiries in that they require an accurate and timely answer after careful research and evaluation. It is always important to document everything that you do, but for legally oriented enquiries it is more likely that you will have to justify what you do. You will not be able to do this if you have not kept careful records.

You should have a clear policy, ratified by your organisation, on how to deal with enquiries that have overt legal overtones. Make this policy clear at the time of the initial request. If the enquiry does not meet the criteria for acceptance, it is helpful to be able to direct the enquirer to an alternative resource.

### Enquiry answering relating to legal proceedings

- In preparing a written answer to an enquiry, structure your answer as outlined in 'Letter writing examples' (see page 293).
- Avoid going beyond your personal sphere of expertise, and specify any limitations to your resources.
- Keep a record of what resources were used.
- Differentiate clearly between your opinion and the facts, and support everything you say with references.

- If it is not possible to provide an answer to certain questions, you should say so, and why.
- Document everything.

### Third-party enquiries

Although this chapter does not cover writing information for the public and patients, in the context of ethical dilemmas it is necessary to provide a brief comment on third-party enquiries.

A third-party enquiry is where someone asks a question about medication being taken by another person. In the case of a health professional asking about a patient, they are working within their professional capacity in the best interests of their patient. However, if a member of the public or a non-health professional is asking, you should consider whether providing an answer could breach patient confidentiality and how appropriate it would be (see also page 385 for patient consent issues and the law).[13]

Having established the enquirer's identity and their reasons for asking the question, you may decide that it is reasonable to give them an answer. You must ensure that you work within your professional code of ethics when doing so, and thus take responsibility for any issues that may arise. You must document your answer and the reasons for providing it.

### Legislation

Under data protection legislation, individuals have a right to inspect records about them, provided suitable notice is given. The Data Protection Act 1998[14] regulates the processing of personal data. Both computerised and manual records are regulated by this Act, which gives every living person, or his or her authorised representative, the right to apply for access to their health records to obtain copies. This applies equally to the private health sector and to health professionals' private practice records. The Access to Health Records Act 1990 still governs access to the health records of deceased people.[15]

The Freedom of Information (FOI) Act[16] came into effect in the UK in January 2005. This gives people a general right of access to recorded information held by public bodies. Scottish bodies are covered by the Freedom of Information (Scotland) Act 2002[17] (see also Chapter 19). Management systems for medicines information services should therefore not only meet operational needs but also comply with these legal requirements.

---

**In summary**

Written medicines information for health professionals must reflect the standard of the content, which should be:

- reliable
- relevant
- robust
- retrievable
- referenced
- up to date.

Know your audience.
Know your limits.
Above all, grasp the opportunity to learn and develop your medicines information skills and competencies!

---

## Letter writing examples

The following are example letters and intended as a guide only.[18] The response is not a definitive answer to this or similar enquiries.

> You receive a letter from a GP who has a patient who has been convicted of drink-driving. The patient has blamed her medication (reboxetine and sodium valproate) for raising her blood alcohol levels above the legal limit. The patient has read that some drugs interact with alcohol. The GP asks if the patient's medication could affect alcohol metabolism, and whether it has been reported to increase blood alcohol levels.
>
> Have a look at the following reply and consider what you think needs to be changed:

*Southshire University Hospitals NHS Trust*
*Medicines Information Centre*
*Southshire General Hospital*
*Southplace SO97 3ZT*
*Tel (026) 7879 9106 Direct*
*Fax (026) 7813 1421*

*29th November 2002*

*Dear Dr Smethurst*

*Thankyou for your enquiry. A large number of medicines interact with alcohol to cause drowsiness.*

*Alcohol is metabolised via alcohol dehydrogenase, cytochrome p450 and catalase, and prescribed medicines are not known to potentiate or inhibit the activity of alcohol dehydrogenase or catalase. However, many prescribed medicines are metabolised with the cytochrome p450 enzyme system and some of them can potentiate or inhibit the enzymes' activity, but interaction between medicines and alcohol via cytochrome p450 is unlikley. However, sodium valproate is not known to affect alcohol levels in the blood: in fact, it induces cytochrome p450. However, the route of metabolism for reboxetine is not known and, unlike a lot of centrally acting drugs, it does not appear to potentiate the affects of alcohol, and this has even emboldenned the manufacturer to state in it's SPC that 'Reboxetine does not appear to potentiate the effect of alcohol on cognitive functions in healthy volunteers'.*

*Yours faithfully*
*Ann Brown*

## Notes on Letter 1

*The content*

- This letter does not answer the actual question very well.
- The letter introduces themes and ideas but does not expand upon them in a way that will be meaningful to the enquirer.
- There is some jargon. Specialist words such as 'induces' and 'SPC' may not mean much to the reader: at the very least they might not understand the implications.
- Given the importance of the enquiry, the answer is not detailed enough and there are no references.
- At the end of the letter there is no offer to provide further support if required.
- Relevant facts are produced but not put into context. See below.

Examples of themes introduced but not explained are:

1. *'A large number of medicines interact with alcohol to cause drowsiness.'*
Is this relevant? If not, why refer to it?

2.   *'Alcohol is metabolised via alcohol dehydrogenase, cytochrome p450 and catalase.'*

A crucial part of the answer is the relative importance of these three enzymes in metabolising alcohol.

3.   *'... interaction between medicines and alcohol via cytochrome p450 is unlikely.'*

Why is this? It seems fairly important, but is glossed over.

## The presentation

- The text of the letter is concentrated at the top of the page and so the presentation is not very eye-catching.
- Major, different themes are all lumped together into one big paragraph. It is best to split these to provide some clarity, as well as for presentation.
- Most of the sentences are too long.
- There is no punctuation other than full stops, so the letter does not read well.

There are some poor uses of English:

- 'effect' instead of 'affect'
- 'it's' instead of 'its'
- 'metabolised with' instead of 'metabolised by'
- needless repetition of certain words, e.g. 'however' and 'potentiate'.

There are spelling errors:

- 'emboldenned' ('emboldened' is also an inappropriate word: there is no need to use elaborate language.)
- 'thankyou'
- 'unlikley'.

## Basic letter writing requirements

- The address of Dr Smethurst is missing from the beginning of the letter.
- There should be a summary of the enquirer's request and a summary of the writer's conclusions.
- There is no header to the letter identifying the patient, the subject of the letter, or the enquirer's original reference number. The enquirer needs to be able to identify immediately which patient is concerned.
- Letters to a named individual should conclude with 'Yours sincerely'. The alternative, 'Yours faithfully', is reserved for letters to unnamed individuals, i.e. letters that might begin with 'Dear Sir/Madam' or 'Dear Colleague', for example.

- The writer of the letter is not identified by her job title. You can add your qualifications, but that is a matter for personal preference.

The revised version of the letter is written in a traditional style, starting with an Introduction, followed by Method, Research and Discussion (IMRAD). Some people prefer an inverted pyramid style, starting with the main conclusion and getting progressively more detailed, i.e. conclusion, supporting information, and then background and technical details. The key point here is that whichever method you choose, you must answer the question and present your answer in a clear, logical and professional manner.

**Revised letter**
*Southshire University Hospitals NHS Trust*
*Medicines Information Centre*
*Southshire General Hospital*
*Southplace SO97 3ZT*
*Tel (026) 7879 9106 Direct*
*Fax (026) 7813 1421*

*29 November 2002*

*Dr S. Smethurst*
*The Fairweather Practice*
*Southampton SO16 2BG*

*Dear Dr Smethurst,*
**Elizabeth Edwards DoB 18/12/1965 26, Belvue Rd SO17 5DR**
*Thank you for your enquiry concerning this patient, who claims that her raised blood alcohol levels, taken by the police as part of a possible conviction, were caused by her medication.*

*A large number of medicines interact with alcohol — something that the patient may have picked up from patient information leaflets. However, this interaction is usually due to the medicine and alcohol having similar effects — namely depression of the central nervous system leading to drowsiness and so forth.*

*The main route for the metabolism of alcohol is via the enzyme alcohol dehydrogenase. A small part is metabolised via two other enzymes — the cytochrome p450 system and catalase. I could find no evidence from a search of the medical literature that prescribed medicines affect the activity of alcohol dehydrogenase or catalase.*

*Many prescribed medicines are metabolised via the cytochrome p450 enzyme system, and some of them can affect the way that the enzymes work, so that they become more or less effective. However, a clinically significant interaction between medicines and alcohol via cytochrome p450 is unlikely because the dehydrogenase enzyme destroys the majority of alcohol first, and alcohol has such a short half-life.*

*Sodium valproate is not known to adversely affect alcohol levels in the blood. In fact, it makes certain elements of cytochrome p450 more active, so even if there was a metabolic interaction, the valproate might tend to lower alcohol levels.*

*The route of metabolism for reboxetine is not known. Unlike many centrally active drugs it does not appear to potentiate the effects of alcohol, as the attached paper suggests.[1] This has led the manufacturer to state in its Summary of Product Characteristics (SPC or 'data sheet') that: 'Reboxetine does not appear to potentiate the effect of alcohol on cognitive functions in healthy volunteers'.[2]*

*In summary, I could find no evidence that either drug would increase blood alcohol levels.*

*I hope that this information is helpful. Please contact me again if you require any further information.*

*Yours sincerely,*
*Ann Brown MRPharmS*
*Southshire Medicines Information Centre*

[1] *Kerr JS et al. The effects of reboxetine and amitriptyline, with and without alcohol on cognitive function and psychomotor performance. Br J Clin Pharmacol 1996 Aug; 42(2): 239–41.*
[2] *Reboxetine SPC. Accessed via eMC http://emc.vhn.net/ 29th November 2001.*

## Useful resources

### UK Medicines Information Services
You can find details of your nearest UK Regional Medicines Information Service in the *British National Formulary*. They will be able to give details of a local centre near you. Non-NHS organisations or individuals are welcome to use the service, but may incur a charge.

### National electronic Library for Health (NeLH)
*www.nelh.nhs.uk*
The aim of NeLH is to provide clinicians with access to the best current expertise and knowledge to support healthcare-related decisions. 'Hitting the Headlines' can be found on the homepage of NeLH.

### National electronic Library for Medicines (NeLM)
*www.nelm.nhs.uk*
The (NeLM) is a comprehensive medicines knowledge base within the National electronic Library for Health and acts as a conduit for the dissemination of both national and local medicines information.

### UKMI website
*www.ukmi.nhs.uk*
This website contains information on courses and resources in medicines information, such as a training workbook and competencies. Website resources include a list of minimum resources required for a medicines information service and details of UK medicines information centres, including specialist advisory services in selected areas of therapeutics such as pregnancy and breastfeeding.

### UK Medicines Information Training Workbook
A basic-level self-directed learning package, *UK Medicines Information Training Workbook* is available to buy. Apply in writing to Wessex Drug and Medicines Information Centre, Mailpoint 31, Southampton General Hospital, Southampton SO16 6YD, UK.

### MiCAL
A computer-assisted learning package for pharmacists in medicines information. This complements the *UKMI Training Workbook* and introduces pharmacists to MI services, concentrating on enquiry answering. It comprises a series of training modules based on a paper-based medicines information system used in the UK. Contact *coacs@coacs.com* for more details.

### MiDatabank
A Windows software application that enables medicines information pharmacists to record, manage and store their enquiries. The UK Medicines Information Network has adopted this as its national storage and retrieval system. It allows medicines information staff throughout the UK to share answers to queries via a central website. Contact *coacs@coacs.com* for more details.

## Further reading

American Society of Health-System Pharmacists (1996) ASHP guidelines on the provision of medication information by pharmacists. *Am J Health-Syst Pharm* 53: 1843–5.

Department of Health (2004) *Better Information, Better Choices, Better Health: Putting Information at the Centre of Health.* London: The Stationery Office.

Department of Health (2004) *Standards for Better Health.* London: The Stationery Office.

Department of Health (2006) *Medicines Matters: A Guide to the Mechanisms for the Prescribing, Supply and Administration of Medicines.* London: The Stationery Office.

National Patient Safety Agency (2004) *Seven Steps to Patient Safety — the Full Reference Guide.* London: Department of Health.

## References

1. UK Medicines Information (2000) *Better Information for Managing Medicines, a Strategy for Pharmacy's Medicines Information Service in the NHS.* [cited October 2005] Available at URL: *http://www.ukmi.nhs.uk/Policy_product/strat.asp*

2. Scott J, Bond CM, Winfield AJ and Kennedy EJ (2005) A pharmacist-led information and advice service based within a voluntary sector drugs service. *Int J Pharm Pract* 13: 1–7.

3. Larkin C, Murray R (2005) Assisting Aboriginal patients with medication management. *Aust Prescriber* 28: 123–125.

4. Alexander K, Banfield S, Gent L and El-Beik S (2003) How do general practitioners solve medicine-related problems? *Int J Pharm Pract* R35.

5. Ward S (2005) Pharmacy practice overseas: bringing medicines information to Uganda. *Pharm J* 274: 369.

6. Joshi M (2004) *Thinking Ahead.* Southampton: Wessex Drug and Medicines Information Centre.

7. Royal Pharmaceutical Society of Great Britain (2006) *Medicines Ethics and Practice — A Guide for Pharmacists and Pharmacy Technicians,* 30th edn. Oxford, UK: Royal Pharmaceutical Society of Great Britain.

8. National Standards for Medicines Information Services. United Kingdom Medicines Information Clinical Governance Working Group. [cited October 2005] Available at URL: *http://www.ukmi.nhs.uk/Policy_product/CGServ Stand.asp*

9. Reason J (2000) Human error: models and management. *BMJ* 320: 768–70.

10. Anon (2005) Medicines information error and near miss database set up. [News]. *Hospital Pharmacy* 12: 48.

11. Electronic Medicines Compendium. Datapharm Ltd. [cited October 2005] Available at URL: *http://emc.medicines.org.uk/*

12. Department of Health (1999) *For the Record: Managing Records in NHS Trusts and Health Authorities.* London: HSC 1999/053.

13. Royal Pharmaceutical Society of Great Britain (2005) *Confidentiality, the Data Protection Act 1998 and the Disclosure of Information.* [Fact Sheet].

14. Information Commissioner's Office. Data Protection Act 1998. [cited October 2005] Available at URL: *http://www.informationcommissioner.gov.uk/eventual. aspx?id=34*

15. Information Commissioner's Office. Access to Health Records Act 1990. [cited October 2005] Available at URL: *http://www.informationcommissioner.gov.uk/eventual.aspx?id=34*

16. Information Commissioner's Office Freedom of Information Act 2000. [cited October 2005] Available at URL: *http://www.informationcommissioner.gov.uk/eventual.aspx?id=33*

17. Scottish Information Commissioner's Office. Freedom of Information Act Scotland. [cited October 2005] Available at URL: *http://www.itspublicknowledge.info/yourrights/index.htm*

18. Emerson A, Wills S (2005) *United Kingdom Medicines Information Training Workbook*, 3rd edn. Ashford, UK: Open Learning Ltd.

# **17**

## Writing and implementing procedures

*Paula Hayes*

> *'Grandma, this is the most divine chocolate cake I've ever tasted' said Grace. 'Please tell me how I can make one just like it'.*
>
> *Grandma handed Grace her recipe book containing a tidy list of instructions written in clear, neat handwriting — it also had photographs of what the finished cake should look like.*
>
> *'In this book you will find all you need to know about how to bake one just like it', she said. 'I've tested out the instructions with many people over the years. Just follow the words and the pictures . . .'*

In their simplest terms, procedures are instructions that enable others to successfully complete a task. Just like a recipe to bake a cake, they aim to:

* deliver the normal method of approaching a task
* tell us how to perform an activity
* give a clear picture of how to get to the end point.

This chapter covers why you need to know about procedures and provides an understanding of the best ways to develop and write them. It will also show you how they can be applied to your current role.

### What is a standard operating procedure (SOP)?

In the workplace there is usually a standard way to undertake most tasks. New staff members are usually trained to follow the same procedures as all the other staff to enable the task to be completed consistently. SOPs save you repeatedly explaining how to do each particular task and provide a written reference for staff to follow.

SOPs can range from simple ones such as describing the process of booting up the dispensary computer in a community pharmacy, to more complex ones such as for the preparation of a batch of paracetamol tablets in a pharmaceutical industry laboratory. SOPs may be developed for setting up and using equipment, or for everyday activities such as hand-washing procedures in a clinical environment.

**SOPs describe in detail in writing:**

- what should be done
- when it should be done
- where the activity should be undertaken or what device used
- who should do the task
- who could do the task.

## Procedures and policies: the same or different?

It is important to understand some of the basic working definitions and applications of procedures in order to maintain consistency when writing these documents.

In my experience, the word 'procedure' usually appears interchangeably with the word 'policy'. However, there is the following difference:

- **Policy** — this is the objective or goal an organisation is working towards. It gives general guidance on acceptable ways of working to achieve that objective or goal.
- **Procedure** — this a detailed, step-by-step method through which a policy can be implemented and actioned.

The following terms are also often used to describe procedures:

- standard operating procedure (SOP)
- department operating procedure (DOP)
- quality operating procedure (QOP).

Individual professions tend to use unique terms when referring to procedures. The list above was compiled from personal observation, and in practice the terms are interchangeable. 'Standard operating procedures' (SOPs) is the term most commonly used and accepted in the professional healthcare setting.

Policies and procedures form the framework for the daily operation of any organisation. Without them, day-to-day running would be hectic and staff would become confused and frustrated.

## Why do we need SOPs?

Clinical governance requires that all healthcare professionals have plans, policies or schemes to manage risk and minimise harm to patients. As a healthcare professional you should ensure that you work within these guidelines. Managers or those responsible for other staff should ensure that all staff work within the same guidelines.

▶ Clinical governance is about improving quality and standards. It's also about achieving things in the correct way, with the right people, at the right time and in the right place.

SOPs are one way to ensure that you maintain safe working practices whereby risk and harm to patients are minimised. Written SOPs provide evidence that you work within the requirements of clinical governance.

On 1 January 2005, the Royal Pharmaceutical Society of Great Britain introduced a requirement for pharmacies to establish and operate written SOPs covering the dispensing process. The dispensing process is defined as all the activities that take place from when the prescription is handed in at the pharmacy, to when the medicines are given to the patient. This requirement applies to all pharmacies dispensing medicines to patients, whether privately or in the NHS. It also applies to pharmacies in prisons and in the armed forces.

Similarly, following the publication of the Farwell Report *Aseptic Dispensing for NHS Patients* in 1995,[1] many unlicensed aseptic facilities in NHS hospitals were required to implement SOPs for activities ranging from staff training to the use of approved cleaning products. These SOPs now provide a routine way of working in aseptic units and are used as the basis for quality control audits.

Hospital laboratories will have SOPs for the use of machinery such as autoclaves, centrifuges and electron microscopes. The procedures ensure that the machinery is used correctly at all times and the safety of the staff using them is assured.

**SOPs are important because they:**

- document the best way to perform a task
- can manage risk and reduce harm to patients
- provide evidence of compliance with clinical governance requirements.

The benefits that SOPs bring to a healthcare organisation are outlined below.

**Benefits of SOPS**

- An efficient, safe and controlled service provision
- Good practice at all times
- Allow for effective skills mix through appropriate delegation of duties
- Valuable training tool
- Provide advice and guidance for locum and part-time staff
- Permit confident delegation while allowing the pharmacist to maintain professional control
- Avoid confusion over who does what, i.e. role clarification
- Contribute to the audit process
- Maintain high standards at all times
- Useful in identifying further training needs
- Can be first line of defence in any litigation process
- If things go wrong or errors are made they provide a way of finding out if there is a problem with your system or a problem at some other level of practice
- Allow sharing of best practice

## Limitations of SOPs

It is important to consider some of the limitations of SOPs. I consider these to be few and that they can be overcome if the correct approach is taken when writing and implementing.

Many of us do not have the time to develop and write procedures: good SOPs demand dedicated time and cannot be constructed in a few minutes. However, one way around this is to delegate the task to one of your support staff. In my experience, pharmacy technicians are suitably trained to produce SOPs to a very high standard, given initial guidance and support by someone with practical experience in developing them.

SOPs cannot always deal with unusual circumstances, which may be seen as a limitation. My view is that SOPs are intended to allow all staff to deal with everyday circumstances, which leaves the manager free to become involved in resolving more unusual problems.

SOPs are only effective if everybody buys into them: you may have worked in organisations where the SOP folder gathers dust on the shelf and everybody has their own variation on the way things are done. This can be avoided by involving all staff from the beginning — encourage them to contribute, and seek their opinions. This way, ownership of the

SOPs is given to the staff, which increases the chance of their being implemented.

Some healthcare professionals assume that SOPs restrict their professional judgement. Personally, I prefer to have guidance on which to base my professional judgement. If you experience particular problems with SOPs, then it is your responsibility to discuss this with the writer/developer and propose alternatives (see below).

**Limitations of SOPs**

- Time-consuming to develop and write
- Do not deal with unusual circumstances
- Require buy-in from the whole staff team
- Limit professional judgement

## Before writing SOPs

### Plan your time

It is important to plan and prepare for writing SOPs in the same way as for any new project or development. Start by planning your time and be realistic about timescales. It may take a full day, or even more, to develop and write an accurate and useful SOP.

### Prioritise which SOPs to write

Do not write SOPs just for the sake of it. Always consider the current legal and professional practice issues when prioritising your work. For example, since 1 January 2005 it has been mandatory for all pharmacies to have SOPs for the dispensing process, so most pharmacies should already have these in place. Since then, pharmacies have also been required to develop SOPs for the delivery of essential repeat dispensing services.

Consider developments or changes in your service where SOPs will facilitate successful implementation and sustainability. If you are working in the pharmaceutical industry or in a hospital laboratory and you are about to receive a new piece of equipment, then it may be a priority for you and your staff to have a comprehensive SOP for its use.

### Get 'buy-in' from your team

Consider getting a team of people to work with you. These are most likely to be the people who already carry out the task(s) you are writing the SOPs for, or those who use or will use the equipment in question. In this way you will get input from those directly involved and begin to get buy-in and ownership from the team. This can only lead to improved success during the implementation and continuation stages of the SOP.

You may want to think about delegating the full process of developing and writing certain SOPs to certain members of staff, particularly if they undertake the task more often than you do. For example, if you are the manager in a hospital pharmacy where the technicians prepare a lot of extemporaneous products, you could delegate the task to one of those familiar with the practical processes and use of the equipment. You could then check and sign off the document before it is used in practice.

### Consider your goals and timescales

Determine the required outcomes for the procedure and be clear about why an SOP is needed. Consider the target audience and how they will use the SOP in practice. Set a deadline for completion of the SOP, and plan the time needed to finish the task.

### Do your research

Research the legal and ethical requirements for the area you are considering, using up-to-date sources. Discuss with your team any controversial or challenging issues you encounter.

When considering the content to include, 'brainstorming' may facilitate the process. Whichever method you use, ensure that all of the key stages of the process have been thoroughly considered. Involving your team at this stage will ensure that all aspects are addressed in a way that makes the SOP most useful to them.

### What to include in a SOP

There are five key elements that any SOP must include:

- objectives or purpose
- scope
- process

- responsibility
- audit or review.

This is easy to remember as **OSPRA.**

### Objective or purpose

This is a statement that describes what you set out to achieve, including the standards to be met.

---

➤ Make sure that the objectives reflect your priorities and that they adhere to any necessary protocols.

---

### Scope

This gives details of the precise area of work that the procedure applies to; it may also specify what the procedure does not apply to. It sets clear parameters, avoids misunderstandings, and makes it easier to write the process stages.

---

➤ Limit the scope so that the procedure does not become over-complex, but ensure that it addresses the activities crucial to the success of your organisation.

---

### Responsibilities

This states who is responsible for carrying out each stage of the process. It can include who takes responsibility under normal operating conditions, and what should happen in different circumstances. This section should include a clear indication of the level of qualification required to carry out each stage or activity.

---

➤ Avoid confusion over who will be responsible for each task. Be sure to note that suitably trained staff should be used where necessary.

---

### Process stages

This section should be an accurate step-by-step description of how the task will be carried out in order to achieve the stated objective. To ensure that this section becomes a useful learning tool, make the steps clear, unambiguous, and jargon free.

---

➤ When writing this section, ask yourself and others:

- Is this the best way to do the task?
- Will doing it this way ensure that the objectives are achieved and standards met?

---

## Audit or review

This section should enable a comprehensive check to be carried out once the SOP is in place, to determine whether the stated objectives are being achieved and to identify problems. It should enable any necessary changes or improvements to the SOP to be identified.

---

➤ Encourage the involvement of all staff to measure the success of the SOP after it has been established. This will help to maintain standards and identify ways to improve work practices.

---

## Additional and variable elements

The five key elements discussed above may be considered the essential ingredients. Creating an SOP is like baking a cake. The essential ingredients are necessary for the basic cake, but in some cases we want chocolate frosting, cream in the middle, or decorations on the top. With SOPs the additional components will make the procedure even more comprehensive. Additional instructions covering circumstances that have variable outcomes may be added. Other things to consider include:

- date of writing and/or date of approval
- date for review
- approving committee (for example, in NHS organisations such as hospitals and primary care trusts this may be the Drug and Therapeutics Committee)
- version number
- circulation list
- references.

Figure 17.1 is an example of a blank template that may provide a useful framework within which to develop and structure your SOPs.

| Pharmacy Name |
| --- |
| Standard Operating Procedure for |
| Purpose |
| Scope |
| Process |
| Responsibility |
| Audit Process |
| Additional Information |

Written by: _____

Signature: _____

Name of authorising personnel: _____

Signature: _____    Version number: [        ]    Review date: [          ]

**Figure 17.1**  Blank SOP template.

## How to write SOPs

### Keep it simple

We began this chapter by explaining that SOPs are a set of instructions. The key to writing an effective instruction is to keep it simple in format, structure and language. Forget fancy vocabulary — throw out all those long complex sentences and don't try to impress your audience with your use of language. Keep it simple in order to make it useful. You want to deliver easily and quickly understood information so that the reader can complete the task successfully.

### Narrative versus step by step

The most straightforward way to write procedures is as a series of simple steps rather than as a narrative. Consider the examples below: they both give the same instructions for taking in prescriptions at a pharmacy dispensary, but which is easier to read?

**Example 1. Narrative procedure**

Confirm that patient's details are recorded, including name, address and date of birth. Any illegible or incomplete details should be clarified where necessary. Ensure that the reverse of the prescription has been completed correctly and that the declaration has been signed. If the repeat side is still attached then hand it back to the patient. Collect the correct number of charges or check the evidence if the patient is claiming exemption from charges (refer to SOP No 7 Prescription Exemptions) . . .

**Example 2. Step-by-step procedure**

- Confirm that patient's details are recorded, including name, address and date of birth. Clarify any illegible or incomplete details where necessary.
- Ensure that the reverse of the prescription has been completed correctly and that the declaration has been signed.
- If the repeat side is still attached, then hand it back to the patient.
- Collect the correct number of charges or check the evidence if claiming exemption from charges (refer to SOP No 7 Prescription Exemptions) . . .

## Making your SOP user friendly

*Format*

Wherever possible, try to keep to a standard format for all your SOPs: consider using the template in Figure 17.1 and adapting it to meet your needs. A standard format will lead to a clear structure. However, a standard format must work for all those who will use it, so get agreement on the structure and format from all your team before you start to write.

*Bullets and numbering*

To further enhance clarity, consider numbering each step or use bullet points.

*Subheadings*

Use headings to break down the information into easy-to-handle chunks and to signpost the SOP to other SOPs, reference sources or additional information.

*Colour*

Think about using colour and different fonts to highlight differences or to emphasise important points. Remember that this is not to make the SOP more impressive, but rather to make it simpler to follow, read or understand.

*Space*

Include plenty of blank space on the page. This helps the reader find their way around the information more quickly and easily. Too much white space will make your SOP appear disorganised, however.

*Lists*

Consider using lists to reduce the number of words and keep the sentences shorter. This will make the SOP easier to follow.

*Diagrams and pictures*

These can help to clarify information. Illustrations can reduce the amount of explanatory text you need and make your instructions more explicit. For example, rather than describing the areas of the hands to concentrate on for a hand-washing procedure in a clinical environment, use pictures of hands and arrows pointing to the specific areas.

Flowcharts are a graphical alternative to written procedures. They are particularly useful for procedures that involve many decisions, such as diagnostic procedures. Flowcharts may also be helpful to depict decision-based elements in an SOP (see Figure 17.2).

*Language*

Keep the language simple and understandable. Aim to avoid jargon and abbreviations, particularly those with several meanings, as this will cause misunderstanding and frustration to the reader. To make your SOP accessible to all, assume that the level of knowledge and understanding of your audience is minimal. Be sure to always explain any jargon or abbreviations at first mention.

*Accuracy*

Ensure that the content of your SOP is precise, accurate and up to date. If necessary, cross-refer to other SOPs to avoid duplication and confusion. The only assumption you can make when writing SOPs is that the audience knows nothing about your process.

**Checklist**

☑  Use a standard format/template
☑  Use numbered or bullet-point steps
☑  Use simple, everyday language that the user is familiar with
☑  Use headings to separate the information into chunks
☑  Use colours and different fonts to highlight differences and emphasise points
☑  Use lists to reduce wordy explanations
☑  Use diagrams to provide clarity
☑  Use flowcharts for decision-related SOPs
☑  Avoid jargon
☑  Avoid abbreviations
☑  Be precise
☑  Make reference to other SOPs where necessary

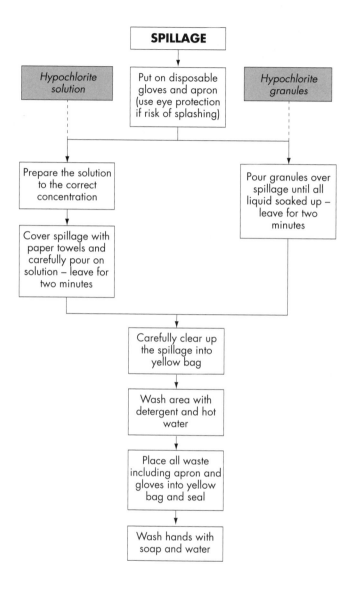

**Figure 17.2**  Example of a flowchart for a procedure.

## Making SOPs work in practice

You now have all the basic information and the beginnings of a toolkit for writing effective SOPs. However, these will be useless if they are not implemented by your staff on a day-to-day basis. You must now consider how you can facilitate the process to ensure that your staff buy in to the concept of SOPs and implement them as part of their normal routine.

## Team 'buy-in'

Getting buy-in from the team is a very important part of implementing your SOP — without it, the procedure will not be carried out effectively. You must take the time to explain:

- why the SOP is necessary
- what the procedure is
- how it is to be carried out.

Getting your team to contribute to the development of the SOP in the early stages will be key in ensuring that they understand how to implement it once it is written. 'Walking through' and testing the procedures while they are in draft stage is another good way to engage staff in the process.

## Ensure SOPs are readily accessible

Once SOPs are written, they must be easily accessible to those who need to use them. Ensure that all staff know where to find the SOPs when they need them. SOPs can be a very effective training tool for new staff, and can be invaluable when locums work in a community pharmacy for the first time.

It is a good idea to keep all your SOPs together in one file that has a clear and easy-to-understand contents page. The file and its contents need to be kept in good condition by replacing any torn or faded documents, and it should be easily identifiable from the cover. The file must be kept in a location where it is easily accessible, for instance on the shelf in the dispensary with all the reference texts, or in the bookcase by the nurses' station on the ward. In larger NHS trust departments it may be necessary to have duplicate copies of the file in different locations — it is important that all copies are checked and updated with any changes or amendments.

## Ensure SOPs have been read and understood

You should make sure that all your staff have read and understood the relevant SOPs. You may like to consider using a list that people sign to confirm that they have done so. In addition, to test their understanding you could develop a quiz for staff that relates to the content of the SOPs. This is another very useful training tool for new staff.

## Non-compliance with SOPs

Some healthcare professionals choose to ignore or work outside the guidance of SOPs for various reasons. The issue of non-compliance can be put into the two broad categories of appropriate or inappropriate.

### Appropriate non-compliance

This usually occurs in exceptional circumstances where there is a requirement for the person to make a professional judgement to work outside the SOP. For example, in the event of a power failure in a dispensary the pharmacist may choose to work outside the *Assembling and Labelling of Medicines* SOP that requires a computer-generated label to be put on each dispensed medicine. They may therefore choose to produce a label on a typewriter, because in their professional opinion it is more important for the patient to receive their drug in a timely manner than to wait for the computer to function before issuing the drug.

### Inappropriate non-compliance

This usually means that the person simply ignores the SOP. Such situations are likely to result in increased risks and possible harm to patients, for example where an SOP for *Prescription Accuracy Checking* stating that all prescriptions should have a second check, is not followed.

The best way to handle such situations is to discuss the issue either with the person involved or with their line manager.

It is good practice to report and record all incidences of non-compliance with SOPs, as these will be useful when reviewing and updating them.

## The importance of good communication

One final consideration for successful SOPs is good communication between the developer/writer and the user at all times. You must establish who you need to communicate with, what you must communicate, and how you will communicate it. Effective communication will provide your staff with answers to the following questions:

- **What** are SOPS; what do they do; what do they mean?
- **Why** should we use them; why are you doing it now?
- **How** will they work; how will they affect us?
- **What if** we don't have them; what if we don't use them?

➤ 'To effectively communicate, we must realise that we are all different in the way we perceive the world and use this understanding as a guide to communication with others.' (Anthony Robbins)

Be creative in the way that you communicate with your team about SOPs. Communication methods could be:

- one-to-one conversations
- formal meetings
- interactive presentation event for the team
- a regular SOPs newsletter
- posters to remind staff about the procedure.

Using more than one approach will have added impact and help to reinforce the importance of SOPs to your staff.

---

**In summary**

- A standard operating procedure (SOP) specifies in writing what should be done, when, where, and by whom.
- SOPs are evidence of working within the requirements of clinical governance.
- There are many benefits and very few limitations to using SOPs in healthcare.
- Before you start, plan your time, prioritise which SOPs, get team buy-in and do your research.
- Remember OSPRA.
- Use step-by-step lists rather than narrative.
- Make your SOPs user friendly.
- Consider all the issues that will facilitate successful implementation.
- Communicate with your team.

---

## Reference

1.  Farwell J (1995) *Aseptic Dispensing for NHS Patients* [Farwell report]. London: Department of Health.

# 18

# Writing marketing authorisation applications for medicinal products

*Tania Thomas*

This chapter is intended to provide a step-by-step guide to writing and assembling a marketing authorisation application in the European Union. It will be useful to pharmacists working either in regulatory affairs or the registration sector in industry, or in a consultancy capacity.

For a medicinal product to be commercially available it must possess a 'licence' known as a 'marketing authorisation'. This is obtained by applying to the responsible regulatory authority of the country where you would like to sell your product. The application consists of a 'life story' of the product, from the first stages of its formulation and development through to its manufacture and quality control. It concludes with the results of all relevant pharmaceutical (physicochemical, biological or microbiological), preclinical (toxicological and pharmacological) and clinical trials performed.

This chapter covers writing marketing authorisation applications for submission to regulatory authorities in the European Union. You should be aware that pharmaceutical legislation on which the marketing authorisation is based is extensive, complex, and constantly changing. This chapter should not therefore be taken as definitive. However, it will be a good basis for any regulatory affairs professional who is starting out, or any other healthcare professional seeking a 'taster' on writing applications for marketing authorisations. All information contained in this chapter is the author's personal view and does not reflect official policy unless indicated by references.

## The basics of marketing authorisation applications

The instructions for writing a marketing authorisation application are included in a document titled the *Notice to Applicants*, which is published in three volumes. Volume 2A deals with the procedures in which you can obtain a marketing authorisation, Volume 2B deals with the presentation and format of the application (the 'dossier'), and Volume 2C deals with regulatory guidelines that should be followed. The *Notice to Applicants* can be found on the European Commission's pharmaceuticals website at *http://ec.europa.eu/enterprise/pharmaceuticals/eudralex/index.htm*.

The three main aspects of a medicinal product that need to be addressed in an application are its:

- **quality** (is it of consistent quality for human consumption?)
- **safety** (is it safe to consume at the doses at which it is recommended?)
- **efficacy** (does it work for the condition for which it is indicated?).

An applicant company should always take into account the scientific guidelines regarding the quality, safety and efficacy of medicinal products for human use, as adopted by the Committee of Human Medicinal Products and published by the European Medicines Agency (EMEA). Medicinal products should also comply with the tests from both specific and general monographs of the European Pharmacopoeias and any relevant national pharmacopoeia.

A reviewer at the relevant licensing authority will be in a position to approve or reject your application for a marketing authorisation, based on the information you provide about the product. Therefore, the manner in which you present this information should be clear and not subject to misinterpretation. Luckily, there is an internationally accepted format that you must use entitled the Common Technical Document. This is the standard format for the presentation of applications to be submitted to regulatory authorities in Europe, the USA and Japan. These three regions were brought together under the International Conference on Harmonisation (ICH) in order to provide guidelines for applicant companies to follow when preparing a marketing authorisation application.

The Common Technical Document format comprises five modules that relate to different aspects of the medicinal product:[1]

- Module 1 — administrative, regional or national information
- Module 2 — summaries (the quality overall summary, the non-clinical overview/summaries, and the clinical overview/summaries
- Module 3 — quality chemical, pharmaceutical and biological information
- Module 4 — non-clinical study reports (toxicological and pharmacological tests)
- Module 5 — clinical study reports.

Each of the modules is associated with specific International Conference on Harmonisation guidelines, which must also be taken into consideration when you are preparing the EU marketing authorisation dossier. These guidelines are constantly being revised by the European Commission, and you should therefore always check for any updates. With respect to the quality (chemical, pharmaceutical or biological) part of the dossier, all monographs, including general monographs and general chapters of the *European Pharmacopoeia*, are applicable. In addition, the manufacturing process should comply with the principles and guidelines of good manufacturing practice (GMP).

The Common Technical Document is a general outline of the presentation and format of the application, but gives no information on the content required in order to gain approval.

---

▶ Remember: The regulatory background is complex and multi-layered; the Common Technical Document guideline always should be read within the framework of the International Conference on Harmonisation and further documents published by the European Commission.

---

## Regulatory procedures

Different procedures may be used to apply for a marketing authorisation.[2] These include the following:

- national procedure (whereby the authorisation is applied for and granted in only one EU member state)
- mutual recognition procedure (whereby the authorisation in one member state is mutually recognised by other member states)
- centralised procedure (whereby the European Commission authorises a medicinal product for the EU market)
- decentralised procedure (whereby one member state, with the contribution of the other member states involved, authorises the medicinal product for all involved member states).

The procedure selected usually depends on the aims of the applicant company to gain marketing authorisation for their product in Europe.[2]

### The centralised procedure

The centralised procedure[3] is run by the European Commission and results in a medicinal product being issued with a marketing authorisation valid throughout the EU. This procedure is mandatory for biotechnology and other innovative products, including those with a new active ingredient and for which the therapeutic indications are acquired immune deficiency syndrome (AIDS), cancer, neurodegenerative disorders or diabetes. From 20 May 2008 this procedure is also compulsory for medicinal products containing new active substances indicated for the treatment of autoimmune diseases and other immune dysfunctions and viral diseases. In this procedure, you should submit the dossier to the European Medicines Agency rather than the national regulatory authority. Instructions for how to submit the dossier can be found on the European Commission's website. The centralised procedure assessment process takes 210 days to complete.[3]

## The mutual recognition procedure

When the centralised procedure is not mandatory and the intention is to market a product in more than one European country, the mutual recognition procedure (MRP)[4] can be used. This involves taking a nationally approved product and submitting applications in the other concerned member states (CMS), requesting them to mutually recognise the national marketing authorisation already granted. The mutual recognition procedure is complete within 90 days.[4]

## The national procedure

If you intend to market in only one country, or if you intend to use this country as the reference member state (RMS) for a mutual recognition procedure, then you should use the national procedure. An application should be submitted to the relevant regulatory authority of the country in question. The timelines for a national application vary across countries.

## The decentralised procedure

The decentralised procedure[2] is an alternative to the mutual recognition procedure to obtaining marketing authorisations in a number of selected European member states, the difference being that the product cannot be authorised in any European member state before the start of the procedure. The application is submitted to the reference member state and concerned member states, and the reference member state assesses the application with comments from the concerned member states. On acceptance the procedure switches to the national phase for granting of the marketing authorisations. The decentralised procedure has a maximum of 210 days to completion.[2]

## The legal basis of submission

Apart from the different types of application procedure that you may go through to obtain a marketing authorisation, there are also different legal claims under which you can submit an application.[2] This is referred to as the legal basis of the application, and is the most important piece of information that you should possess at the beginning of writing a marketing authorisation application as this will govern the data to include in your dossier, and the angle you should present it from. The different types of legal basis are described below.

### A complete and independent/standalone application

If you wanted to apply for a marketing authorisation for a new medicinal product (new chemical entity) you would need to submit your application under the heading of 'complete and independent application' (otherwise known as a 'standalone' application). As can be assumed from the title, this is a complete dossier and you would have to provide full administrative, quality, preclinical and clinical data for such a submission.[5]

### Generic application

In line with current pharmaceutical legislation (EC Directive 2001/83/EC[5]), this claim basically cross-refers to a product that has already been available on the EU market for a period of 8 years. The dossier should contain the complete administrative and quality data and relevant preclinical and clinical data.

Generic applications may be achieved using data generated by the original applicant company, data published in the literature ('well-established use'), or a combination of the two (hybrid application). For generic products the applicant can refer to the preclinical and clinical data of the reference product in support of the application. However, under the 'well-established use' claim, the information submitted should still reflect the content of a full application, including preclinical and clinical data.[5]

## Fixed combination applications

These are medicinal products that contain two or more active substances as a combination product (e.g. co-amilofruse, which consists of amiloride hydrochloride and furosemide). The dossier should contain complete administrative and complete quality, preclinical and clinical data on the combination only, rather than on the different active substances.[5]

## Informed consent applications

Informed consent applications are simple applications for a medicinal product that is identical to one that already has an existing marketing authorisation, and for which the current marketing authorisation holder has given permission for their data to be used in support of this application. You should provide complete administrative data for such applications.[5]

▶  Remember: The legal basis is vitally important to the content of the dossier that you will be preparing. You should always seek regulatory advice from the regulatory agency in the country where you are planning to submit your application if you are not sure under which legal basis it should be submitted.

## Additional legal basis issues

### Data exclusivity and patents

A generic medicinal product cannot be placed on the market until 8 years after the date of first authorisation in the EU for that active substance.[5] This is referred to as 'data exclusivity', and patents exist to protect the original product from this type of competition. As a result, if a marketing authorisation is obtained for a product that claims essential similarity to a reference product that has not been licensed for a period of 8 years, the placement of that product on the market would constitute an illegal act on the part of the company. This period of data exclusivity may also be extended beyond 8 years if it is supported by data submitted by the original company,[5] for example new clinical studies claiming the use of the product for one or more new therapeutic indications considered to bring significant clinical benefit compared to existing therapies.

➤ Regulatory authorities are not concerned with patent issues, and you as the applicant company are responsible for not breaching patent laws.

➤ Remember: always check the data exclusivity period of the reference medicinal product — you do not want to waste your time working on an application if you will not be able to place the product on the market for a significant period.

### Line extension

An additional issue to legal basis is the concept of a line extension, which occurs when certain fundamental changes are made to a medicinal product, e.g. a change in the strength of the product (10 mg as opposed to 5 mg), or a change in the pharmaceutical form (e.g. modified-release tablet).[5]

➤ For a line extension product you should always use the same legal basis as for the original product.

## Presentation

Presentation is key in getting the information across in a simple and direct manner.[1] You do not want the reviewer to have to search through all the documentation provided to obtain the information they require in order to decide on the quality, safety and efficacy of the product. Nor do you want them to make an unfavourable decision on your product because they cannot find the correct information in the dossier!

The information on style and plain English in Chapters 1 and 2 should be taken into consideration when writing marketing authorisation applications.

### Contents page

You should always include a contents page and label individual dossiers as '$x$ of $y$', so that the reviewer knows how much documentation is being submitted.

## Font style and size

Although we are moving towards a 'paperless' state, many documents included in the submission will still be scanned, printed or photocopied, so you should make sure that the font sizes for text and tables are easily legible. I would recommend using Times New Roman 12-point for narrative text. You should also use your common sense, for example using margins wide enough that the text can be easily read after binding, and preparing both text and tables with margins so that the entire document can be printed on A4 paper.

## Information about national administrative requirements

It goes without saying that your application should be sent to the correct address and in the correct language. All logistical information on where to send dossiers (addresses of national authorities), the numbers of copies of dossiers and modules required, and which languages should be used and further national requirements are published by the European Commission in the *Notice to Applicants*, Vol. 2A, Chapter 7 'General Information'.

## Further issues

When you include published literature with your application, it is good practice to provide a detailed description and justification of the search strategy used to find it. A review of the literature is also very helpful in supporting your application. You should include all documentation, whether favourable or unfavourable, and give justification for any document that is not included in order to present a non-biased summary of published literature.

▶ When including published literature, give the full article as well as any necessary translations.

At this point, you have obtained all of your information on the product from the relevant sources and are ready to start writing. The Common Technical Document (CTD) is a format in which you can present information about your product to the reviewer in a clear and structured manner. As already mentioned, the CTD format consists of five modules, which are described further under each heading.

# Common Technical Document format — Module 1

Module 1 is the administrative part of the application and contains the marketing authorisation application form (MAA form)[6] and relevant appendices, additional national information, labelling, package leaflet and the Summary of Product Characteristics.[7]

## How to complete an MAA form

The MAA form sets out the main particulars of the application, including the legal (legal basis of submission), medical (e.g. therapeutic category, indications) and pharmaceutical particulars (e.g. shelf life, pack sizes). You can usually obtain a copy of the form electronically via the website of the authority to which you are submitting the application. You should complete an application form for each proposed marketing authorisation, in other words, a separate form is required for each pharmaceutical form and strength of the medicinal product. The application should always be completed in English unless the relevant national language is requested. You should note that electronic applications will be the way forward, and a version of the electronic submission document can be found in the *Notice to Applicants*, Volume 2B, Electronic Common Technical Document (eCTD).

The main sections of the marketing authorisation Application form are as follows.[6]

### *Declaration and signature*

This section includes the basic details of the product, including:

- proposed name
- active substance
- strength
- pharmaceutical form
- name and address of the proposed marketing authorisation holder
- signature of contact person on behalf of the applicant.

---

▶ Ensure that the regulatory authority is informed if the contact person is changed, as they will be contacting this person directly for any issues to do with the application.

---

*Type of application (Section 1)*

The legal basis of the application should be stated here.

For all but 'well-established use' applications, you should include name, country of registration and date of authorisation for the:

- original reference product (which has been marketed in the EU for more than the requested 8 years)
- medicinal reference product (a similar generic product already marketed in the country to which you are submitting the application).

You should include the name, and the country of source for the reference product used in the bioequivalence studies if this is different from the original medicinal product.

For a mutual recognition procedure application, state the countries you intend to include. If this is a repeat use mutual recognition procedure you should include the countries that recognised the marketing authorisation during the previous use of the procedure.

If the application is considered to be a line extension (as described above) you should detail the original marketing authorisation (name, marketing authorisation number) and the differences between the original product and the one that you are submitting.

You are also required to give a declaration on whether your medicinal product possesses orphan medicine status in this section.

*Marketing authorisation particulars (Section 2)*

Section 2 of the form is split into different parts. The relevant information to include in each part is as follows.

Part 1

- Proposed name of the product (brand name)
- Active substance
- Pharmacotherapeutic category

The active substance should be expressed as the international non-proprietary name (INN) with its accompanying salt or hydrate form, and pharmacotherapeutic category is expressed as the ATC code, which you can obtain from the WHO website (*www.who.int*).

## Part 2

- Strength
- Pharmaceutical form
- Route of administration
- Proposed packaging
- Pack sizes

For the pharmaceutical form, route of administration and container, you should use the standard terms, which are defined in the *European Pharmacopoeia*.

## Part 3

- Legal status for supply

In other words, is the medicinal product to be supplied on prescription only (or not), and the availability of supply (e.g. will it be restricted to certain patients only?).

## Part 4

- Marketing authorisation holder's name
- Address
- Phone number
- Email address
- Contact person details

## Part 5

- Site name(s)
- Address
- Phone number
- Email address

You should list all sites involved in any stage of the development, manufacture or testing of the product and its active substance, including distributors (with reference to relevant manufacturers' licences). The actual site address should be given for each site specifically, rather than the headquarters address.

> The authorised manufacturer or importer responsible for batch release of the medicinal product should be based in the European Community.

Part 6

- Formulation
- Transmissible spongiform encephalopathy (TSE) declaration

You should refer to the relevant pharmacopoeial reference for each component of the formulation.

## Scientific advice (Section 3)

You should declare whether you have obtained any scientific advice or recommendations from any EU member state for this application.

---

➤ You should request scientific advice when you want clarification on any part of your application, or an area that is not clear in the guidelines. Although this carries an expense in most regulatory authorities it can be extremely beneficial in the long run, in reducing processing timelines and time to getting the product on to the market.

---

## Paediatric Development program (Section 4)

You should provide details on any studies performed or to be implemented, in order to support the use of the medicinal product in children.

## Other marketing authorisations (Section 5)

If you have submitted an application for the same product in other countries, you should declare all relevant details in this section, whether this has been authorised, pending, refused, withdrawn, suspended or revoked, and whether different therapeutic indications have been granted in those member states. Duplicate applications should also be included in this section, stating the product name and marketing authorisation number for each application.

---

➤ If a product has already been authorised in a European member state, you must use the mutual recognition procedure. A national application for such a product will be deemed invalid if it is used to place this product on other markets of the European Union.

---

## Annexed documents (Section 6)

The annexed documents[6] (appendices) that you must include to support the application are as follows:

- proof of payment to the relevant authority, e.g. a photocopy of the cheque sent to the finance division of the authority or bank transfer receipt
- an informed consent letter from the original company granting the applicant company access to product data (in the case of informed consent applications)
- proof of establishment of the applicant in the European Union or European Economic Area, i.e. a company registration document
- letter of authorisation for communication on behalf of the applicant, in cases where the applicant is not the contact person for the application (e.g. when a regulatory consultant is used)
- curriculum vitae of the qualified person for pharmacovigilance
- manufacturing authorisation. A current valid manufacturer's licence or good manufacturing practice certificate should be provided
- justification for more than one manufacturer being responsible for batch release in the EEA, if appropriate. You should explain why several sites are required, but this will be mostly for marketing reasons in different countries
- flowchart indicating the different sites involved in the manufacturing process of the product (including the sites involved in sampling and testing for batch release of products manufactured in non EEA-EFTA states and candidate countries for accession to the European Union
- statement from the competent authority that inspected the manufacturing site(s) or, where applicable, a summary of other good manufacturing practice inspections performed in the last 3 years
- a letter from the active substance manufacturer granting access to its drug substance data via a Letter of access to Drug Master File, or a copy of the *European Pharmacopoeia* Certificate of Suitability with access granted to the applicant
- copy of written confirmation from the manufacturer of the active substance to inform the applicant (in cases where there may have been modifications to the manufacturing process or specifications)
- *European Pharmacopoeia* Certificate of Suitability for the active substance and/or risk materials of animal or human origin
- written consent of the competent authorities regarding GMO release in the environment, if relevant
- scientific advice given by CHMP (The Committee on Medicinal Products for Human Use). A copy of the report should be provided if appropriate
- copies of any marketing authorisations for the specific product already obtained in other countries

- list of product labelling or leaflet mock-ups
- copy of the Orphan Designation Decision
- list of proposed (invented) names and marketing authorisation holders in the concerned member states
- copy of EMEA certificate for a Vaccine Antigen Master File (VAMF), if appropriate
- copy of EMEA certificate for a Plasma Master File (PMF), if appropriate.

### Additional data requirements

Additional data requirements are different for each country and are detailed in the *Notice to Applicants*.

---

➤ 'Questions and Answers' documents are a type of 'frequently asked questions' document and should be used as your first port of call in situations that are unclear.

---

## How to write the Summary of Product Characteristics

The Summary of Product Characteristics (SPC) is a document containing all of the information on the safe and effective use of a medicinal product and is written for health professionals.[8] The SPC is also the basis upon which the package leaflet and labelling are constructed, and therefore should be accurate to the product's particulars. In certain countries, including the UK, you are required to provide separate SPCs for each strength and pharmaceutical form of the product.

The SPC should be written in line with the relevant guidelines,[8] including the *Guideline on Summary of Product Characteristics*.[8] It should be in line with data generated in the quality, clinical and toxicological studies performed on the product, and for European procedures, as outlined in the Quality Review of Documents (QRD) Group publications.[9]

The Summary of Product Characteristics should contain the following sections:

1. Name of medicinal product
2. Qualitative and quantitative composition
3. Pharmaceutical form
4. Clinical particulars:
   4.1 Therapeutic indications

4.2   Posology and method of administration
4.3   Contraindications
4.4   Special warnings and precautions for use
4.5   Interactions with other medicinal products and other forms of interaction
4.6   Pregnancy and lactation
4.7   Effects on ability to drive and use machines
4.8   Undesirable effects
4.9   Overdose
5.   Pharmacological properties:
   5.1   Pharmacodynamic properties
   5.2   Pharmacokinetic properties
   5.3   Preclinical safety data
6.   Pharmaceutical particulars:
   6.1   List of excipients
   6.2   Incompatibilities
   6.3   Shelf life
   6.4   Special precautions for storage
   6.5   Nature and contents of container
   6.6   Special precautions for disposal
7.   Marketing authorisation holder
8.   Marketing authorisation numbers
9.   Date of first authorisation/renewal of the authorisation
10.   Date of revision of the text
11.   Dosimetry (for radiopharmaceuticals)
12.   Instructions for preparation of radiopharmaceuticals

## How to write the package leaflet

The package leaflet should be a reflection of the SPC, written for the public. As such, no additional information can be written in the leaflet that is not contained within the SPC.[1]

For the layout and standard text of the leaflet, you should refer to the Quality Review of Documents Group Product Information Templates which can be found on the EMEA website[9] (*www.emea.eu.int*).

The text should be written in patient-friendly language, the acceptability of which has been approved through user testing and which complies with guidelines on readability.[10] It should be clear and easy to understand, and follow the principles of plain English (see Chapter 2). You should use a print size of at least 8-point Didot (or at least a font where the lower case of the character 'x' is 1.4 mm in height), and a space between lines of at least 3 mm. No promotional content is allowed in the package leaflet. Avoid using long sentences (i.e. more than 20 words). A minimal number of words should be used in the bullet points, and never more than one sentence. Abbreviations should be avoided.

The sections should be as follows:

1.   What X is and what it is used for
2.   Before you [take] [use] X
3.   How to [take] [use] X
4.   Possible side effects
5.   How to store X
6.   Further information.

You can use diagrams for additional clarification if necessary, but be aware that these must not be promotional in nature. You should also restrict excessive use of the brand name in the text, as this may also be considered promotional. You may submit a joint leaflet for different strengths of a product if the clinical section is shared for each strength.

Although there is no legal requirement, technical leaflets should usually be provided for products intended for administration by health-care professionals (e.g. intravenous products). If written clearly and comprehensively, you can usually provide the main body of the SPC as the technical leaflet.

The availability of package leaflets in formats for the blind and partially sighted is another European legal requirement you should take into consideration when constructing the leaflet.

▶   Faithful translations are vital! It is worth spending more for a translations company that is experienced in pharmaceutical translations.

**Useful guidelines for this section**

- *Notice to Applicants* Volume 3B — *Regulatory Guidelines. Excipients in the label and package leaflet of medicinal products for human use.*
- CPMP/463/00 — *Excipients in the label and package leaflet of medicinal products for human use.*

**Checklist**

☑ Have you ensured that no information additional to that in the SPC is contained in the leaflet?

☑ Have you listed adverse events in decreasing order of seriousness and subdivided them according to frequency?

☑ Have you checked that any translations performed on the SPC are faithful representations of medical terminology?

## How to write the product label

You must include a 'mock-up' of the product presentation as well as the proposed package leaflet with the application.[1] A 'mock-up' is a full-colour copy on paper of the flat artwork design providing a two-dimensional presentation of the inner and outer packaging. This can usually be computer-generated.

You should include the EU minimum legal requirements on the product label, which should be both clear and legible. Print size should be at least 7-point Didot (or at least a size where the lower case of the character 'x' is 1.4 mm in height), and there should be a space between lines of at least 3 mm. Words in full capitals/upper case should be avoided. Figure 18.1 is an example of a simple mock-up.

Since November 2005 it has been a European legal requirement for certain particulars to be expressed in Braille on the secondary packaging of all medicinal products, including the name of the product, its strength, the pharmaceutical form, and whether it is intended for babies, children or adults. Although several Braille formats may be acceptable, the European Commission recommends the use of Marburg Medium. Contracted Braille (an abbreviated form) is not generally accepted.

The following information is required on a product label.

*Outer packaging should have[1]*

- product name, strength and pharmaceutical form, followed by the international non-proprietary name (INN) on three non-opposing sides of the label
- the contents of the pack, e.g. 30 tablets
- a list of excipients
- method/route of administration. These should be detailed in full for over-the-counter (OTC) or pharmacy products

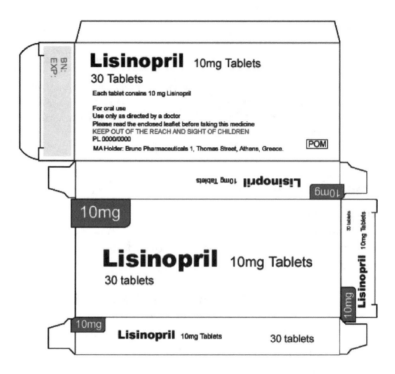

**Figure 18.1** Example of a simple mock-up.

- for POM (prescription-only) products the instruction '*Use as directed by the physician*'
- for OTC medicines, indication(s), dosage recommendations, contraindications and warnings
- the standard warning '*Keep out of the reach and sight of children*'
- any special warnings for use of the product or special precautions for disposal
- storage precautions
- name and address of MA holder
- PL number
- batch number
- expiry date
- legal status (for prescription-only products a boxed POM and for pharmacy products a boxed P).

All excipients must appear on the label for parenteral, topical, ophthalmic and inhaled products. For other products, the excipients with a recognised effect as stated in the guideline on *Excipients in the Label and Package Leaflet of Medicinal Products for Human Use*[11] should also be stated on the label.

When the immediate packaging is too small to include all of the information it is only necessary to include the product name, strength, method/route of administration, contents, expiry date and batch number. For blister packs the minimum requirements are the product name, name of the MA holder, expiry date and batch number.

---

➤ You should be careful not to include promotional claims on the label that are not supported by clinical data in the application. Some examples of such claims, which are currently not allowed for new product applications in the UK, are 'no artificial colours' or 'suitable for vegetarians'.

---

**Useful guidelines for this section**

- *Notice to Applicants* Volume 2C — *Regulatory Guidelines*. Guidelines on the packaging information of medicinal products for human use authorised by the European Community
- CPMP/463/00 — *Excipients in the Label and Package Leaflet of Medicinal Products for Human Use*
- *Notice to Applicants* Volume 2C — *Regulatory Guidelines*. Guidelines on the readability of the label and package leaflet of medicinal product for human use.

## Common Technical Document format — Module 2

Module 2 consists of summaries of the entire documentation.[1] These should be clearly written so that the reviewer may gain an initial understanding of the entire application and be able to pinpoint its strengths and weakness. The quality expert (usually, but not necessarily, a pharmacist) assumes personal responsibility for the quality overview and quality overall summary (QOS), which is a summary of the quality information submitted in Module 3. It is mandatory that a medical doctor be responsible for the clinical overview and summaries, which outline all studies performed using the proposed product and relevant reference products in support of its therapeutic claims. Finally, a pharmacologist/toxicologist usually assumes responsibility for the non-clinical overview and summary. They would summarise all pharmacological/toxicological issues with the product, including critical issues such as impurity levels. The overviews are exactly that — an overview of the information contained in the summary. The following is a detailed guide on how to write the quality overall summary, but the same principles apply when writing the clinical and non-clinical summaries.

### How to write the quality overall summary

The aim of the quality overall summary is to provide the reviewer with an outline of the key particulars of the product.[1] The QOS should not exceed 40 pages (excluding tables and figures), but may go up to 80 (excluding tables and figures) for products manufactured using more complex processes (e.g. biotech products). Most importantly, the QOS should not include any information that has not already been included in Module 3.

When writing a QOS, you should provide a brief summary on each section of Module 3. Where guidelines have not been followed, you should provide a sound justification for this, including for the lack of documentation. The QOS serves to present the product from the quality aspect, and therefore key aspects of each Module should be integrated in this report, such as:

- the legal application under which the product is being submitted, together with its supporting information
- the relevance of any clinical studies performed with regard to the final formulation or manufacturing process.

The QOS is also where you should discuss any particular critical parameters of the product and emphasise certain sections of the data, according to the type of product submitted. For example, for generic applications you should ask yourself the following questions:

**Checklist**

☑ Have you discussed the grounds for claiming that your product is 'essentially similar' to one already on the market?

☑ Have you provided a summary of any bioequivalence studies performed, or provided justification for claiming a biowaiver?

☑ Have you discussed potential impurities or degradation products that are detected or may be formed in the product?

☑ Are you claiming any additional claims in the SPC over the product already on the market, and have you provided a summary of any relevant studies or data in support of this?

☑    Have you focused on the key critical issues that pertain to the product in question?

☑    Do not exceed 40 pages for a 'simple' product, 80 pages for a complex one (excluding tables and figures).

☑    Do not include any information additional to that mentioned in the relevant modules.

➤ Remember: Keep your information as straightforward and to the point as possible.

## Common Technical Document format — Module 3

You should include all chemical, pharmaceutical and biological information about the product in Module 3 of the dossier. This module is divided into two main parts covering the active substance and the drug product.

### Active substance

You should follow the Common Technical Document guidelines on what information and degree of detail to include in this part.[1] The relevant details of the active substance can be presented in full as part of the dossier, as either a European Drug Master File or as a Certificate of Suitability from the active substance manufacturer. You should always include details on the processing and testing of the substance (obtained from the manufacturer).

**Useful guidelines for this section**

- CPMP/QWP/227/02 — Active Substance Master File procedure.
- CHMP/QWP/297/97 — Summary of Requirements for Active Substances in the Quality Part of the Dossier.

The content of the active substance part of Module 3 is as follows.

*General information*

This includes all details on the nomenclature of the active substance under the relevant headings.[1]

- Recommended INN
- Pharmacopoeial name
- Chemical name
- Company or laboratory code
- Other non-proprietary names
- Chemical Abstracts Service Registry number
- Diagram of the structure
- Molecular formula
- Relative molecular mass
- Physicochemical properties, e.g. solubility

You should also provide short statements on the chemistry of the active substance molecule, covering areas such as chirality and polymorphism.

**Useful guidelines for this section**

- CPMP/QWP/130/96 — Chemistry of the New Active Substance.
- European Pharmacopoeia.

*Manufacture section should have:*[1]

- name, address and role of the manufacturer. It is good practice to include contact phone numbers and email addresses
- manufacturing flow diagram that demonstrates the step-by-step process using the chemical structures of the materials
- description of the manufacturing process (each stage of the process, materials, equipment, and process parameters such as temperature, pH, times)
- reprocessing details if this occurs
- any controls used during the manufacturing process
- information on raw materials.

You should state material amounts and yield ranges of the end product for each step for a standard commercial production batch size (remember to always state the size!). This can be in the form of a summary table or as text in the description of the process.

In-process controls are tests used to demonstrate control of the process at various stages. The methods and appropriate limits should be specified, as well as details on sample selection covering quantity and location.

Information on materials used in the manufacturing process must be given, including their function, at which points they are used, and which quality standards they comply with (e.g. *European Pharmacopoeia*). Materials may include the following:

• starting materials
• solvents
• catalysts
• reagents
• auxiliary materials.

The best way to present this information is in the form of a table. In support, you should also give specifications for each material, including the relevant limits and details of the test methods. You are also required to provide certification as evidence that no materials with a risk of transmitting TSE/BSE (transmissible spongiform encephalitis/bovine spongiform encephalitis) are included in the manufacture of the drug substance.

During manufacturing there is usually a series of intermediate products that should also be adequately controlled. You should present the specification with the limits used to control all intermediates as a table, with a written description of the methods used.

You should provide relevant details on the development of the manufacturing process, covering changes to the process parameters, equipment, manufacturing site or scale. This should be in the form of a discussion providing information on the changes made, the reasons for them, and any consequences they had on the finished active substance.

➤ A simple way of constructing the manufacturing flow diagram is by linking the starting material with the various intermediates and the finished active substance using a series of process arrows around which the additional raw materials, solvents, catalysts and reagents should be listed, with any relevant process parameters.

**Useful guidelines for this section**

• CPMP/ICH/4106/00 — Good Manufacturing Practice for Active Pharmaceutical Ingredients.
• CPMP/QWP/227/02 — Active Substance Master File procedure.

*Characterisation*[1]

Data to confirm the structure of the molecule produced using the proposed manufacturing process should be discussed in this section. You should support the discussion with copies of a range of spectral analyses used to confirm the structure, including ultraviolet (UV), neutron magnetic resonance (NMR), mass spectrometry (MS), X-ray diffraction (XRD), differential scanning calorimetry (DSC) and infrared (IR).

---

➤    Present the peaks of the spectra in a tabular format, with cross-reference to a labelled diagrammatic representation of the structure. It is good practice to provide a discussion document on how the spectra and synthetic route confirm the structure of the molecule.

---

You should discuss the potential for isomerism, identification of stereochemistry and polymorphism of the molecule in relation to its chemistry and the synthetic route used. It is best to use a diagram of the molecule in the discussion.

Sufficient details of the impurities that might be present in the active substance should be provided. This can easily be represented by a flow diagram using the chemical structures involved.

*Control of active substance*

The final quality specification with which the drug substance complies should be given in the form of a table with the specific test and accompanying relevant limit.[1] This provides easy reference to the specification at any point. It should be associated with the analytical procedures used for each test, providing sufficient detail to enable the method to be replicated, including reagents with quantities, equipment and test parameters.

You should provide analytical method validation obtained from the relevant quality control department for all tests included in the dossier, excluding simple routine pharmacopoeial or other methods. You should always provide full validation data as detailed in the guidelines on analytical method validation for complex non-pharmacopoeial methods. This is described in more detail in the drug product section. You should discuss the results and conclude on the suitability of the method for the purpose intended.

➤ Validation data can be presented in a table, clearly stating the results obtained and relevant acceptance limits.

Provide examples (at least two, and ideally three) of batches tested to the active substance specification. Include 'batch histories' as tables, including the following information:

- batch numbers
- date of manufacture
- site of manufacture
- batch size
- source of drug substance used.

➤ The best way to present the batch analysis data is in a table with the accompanying certificates of analysis directly following it.

**Useful guidelines for this section**

- CPMP/ICH/367/96 — Specifications: Test procedures and acceptance criteria for new drug substances and new drug products: chemical substances.
- CPMP/ICH/2737/99 — Impurities testing: Impurities in new drug substances.

*Reference standards or materials*

In this section you should provide:[1]

- certificates of analysis on the reference standards and working standards
- discussion on how the standards are obtained, generated or standardised.

*Container closure system*

Provide:[1]

- a full description of the container closure system (primary and any secondary packaging)
- construction material
- drawings where relevant
- specifications
- details of the test methods

- certificates of analysis from the active substance manufacturer and the packaging material manufacturer
- compliance with the relevant pharmacopoeia monograph, EC directive on contact with food stuffs legislation, e.g. for plastic materials.

You should comment on the compatibility of the packaging materials with the active substance, covering the possibility of sorption, extractables and leaching.

**Useful guidelines for this section**

- CPMP/QWP/4539/03 Guideline on Plastic Primary Packaging Materials.

*Stability*

Provide:[1]

- batch histories of the stability batches
- type of packaging and pack sizes used
- conditions for long-term and accelerated storage
- stability protocol and duration of the stability study
- characteristics studied
- the proposed shelf life and the recommended storage temperature.

Refer to the drug product part below for further details on information and presentation for this section.

**Useful guidelines for this section**

- CPMP/QWP/122/02 — Stability Testing of Existing Active Substances and Related Finished products.
- CPMP/QWP/609/96 — Declaration of Storage Conditions for Medicinal Products Particulars and Active Substances (Annex to note for Guidance on Stability Testing of New Active Substances and Medicinal Products, Annex to Note for Guidance on Stability of Existing Active Substances and Related Finished Products).
- CPMP/ICH/279/95 — Photostability testing of New Active Substances and Medicinal products.
- CPMP/ICH/420/02 — Evaluation of Stability Data.
- CPMP/ICH/2736/99 — Stability testing of new drug substances and products.

**Checklist for the drug substance part of your application**

☑  Are the drug particle size, residual solvents, organic impurities and active ingredient compatible with the intended route of administration for the proposed product?
☑  Do the data comply with International Conference on Harmonisation guidelines?
☑  Have you attached all relevant documentation, e.g. Good Manufacturing Practice certificate for the manufacturer of the active ingredient?
☑  Have you listed all tests performed by the finished product manufacturer on receipt of the active ingredient?

➤ If no information is available for a specific heading, the title page for that section should still be included in the application followed by the statement 'not applicable'.

## Drug product

### Description and composition

The following should be provided:[1]

• a description of the product
• container closure system used
• composition of the product.

It is desirable to present the composition of the product as a table, including a list of ingredients, quantities per unit (including any over-ages used), and the function the material plays in the formulation, with reference to a pharmacopoeial monograph where appropriate.

### Pharmaceutical development[1]

This section describes how the product was developed for the market. As a result, all properties of the active substance that will ultimately affect the performance of the product should be mentioned here. Discuss the compatibility of the active substance with the chosen excipients, including a discussion of how those excipients were selected at their respective concentrations in the formulation. Summarise the development of the formulation and include the qualitative and quantitative composition and the results of the physical and chemical analyses from key batches during development, along with a discussion on the relevance on the formulation. Formulations and test results can be presented as tables.

In addition to the active substance, the dosage form of the product will also raise critical issues regarding product performance that should be addressed. For low-dose solid products, data should be provided on dissolution and content uniformity, and for multiple-dose liquid or semi-solid products, data on preservative efficacy tests. You should identify critical parameters such as pH, dissolution, particle size distribution or rheology. Include supporting data to demonstrate the influence of critical parameters and the suitability of the process controls used to ensure the consistent manufacture of a well-controlled product.

You should provide details to justify the development of the manufacturing process, including, for example, the selection of the process and the need to include certain excipients in different phases; choice of equipment; and process parameters. This is of particular consequence for sterilised products: the chosen method must be described and justified. In the majority of cases the process used to manufacture the first batches of a medicinal product, which are used in clinical trials (clinical batches), is different from that which is to be used to manufacture the pilot or commercial-scale batches. Therefore the applicant should discuss all differences in the manufacturing process used to manufacture the clinical batches compared to the proposed manufacturing process in the application (which will be used for commercial batches), including a discussion on whether or not these differences influence product performance (for example, for a tablet changes in the manufacturing process may affect hardness or dissolution, and consequently release of the active substance from the dosage form). You should discuss the suitability of the container closure system as regards the selection of the construction material, any environmental protection issues, and compatibility with the drug product. Any performance issues, for example the suitability of an inhaler to deliver the required dose, should be included.

Additional areas that should not be ignored are the microbiological attributes and compatibility of the drug product with any reconstitution diluents or dosage devices.

For generic products claiming essential similarity it is important to provide evidence of this via comparative dissolution, assay and impurity profiles of both the proposed and the reference products. It is good practice to include at least two batches of the proposed product, and batches of the reference product from more than one country's markets if you are planning to submit via a mutual recognition procedure, particularly if the composition of the product differs between countries.

▶ An easy way to find the qualitative composition of a medicinal product from a particular country is from the patient information leaflet.

**Useful guidelines for this section**

- CPMP/QWP/155/96 — Development Pharmaceutics.
- CPMP/QWP/054/98 — Annex to Note for guidance on Development Pharmaceutics.
- CPMP/QWP/155/96 — Decision Trees for Selection of Sterilisation Methods.

## Manufacture

This section should consist of the following:[1]

- name, address and role of the manufacturer. It is good practice to include contact phone numbers and email addresses
- batch formulae
- standard and maximum batch sizes
- manufacturing flow diagram demonstrating different steps of the process, critical steps and in-process controls
- description of the manufacturing process
- reprocessing details
- in-process controls
- process validation protocols and data.

You should present batch formulae in a table listing the quantities of each ingredient used in a batch. Batch sizes should reflect any batches already produced, and should be supported by process validation and batch analysis data available at the time of submission of the dossier.

The description of the manufacturing process should consist of an explanation of each stage of the process, including the materials involved, equipment (which should be identified at least by type), and process parameters such as temperatures, pH and time, and the scale of the production. You should provide enough detail to demonstrate the process, but not too much so that any minor amendment would require you to submit an amendment.

You should provide suitable details on the in-process controls, including the methods used and the limits set. The suitability of these tests to control the critical steps of the process should be discussed and justified.

Process validation data for at least two batches representative (minimum 10%, or 100 000 units, whichever is the greater) of the production scale should be included in support of the manufacturing process. This should demonstrate that the proposed process is suitable for the intended purpose and identify the critical steps to be tested during the process to limits suitable to control the quality of the manufactured product.

Sampling details (quantities, location the samples are taken from, and timings) should be included. The results obtained for the validation batches are best presented in tables, and the results discussed in terms of the suitability of the process to produce a controlled product. If the batches used in the process validation are pilot-scale batches then you should provide a commitment to complete process validation on production-scale batches as well as a process validation protocol.

---

➤ The batch sizes permissible (production or pilot scale) are dependent on the actual product, so always check the guidelines! Non-standard methods of manufacture, such as aseptic sterilisation, require validation data on production-scale batches.

---

---

➤ A good way of presenting this part is by providing the 'protocol' (tabulated format of the tests to be performed) and the results obtained. The protocol should provide all details of the manufacturing method and the various tests to be performed, including details of sampling and sample selection. Present the results for the different steps of the process in a tabular format, with relevant discussion and justification of the relevance of the results in relation to process control.

---

---

➤ Remember: The description of the manufacturing process, apparatus and in-process controls is legally binding unless amended by variation. It is therefore in your interest to avoid detailed descriptions and hence unnecessary applications for variations. Unnecessary variation applications can be avoided by, for example, naming the type of equipment used rather than the actual make of the machines.

---

## Control of excipients

Provide the following information:[1]

- list of excipients in the formulation, with relevant details of the quality standards to which they are controlled
- analytical test methods used, including validation for any complex methods
- certificates of analysis for each excipient
- relevant documentation stating compliance with regulatory requirements on TSE and BSE.

Primarily, excipients will be controlled to pharmacopoeial standards, which can be referenced in a table. For non-pharmacopoeial excipients the specification, stating tests, appropriate limits and validation for complex methods, should be given.

---

➤ You can provide TSE/BSE documentation as formal statements from the material manufacturer stating compliance with the relevant guidelines.

---

For novel excipients, full details in line with the format described in the active substance section should be provided, with references to supporting safety data.

---

➤ For water, provide details on the manufacture (even if produced on site) and quality controls.

---

## Control of the drug product

The final quality specification with which the product complies at the time of its release and during its shelf life should be presented in the form of a table, together with the specific test and accompanying relevant limit.[1] The general specification would usually include the following tests:

- a visual description of the product
- two specific identity tests for the active substance(s)
- assay of the active substance(s)
- related substances
- microbial quality
- identification tests for all colouring agents used in the product.

Product-specific tests for different products would be included, such as:

For solid oral dosage forms:

- uniformity of content for the active substance <2 mg or 2% w/w or low-dose products
- dissolution test
- disintegration test (not required if a dissolution test is included).

For dispersible tablets:

- dispersion test.

For parenteral products:

- particulate matter test
- sterility test.

For ointments:

- particle size test for ophthalmic suspensions or ointments.

For pressurised inhalers:

- deposition of the emitted dose test
- number of deliveries per container test.

The tests and limits included in the product specification should be justified, with a brief explanation as to why the test has been included and how the limit was set.

You should supply the analytical procedures used for each test, with full details so that the method can be replicated, including reagents with quantities, equipment and test parameters. As far as possible these tests should comply with the *European Pharmacopoeia* or other relevant pharmacopoeias. Complex non-pharmacopoeial methods should be suitably validated as detailed in the guidelines on analytical method validation. These details can include the following:

- specificity (does the method pick up the specific substance?)
- linearity and range (over what range of concentrations does this method work in the way it is expected to?)
- accuracy (is the method accurate?)
- precision (is the method precise, repeatable and reproducible? e.g. if the analytical scientist working on it is changed, does this affect the results?)
- detection limit (at what level can impurities be detected?)
- quantitation limit (at what level can impurities be measured?)
- robustness (what changes in the method will change the results obtained?).

Microbiological testing on pharmaceutical products, with accompanying validation data, should be provided in compliance with the requirements of the *European Pharmacopoeia*.

To support your drug product specification, provide the results of ideally three batches tested to the specification. These batch analyses should include details of batch numbers, date of manufacture, batch size and test results. The best way to present the data is in a table together with the accompanying certificates of analysis.

You should provide sufficient detail on the potential impurities present in the product, listing their structures and chemical names and a brief discussion on their route of formation. If it can be demonstrated that the manufacturing process does not generate additional impurities, you can reference the characterisation of impurities in the active substance section.

---

**Useful guidelines for this section**

- CPMP/ICH/282/95 — Impurities in New Drug Products.
- CPMP/ICH/367/96 — Specifications: Test Procedures and Acceptance Criteria for New Drug Substances and New Drug Products: Chemical Substances.
- CPMP/ICH/283/95 — Impurities: Residual Solvents.
- CPMP/ICH/281/95 — Validation of Analytical Procedures: Methodology.
- CPMP/ICH/381/95 — Validation of Analytical Methods: Definitions and Terminology.

---

▶ You should provide analytical test method validation for each test that has been performed on the product for which the application is made.

*Reference standards or materials*

In this section you should provide:[1]

- certificates of analysis on the reference standards and working standards
- discussion on how the standards are obtained, generated or standardised.

If these are the same as those used for the active substance you can refer to the reference standards used in the active substance section.

*Container closure system*

Provide:[1]

- a full description of the closure system (primary and any secondary packaging)
- material of construction
- drawings where relevant
- specifications
- details of the test methods used
- certificates of analysis from the active substance manufacturer and the packaging material manufacturer
- compliance with the relevant pharmacopoeia, or EC directive on contact with food stuffs legislation, e.g. for plastic materials
- data on migration and extraction studies performed in relation to semi-solids and liquids in plastic primary packaging.

Some medicinal products also require certification to prove compliance with the Medicines Regulations on Child Safety for relevant products (e.g. paracetamol-containing products in the UK).

---

**Useful guidelines for this section**

- CPMP/QWP/4539/03 — Guideline on Plastic Primary Packaging Materials
- European Commission Directive 2002/72/EC.

---

*Stability*

Provide:

- batch histories of the stability batches
- type of packaging and pack sizes used
- conditions for long-term and accelerated storage
- stability protocol and duration of the stability study

- characteristics studied
- the proposed shelf life and the recommended storage temperature.

The stability batches should ideally be production-scale batches; however, you may provide data from pilot-scale batches that are at least 10% of the size of a proposed production-scale batch. Batches of product should contain at least two different batches of active substance. Storage conditions should be in line with ICH requirements.

Stability results should be discussed, with an explanation of any trends observed and the influence these have on the quality of the product. The proposed shelf life and accompanying relevant storage conditions are set from these data.

You should state any post-approval stability commitment, including details on the batches to be tested, storage conditions and test protocols.

If the stability studies have been performed on pilot-scale batches, a post-approval stability commitment is required, with data on three production-scale batches under long-term and accelerated storage conditions, and at least one batch per year under long-term conditions.

---

➤ Present results in a tabulated format using actual numerical values to give an indication of the product's stability profile or trend.

---

➤ Present each batch at each specific storage condition studied, and each test at each time point analysed.

---

For certain products it may also be necessary to present the results of photostability testing, in-use stability studies, preservative efficacy testing, and/or determination of shelf life for sterile products after first opening or following reconstitution.

Storage conditions for the product should be in line with guidelines on the declaration of storage conditions.

**Useful guidelines for this section**

- CPMP/QWP/609/96 — Declaration of Storage Conditions for Medicinal Products Particulars and Active Substances.
- CPMP/QWP/122/02 — Stability Testing of Existing Active Substances and Related Finished products.
- CPMP/QWP/072/96 — Start of Shelf Life of the Finished Dosage Form.

- CPMP/QWP/2934/99 — In-Use Stability Testing of Human Medicinal Products.
- CPMP/QWP/159/96 — Maximum Shelf Life for Sterile Products after First Opening or following Reconstitution.
- CPMP/ICH/420/02 — Evaluation of Stability Data.
- CPMP/ICH/421/02 — Stability Data Package for Registration in Climatic Zones III and IV.
- CPMP/ICH/4104/00 — Bracketing and Matrixing Designs for Stability Testing of Drug Substances and Drug Products.
- CPMP/ICH/279/95 — Photostability testing of New Active Substances and Medicinal Products.
- CPMP/ICH/280/95 — Stability Testing: Requirements for New Dosage Forms.

## Appendices

There is an appendix section in the dossier that covers facilities and equipment (for biotechnological products), adventitious agents safety evaluation (assessment of risk with respect to potential contamination) and novel excipients.[1]

## Regional information

This section should include the supporting documents for Module 3, as follows:[1]

- process validation protocol
- details on any medical device that has been used in the product
- certificates of suitability
- certification on compliance with the requirements on materials that contain or use in the manufacturing process materials of animal and/or human origin.

### Useful guidelines for this section

General guidelines specific to certain dosage forms should also be taken into consideration, such as:

- CPMP/QWP/604/96 — Quality of Modified Release Products: A. Oral Dosage Forms; B. and Transdermal Dosage Forms; Section I (Quality).
- CPMP/QWP/158/96 — Dry Powder Inhalers.
- CPMP/QWP/2845/00 — Requirements for Pharmaceutical Documentation for Pressurised Metered Dose Inhalation Products.
- CPMP/ICH/365/96 — Specifications: Test Procedures and Acceptance Criteria for Biotechnological/Biological Products.

## Common Technical Document format — Module 4

Module 4 comprises all pharmacological, pharmacokinetic and toxicological studies performed with the medicinal product. There are several guidelines that should be followed for the format and presentation of all non-clinical studies, and these can be found in the relevant CTD guidelines.[1]

## Common Technical Document format — Module 5

In Module 5 you should include all clinical studies performed using the product you are submitting. There are some cases where studies are not required: for example, for generic medicinal products bioequivalence studies are not mandatory for simple oral solutions or aqueous solutions that are administered intravenously or intramuscularly. In these cases, cross-referral can be made to the original reference product (see 'The Legal Basis of Submissions' above).

---

**Useful guidelines for this section**

- CPMP/EWP/QWP/1401/98 — Investigation of Bioavailability and Bioequivalence.

---

➤ If you are dealing with a particularly complex product, or are not sure which guidelines apply to you, remember that most regulatory authorities will provide regulatory or scientific advice prior to submission. Paying for advice may save your company a huge amount of money, preventing the wrong studies being performed and/or the product being rejected.

---

**Final checklist**

- ☑ Ensure that you are submitting under the correct legal basis for the application.
- ☑ Present a legible and clearly written marketing authorisation application.
- ☑ Follow the recommended *Notice to Applicants*, CTD format and guidelines.
- ☑ Check the relevant websites for the latest versions or additions to guidelines.
- ☑ Provide all necessary documentation for the marketing authorisation application.
- ☑ Justify any lack of relevant information in the application.
- ☑ Always check the documentation before submission.

## Further information

The guidelines referred to above under 'Useful Guidelines' are available on the EMEA website at *http://www.emea.eu.int* or in Volume 3A of the *Rules Governing Medicinal Products in the EU* — Eudralex, available on the website of the European Commission at *http://ec.europa.eu*.

The *Notice to Applicants* can be found online on the European Commission's pharmaceuticals website at *http://ec.europa.eu/enterprise/ pharmaceuticals/eudralex/index.htm*.

## References

1.  European Commission Website. European Commission — Enterprise and Industry Directorate General — Consumer Goods — Pharmaceuticals. Volume 2 — Notice to Applicants, Volume 2B, incorporating the Common Technical Document (CTD). (April 2006) Available from: *http://ec.europa.eu/enterprise/ pharmaceuticals/eudralex/vol-2/b/ctd_05–2006.pdf*

2.  European Commission Website. European Commission — Enterprise and Industry Directorate General — Consumer Goods — Pharmaceuticals. Volume 2 — Notice to Applicants, Volume 2A — Procedures for marketing authorisation, Chapter 1. (November 2005) Available from: http://ec.europa.eu/enter prise/pharmaceuticals/eudralex/vol-2/a/pdfs-en/intr2[1] European Commission Website. European Commission — Enterprise and Industry Directorate General — Consumer Goods — Pharmaceuticals. Volume 2 — Notice to Applicants, Volume 2B, incorporating the Common Technical Document (CTD) (April 2006). Available from: *http://ec.europa.eu/enterprise/pharmaceuticals/ eudralex/vol-2/b/ctd_05–2006.pdf* aen.pdf

3.  European Commission Website. European Commission — Enterprise and Industry Directorate General — Consumer Goods — Pharmaceuticals. Volume 2 — Notice to Applicants, Volume 2A — Procedures for marketing authorisation, Chapter 4. (April 2006) Available from: *http://ec.europa.eu/enterprise/ pharmaceuticals/eudralex/vol-2/a/chap4rev200604%20.pdf*

4.  European Commission Website. European Commission — Enterprise and Industry Directorate General — Consumer Goods — Pharmaceuticals. Volume 2 — Notice to Applicants, Volume 2A — Procedures for marketing authorisation, Chapter 2. (November 2005) Available from: *http://ec.europa.eu/ enterprise/ pharmaceuticals/eudralex/vol-2/a/vol2a_chap2_2005–11.pdf*

5.  European Commission Website. European Commission — Enterprise and Industry Directorate General — Consumer Goods — Pharmaceuticals. Volume 1 — Pharmaceutical Legislation. (November 2005) Available from: *http:// ec.europa.eu/enterprise/pharmaceuticals/eudralex/homev1.htm*

6.  European Commission Website. European Commission — Enterprise and Industry Directorate General — Consumer Goods — Pharmaceuticals. Volume 2 — Notice to Applicants, Volume 2B — Presentation and content of the dossier, Updated Version — October 2005. Available from: *http://ec.europa.eu/ enterprise/pharmaceuticals/eudralex/vol-2/b/partia_20051028.pdf*

7. European Commission Website. European Commission — Enterprise and Industry Directorate General — Consumer Goods — Pharmaceuticals. Volume 2 — Notice to Applicants, Volume 2B — Presentation and content of the dossier, User guide for the application form March 2005. Available from: *http:// ec.europa.eu/enterprise/pharmaceuticals/eudralex/vol-2/b/part1a_userguide_ 03-2005.pdf*

8. European Commission Website. European Commission — Enterprise and Industry Directorate General — Consumer Goods — Pharmaceuticals. Volume 2 — Notice to Applicants, Volume 2C — Regulatory Guidelines. Guideline on Summary of Product Characteristics (October 2005). Available from: *http://ec.europa.eu/enterprise/pharmaceuticals/eudralex/vol-2/c/spcguidrev1- oct2005.pdf*

9. European Medicines Agency website: Quality Review of Documents Group (QRD), Product Information Templates, Human Medicinal Products The Product Information Templates. (July 2005) Available from: *http://www.emea. eu.int/htms/human/qrd/qrdplt/24530905en.pdf*

10. European Commission Website. European Commission — Enterprise and Industry Directorate General — Consumer Goods — Pharmaceuticals. Volume 2 — Notice to Applicants, Volume 2C — Regulatory Guidelines. Guideline on the readability of the label and package leaflet of medicinal product for human use. (September 1998) Available from: *http://ec.europa.eu/enterprise/ pharmaceuticals/eudralex/vol-2/c/gl981002.pdf*

11. European Commission Website. European Commission — Enterprise and Industry Directorate General — Consumer Goods — Pharmaceuticals. Volume 3B — Medicinal Products for Human Use: Guidelines — Excipients in the Label and Package leaflet of Medicinal Products for Human Use, Updated Version — July 2003. Available from: *2005.http://ec.europa.eu/enterprise/ pharmaceuticals/eudralex/vol-3/pdfs-en/3bc7a_200307en.pdf*

# Section Six

Medical publishing

# 19

## Medical media and the law

*Robin J Harman*

Legislation affects all aspects of our daily lives, and its influence on medical writing is no less comprehensive. There are also a number of non-legislative aspects governing medical writing that in effect come under the term 'good practice'. Some of these are also briefly considered here.

This text can be no more than an introduction to the many aspects of UK and EU legislative controls that apply to medical publishing. Writers are recommended to consult the most up-to-date documents when confronted with potential legislative issues in their work.

This chapter will consider:

- the law governing the advertising of medicines
- copyright law
- trademarks
- legislative aspects of writing for the internet
- the law governing racist remarks and writing
- patient consent issues
- ethical issues.

## Law governing the advertising of medicines

Those working in medical writing may become involved in creating advertisements for medicinal and related products (e.g. herbal products), or more commonly, writing material that explains how diseases occur and the ways in which medicinal products are used in their treatment.

The advertising of medicines is a complex area of pharmaceutical regulation, combining a potent mixture of statutory requirements and self-regulatory codes. The controls that apply depend upon which medium is being used (e.g. paper-based, or television and radio) and to whom the advertisement is directed (health professionals or the public). For more information on advertising, see Chapter 12.

Most people would agree that there needs to be a carefully controlled balance between, on the one hand, companies' legitimate desire to ensure that the products in which they have invested large sums generate a financial return, and on the other the need to ensure that inappropriate prescribing does not take place, or that people are not encouraged to take or use medicines inappropriately or unnecessarily. When that balance is upset, any one of a number of organisations can implement disciplinary measures against the advertiser.

There are also many specific requirements regarding the content of advertisements, both what can and cannot be included in them. These are to a large extent determined by the type of product being advertised, the size and location of the advertisement, and the target audience. (See also Chapter 12.)

The legislation applying to the advertising of medicinal products relates to advertisements in:

- articles in published journals, magazines and newspapers
- display on posters and public notices
- photographs
- films
- broadcast material
- video recordings
- electronic transmissions
- information posted on the internet
- product claims in point-of-sale materials, leaflets and booklets
- words that are part of a sound track or video recording
- relevant spoken words.

One area of controversy in the advertising of medicines is the boundary between advertising and appropriate educational material. Campaigns for 'disease awareness' and 'health promotion' often play an important part in helping people to understand the conditions from which they are suffering. However, there is a fine line between achieving this and potentially encouraging someone to specifically ask their GP for a particular prescription-only medicine, or to go to their pharmacy for an over-the-counter product. In such cases there is clearly a delicate balance to be struck between the legitimate provision of information and the advertising of a particular product for the treatment of a particular condition.

There is a complex web of UK and European legislation, and UK codes of practice that must be obeyed, that govern how medicinal products can be advertised. In the UK, Acts are Acts of Parliament that have been given the Royal Assent. Bills are legislation that is still going through the parliamentary process. Statutory Instruments (SIs) are secondary or subordinate legislation. They normally consist of an order, regulations, rules or a scheme and are made under powers conferred by primary legislation (an enabling Act). They are normally signed by a Minister and then laid before Parliament. On a given date they come into force and become law. In general, subordinate legislation makes detailed provisions and supplements the enabling Act. Subordinate legislation is also used when frequent or speedy changes in the law are required.

## Legislation governing advertising

As with all other aspects concerning the statutory control of medicinal products, both EU and UK legislation governs the advertising of medicines. Until 2001, there existed a vast panoply of different EU Regulations and Directives covering all aspects of the regulation of medicinal products. As Directives must be implemented into national legislation by each EU member state, various UK Statutory Instruments (SIs) on the advertising of medicines have been introduced.

### European legislation (see also Chapter 12)

In 1992 Council Directive 92/28/EC introduced specific requirements for advertising medicinal products. The scope of the original Directive 65/65/EEC was widened to incorporate requirements for advertising of homoeopathic medicinal products by Council Directive 92/73/EEC. In 2001, these Directives, and many more, were consolidated into a single piece of legislation, Council Directive 2001/83/EC, the 'Community Code Relating to Medicinal Products for Human Use'. The content and control of advertising are covered in Title VIII of this Directive. Since 2001, the Community Code has been further amended by Directive 2004/27/EC. A further amendment to the Community Code provided by Council Directive 2004/24/EC is that, from 30 October 2005, the same controls that apply to all medicinal products also apply to the advertising of herbal medicines.

In addition to specific pharmaceutical legislation, there is other European legislation that regulates the advertising of medicines. The ban on advertising POMs (prescription-only medicines) to the public defined in pharmaceutical legislation is made specific for advertising on television by Council Directive 97/36/EEC, the Television without Frontiers Directive.

### UK legislation (see also Chapter 12)

In the UK, two types of legislation exist: legislation that is directly applicable to medicinal products, and legislation that affects the advertising of medicines. The principal initial legislation, the Medicines Act 1968, controls all matters relating to medicinal products and came into effect on 1 September 1971. Part VI covered the promotion of medicines, but this has largely been superseded by later legislation.

Most of the other controls are operated through SIs and are listed in Table 19.1.

Under the above legislation, most products are classified as 'relevant medicinal products'. In other words, they either claim to or actually do treat or prevent disease in humans or animals. Other products that fall outside this definition include homoeopathic medicines, which are covered by Product Licences of Right, and unlicensed herbal medicines.

Such products are also governed by legislation that controls their advertising. The Medicines (Advertising of Medicinal Products) (No 2) Regulation 1975 (SI No 1326) applies to products such as Product Licences of Right. Under its provision, the information relating to advertising of such products issued to health professionals must be consistent with the data sheet, and the advertisement must state that a data sheet will be sent on request to any doctor or dentist.

Also applicable to Product Licences of Right are The Medicines (Labelling and Advertising to the Public) Regulations 1978 (SI No 41), which had previously also applied to 'relevant medicinal products' but were amended to no longer do so.

Other indirect legislation also has an impact on the advertising of medicines. The Cancer Act 1939 prohibits certain advertisements relating to cancer (as opposed to the restrictions on medicinal products used to treat cancer, which are described below).

Advertising in general, including that of medicines, is also subject to control by the Trade Descriptions Act 1968 and the Control of Misleading Advertisements Regulations 1988 (SI 1988/915; see Table 19.1). The legislation is administered by the Department of Trade and Industry.

As so much advertising of non-prescription medicinal products now takes place on television, it is unsurprising that there are separate parts of the legislation governing broadcasting that control such advertising. The relevant legislation comprises the Broadcasting Acts of 1990 and 1996, and the Communications Act 2003, which are administered by the Office of Communications (OFCOM) (see also page 191). The

**Table 19.1** Statutory Instruments (SIs) that control the promotion and advertising of medicinal products in the UK

| Statutory Instrument | Action |
|---|---|
| Control of Misleading Advertisement Regulations SI 1988/915 | Implement Council Directive 84/450/EEC. Require the Director-General of Fair Trading to review complaints about misleading advertisements (that are not broadcast on television or radio) and where they have not already been adequately considered by local trading standards departments or the profession's self-regulatory bodies. Also cover comparative advertising. Administered by the UK Department of Trade and Industry |
| Medicines (Advertising) Regulations 1994 SI No 1932 (the 'Advertising Regulations') | Implement Title VIII of Directive 2001/83/EC (previously Directive 92/28/EC) into UK law. Covers advertising of medicines (including homoeopathic medicines) to the public and to health professionals. Breaches are criminal offences, and penalties are specified |
| Medicines (Monitoring of Advertising) Regulations 1994 SI No 1933 (the 'Monitoring Regulations') | Implement Articles 97, 98 (part), and 99 of Directive 2001/83/EC. Specifies procedures whereby advertisements are considered to be inconsistent with the advertising regulations can be acted upon, either by reference to an administrative body or by civil proceedings |
| Medicines for Human Use (Marketing Authorisations Etc) Regulations 1994 SI No 3144 | Implement various European Directives covering medicines for human use. Schedule 7 of these Regulations amends some aspects of SI 1994/1932 |
| Medicines (Advertising) Amendment Regulations 1996 SI No 1552 | Amend SI 1994/1932 to allow advertising of products for prevention of neural tube defects and for the treatment of symptoms of strains or sprains, or the pain or stiffness of rheumatic or non-serious arthritic conditions |
| Medicines (Advertising and Monitoring of Advertising) (Amendment) Regulations 1999 SI No 267 | Further amends SI 1994/1932 and SI 1994/1933. Introduces a statutory procedure for making decisions on alleged breaches of the legislation on advertising, and permits written representations to Health Ministers before they reach a decision on alleged breaches and a procedure to publish corrective statements |

(continued)

**Table 19.1**  *Continued*

| Statutory Instrument | Action |
| --- | --- |
| Medicines (Monitoring of Advertising) Amendment Regulations 1999 SI No 784 | Amend SI 1994/1933 and SI 1999/267 and clarify the maximum penalty for summary conviction of an offence under advertising legislation |
| Communications Act 2003 (Amendment of the Medicines (Monitoring of Advertising) Regulations Order 2003 SI 3093 | Amend SI 1994/1933 as a result of the Communications Act 2003 and the regulatory functions taken on by OFCOM, which were previously the responsibility of the Independent Television Commission, the Radio Authority, and the Welsh Authority (for Channel S4C) |
| Medicines (Advertising) Amendment Regulations 2004 SI No 1480 | Amend SI 1994/1932 and remove the prohibition on advertising to the public of medicinal products for the treatment, prevention, and diagnosis of certain diseases. The ban on advertising medicinal products for chronic insomnia, diabetes and other metabolic diseases, malignant diseases, serious infectious diseases, and sexually transmitted diseases remained in force until October 2005 |

most recent legislation delegates to OFCOM the regulatory functions previously held by the Independent Television Code and the Radio Authority, and in particular the ability to regulate advertising standards.

Some of OFCOM's regulatory functions, including that relating to advertising of medicinal products, are delegated to self-regulatory bodies under the Contracting Out (Functions Relating to Broadcast Advertising) and Specification of Relevant Functions Order 2004, SI 2004/1975. This covers both television and radio advertising. For more information on regulatory bodies in advertising, see page 190.

### Statutory controls

To understand how the EU and UK legislation controls the advertising of medicinal products, a primary prerequisite is a legal definition of 'advertising'. Under Title VIII, Article 86 of the EU Community Code, Council Directive 2001/83/EC, 'advertising' includes:

*'. . . any form of door-to-door information, canvassing activity or induce-ment designed to promote the prescription, sale, supply or consumption of medicinal products'.*

The definition covers advertising to the general public, to persons qual-ified to prescribe or supply medicinal products, visits by medical sales representatives to persons medically qualified to prescribe them, and the supply of samples of medicinal products. It also refers to the contentious issue of inducements that can be offered, be they gifts of money or in kind, sponsorship of promotional meetings or of scientific congresses, and the payment of travelling and accommodation expenses associated with such meetings.

The legislation ensures that advertising of a medicinal product is only allowed if the product has a valid marketing authorisation. It also states that the advertisement must:

- comply with the SPC (Summary of Product Characteristics)
- encourage rational use
- not be misleading.

## Compliance with the Summary of Product Characteristics

An advertisement must comply with all parts of the approved SPC. In other words, it cannot promote a medicine by stating that it works out-side the approved therapeutic indications, nor in a patient group for whom the medicine is not approved. One example of a breach of the leg-islation would be to use an image of a young child in an advertisement when no formal approval has been given for use of the product in children.

## Rational use

An advertisement is also required to encourage the rational use of the medicinal product: how it is taken, the route of administration, who should use it, and when any special precautions should be observed. An advertisement should not imply that the product can cure a condi-tion when in reality it only acts to ameliorate the symptoms. Similarly, comments by others, who may or may not be qualified to make such statements, should be avoided when there is no factual evidence to support them.

*Not be misleading*

Finally, the most 'catch-all' provision of the legislation is the injunction that the advertisement must not be misleading. Potential benefits and the minimisation of possible risks must not be presented in such a way as to confuse or mislead.

*Informing appropriate personnel of future medicines*

'Abridged' advertising of medicinal products that do not as yet have a valid marketing authorisation is allowed in exceptional circumstances. If a company wishes to advise hospital budget holders or health authorities of the future launch of a product that could have a major impact on their expenditure, this is permitted. However, it is unlikely that this material would be addressed to any prescriber: it is solely for financial administration purposes.

## The role of the MHRA

As well as ensuring that all medicinal products in the UK are of an acceptable quality, safety and efficacy, the Agency has a legal obligation to promote the safe use of medicines. This statutory role underpins the system of self-regulation operated by the prescription-only and non-prescription medicines industries.

Four primary tasks are defined within the legislation:

* pre-vetting material for publication (in particular circumstances)
* monitoring published advertisements
* dealing with complaints received about advertising
* ensuring that any necessary sanctions are applied appropriately.

*Pre-vetting of advertising*

Although most companies do not have to submit their advertisements for pre-vetting prior to publication, those that do generally are happy to do so when asked by the MHRA. It is more common for pre-vetting to be applied when a newly approved product is initially placed on the market, when there has been a switch of legal status (e.g. from POM to P), or where previous advertising has resulted in sanctions applied by the MHRA.

The pre-vetting period can last up to 6 months, and usually only applies to a specific product rather than the company's entire portfolio (unless earlier breaches in the advertising regulations were particularly extreme). The advertising material submitted for pre-vetting should in effect be that which is ready for release (i.e. all internal quality assessments will have taken place). The Agency's own assessment will take 5 working days to complete. For further information about the vetting of advertisements by the MHRA, see page 193.

### Monitoring current advertisements

All the health professional and consumer journals are scanned and monitored for the content and format of the published advertisements. If the Agency believes that an aspect of the advertisement does not comply with the regulations, the marketing authorisation holder will be contacted. If the information supplied by the company is less than satisfactory, the procedure for initiating a complaint will be followed.

### Dealing with complaints

All complaints are initially assessed by the MHRA, but any further action depends on whether there has been a statutory breach (i.e. of the legislation) or one of the self-regulatory codes of practice has been broken. The decision on future action is made by the Agency. Complaints that are dealt with by the self-regulatory codes of practice will be considered in later sections that explain in detail the codes for both POMs and non-prescription medicines.

If a complaint about a broadcast advertisement is received solely by the Advertising Standards Authority (Broadcast), or by both the MHRA and the ASA (Broadcast), it is the responsibility of the ASA (Broadcast) to deal with it. When a complaint is received by the MHRA, it is acknowledged and an anonymised copy sent to the advertiser, together with a request for a response and any supporting material to deal with the complaint. Complaints are dealt with at weekly MHRA Advertising Unit meetings, although more rapid action can be taken if the Agency believes that continued use of the advertisement is likely to pose a serious health risk. Responses to any feedback then sent to the marketing authorisation holder company are normally expected within 7 working days of their receipt (unless the company has voluntarily suspended or withdrawn the advertisement, in which case more time would be allowed).

It is unusual for a complaint not to be dealt with quickly and amicably, either because the Agency believes that the complaint has no basis, or because the company recognises its validity and takes appropriate action. If the legislation has been breached, the MHRA will define what those breaches are and recommend the action the company needs to take. This may include amending or withdrawing the advertisement (and submitting the amended copy to the Agency prior to re-issuing it), or issuing a corrective statement. It may also be decided by the MHRA that future advertising needs to be submitted for pre-vetting.

### Application of appropriate sanctions

A misleading advertisement may have resulted in inappropriate prescribing and a potential risk to public health. In more extreme cases, it is necessary for the company to issue a corrective statement to the target audience that would have been likely to see the original advertisement. The MHRA recommends the following format:

- an opening statement, which indicates that the information is a corrective statement issued at the MHRA's request
- a description of the case, detailing the location of the original advertisement, the date(s) of publication, the type of promotional material, and whether it has now been withdrawn
- a statement indicating in what way the advertising regulations were breached (without further repeating the offending text) and what the MHRA has now requested should be stated about the promotion of the product
- an expression of regret and apology
- contact details for any readers who might require further information.

The MHRA is also willing to give any company, advertising agency or trade association advice about a specific advertisement and its suitability for publication prior to its being issued. If, however, any advice regarding suggested amendments is not implemented, and the advertisement is still in breach of the statutory controls, the same sanctions remain applicable.

## Self-regulatory controls

Allied to the statutory controls provided by UK and EU legislation are the self-regulatory controls on advertising, which are frequently used as the primary tool for resolving problems. A considerable number of organisations are involved in implementing self-regulation. Their roles in the control of medicines, pre-vetting of advertising material, and investigation of complaints are summarised in Table 19.2.

## Copyright

Copyright is an essential part of the fabric of society, but the controls on it are frequently ignored or flouted. Copyright is in effect a form of intellectual property. When you undertake medical writing you no doubt expect to be paid for the work you have done (unless it is writing 'original' research papers for publication in a professional journal). Your being paid is a result of the publisher charging those wishing to read your written material, whether in the form of a subscription to a journal or the purchase of a book. (Alternatively, many publications oriented to the medical profession are funded through the advertising they contain.)

Without copyright to prevent people using and photocopying published information (although a certain amount of copying is still legally acceptable, this revenue would not be forthcoming and author payment would not be possible. The principle applies not only to the written word, but also to music (provided on CDs and DVDs), films and computer software.

However, there is rarely anything completely original in the material that anyone writes: there is invariably some source or sources from which the information has been derived. The issue in copyright is in determining how much it is legally permissible to use.

### Private use

Copyright also impinges on the photocopying of source material for current or later use — something that is frequently undertaken with a view to its use solely for 'private study'. However, if the copied material is to be the basis for writing new material, there is some legal debate as to whether that activity constitutes 'private use'.

### Internet copyright

The advent of the internet has also clouded copyright issues. The internet is often mistakenly considered to be a 'copyright-free' zone, but the same national laws apply to material published on the net as to paper-based products. Indeed, many websites contain copyright declarations that require users to abide by their terms. These declarations in effect act as a licence between the copyright holder and the user.

**Table 19.2** Self-regulatory bodies for the advertising of medicines

| Body | Applicability | Functions | Contact details |
|---|---|---|---|
| Prescription Medicines Code of Practice Authority (PMCPCA) | Prescription-only medicines | Operates independently of the ABPI. Administers the ABPI Code of Practice for the Pharmaceutical Industry, which applies to the promotion of medicines to UK health professionals and to appropriate administrative staff, and to information made available to the public about POMs. The Code also applies to some of those areas that are non-promotional (e.g. disease awareness campaigns). The Code is drawn up after consultation with the British Medical Association (BMA), the Royal Pharmaceutical Society of Great Britain (RPSGB), and the Medicines and Healthcare products Regulatory Agency (MHRA). The Code also refers to training of all personnel, including medical representatives | 12 Whitehall London SW1A 2DY Tel: 020 7930 9677 www.pmcpa.org.uk |
| Proprietary Association of Great Britain (PAGB) | Non-prescription (over-the-counter) medicines | The Consumer Code lays down standards for the advertising of over-the-counter medicines to the general public. Also operates a Professional Code of Practice for advertising directed at persons qualified to prescribe or supply medicines. The Codes are drawn up in consultation with the Medicines and Healthcare products Regulatory Agency (MHRA), the Advertising Standards Authority (ASA), Codes of Advertising Practice (CAP), the Office of Communications (OFCOM), Broadcast Advertising Clearance Centre (BACC), and the Radio Advertising Clearance Centre (RACC). Training programmes are also offered | Vernon House Sicilian Avenue London WC1A 2QH Tel: 020 7242 8331 www.pagb.co.uk |
| Health Food Manufacturers' Association (HFMA) | Specialist health products | Operates a Code of Advertising Practice covering advertising to the public and to healthcare professionals | 63 Hampton Court Way Thames Ditton, Surrey KT17 0LT Tel: 020 8398 1819 www.hfma.co.uk |

| Organisation | Sector | Description | Contact |
|---|---|---|---|
| British Dental Trade Association (BDTA) | Dental products | Comprises a group of manufacturers, wholesalers, distributors and suppliers of products and services to the dental profession. Provides a Code of Practice for its members | Merritt House Hill Avenue Amersham HP6 5BQ Tel: 01494 431010 www.bdta.org.uk |
| Office of Communications (OFCOM) | Communications industries | Independent regulatory and competition authority which has a statutory role to ensure that the contents of programmes meet appropriate standards | Riverside House 2a Southwark Bridge Road London E1 9HA Tel: 020 7981 3040 www.ofcom.org.uk |
| Advertising Standards Authority (ASA) and Committees of Advertising Practice | Non-broadcast media | Administers the Code of Advertising, Sales Promotion and Direct Marketing for non-broadcast advertising, and provides a point of contact for all complaints about the content of advertisements. From November 2004 it also assumed the same powers in respect of radio and television advertisements, and works in a co-regulatory partnership with OFCOM for this | Mid City Place 71 High Holborn London WC1V 6QT Tel: 020 7492 2222 www.asa.org.uk |

The primary difficulties arise with the internet because of its use beyond national boundaries, when different countries' laws on copyright may be at variance with each other. However, trying to protect copyright across national borders and claiming a breach of copyright is an even more complex and expensive process than trying to do so within one's own national boundaries. Because of this, many governments (both national and supranational) and international organisations are currently attempting to define the rules by which such activities as breaching copyright can be legally and effectively enforced. (For more information about internet copyright, see page 416.)

### Legislative framework

The current UK legislation covering copyright is under review, following the passing of EU Directive 2001/29/EC that is currently being implemented into UK law by the Department of Trade and Industry. The European legislation will further modify the UK Copyright, Designs and Patents Act 1988 to take account of the advances in electronic publishing and all other forms of presentation of information. The implementing legislation in the UK is the Copyright and Related Rights Regulations 2003, SI No. 2498, which came into force on 31 October 2003.

The most important changes that resulted from the new legislation were to remove some exceptions to copyright, including fair dealing and library privileges, and copying that is carried out for commercial purposes. In other words, the law now prevents any limited copying without the consent of the copyright holder if it is undertaken for a commercial purpose, even if the copies are for research or private study. If the copying is indeed for non-commercial purposes, the rules governing the amount that can be copied, the requirement for it to be 'fair dealing', or the need to sign a declaration remain as always. (This change is discussed in more detail below.)

### Copyright of other's work

There are many copyright issues concerning the information you may use in writing. In essence, all original information created by a company or an individual that shows a degree of labour, skill or judgement is automatically bound by copyright. Copyright protection does not extend to names, titles or short phrases, but does cover other original combinations of such material (e.g. as a logo or other distinctive mark).

The original work is owned by the person who created it or, if that person is employed by a company or organisation, by the body that asked the individual to create the work. Freelance or commissioned work usually belongs to the person who is author; however, if it was written in response to a written contract for service, it will belong to the commissioner.

Under UK law, as defined by the 1988 Copyright, Designs, and Patents Act, copyright applies to any form of 'literary' work. This may be books, journal articles, letters, or, in an electronic age, a table or compilation, a computer program or a database.

The period of copyright protection for literary, dramatic, musical or artistic works is 70 years from the end of the calendar year in which the last of the authors dies. If the author is unknown, copyright protection is also 70 years from the end of the year in which the work was created or made available to the public. The period of protection for sound recordings and broadcasts is set at 50 years.

## Consequences of changes to 'fair dealing' concepts

Under the legislation, it is forbidden to copy work without the consent of the copyright owner. However, various acts concerning the copy-righted work are allowed under the guise of 'fair dealing'. However, this concept has changed significantly with EU Directive 2001/29/EC, which became part of UK law on 31 October 2003. From this date, copying of material for research purposes and for private study is no longer considered to be 'fair dealing' if that research or private study is carried out for commercial purposes.

The criteria for what constitutes 'commercial' purposes will prob-ably encompass far more activities than are normally considered likely, according to guidance notes issued by the British Library and the Copyright Licensing Agency. The term 'commercial' is taken to mean directly or indirectly income-generating, rather than just 'profit-making'. If you are writing for any organisation that expects to generate income from your contributions, this is considered 'commercial' under the legislation. The following would also be considered as being for 'commercial' purposes:

- if you are a research student at a university carrying out research sponsored by a commercial organisation
- publishing a paper in a publication that will earn royalties or other income at a later stage

- research relevant to development in a commercial company
- work done by an information broker for clients.

The legislation has also changed the way in which libraries can copy material and send it to writers for their use. Previously, it was possible to make a single copy and this would fall within the remit of 'fair dealing' for research or private study. The recipient had only to sign a statement that the copy was required for such purposes. Now, however, this can only be done if the copy is definitely to be used only for non-commercial purposes. If a business or a person writing for income generation requests a copy, the library is now bound to charge a copyright fee.

As regards fair dealing and the internet, it is important to remember that downloading and printing material from a website is in effect an act of copying. Many sites have a copyright notice, and it is important for anyone writing for websites to ensure that such notices are prominently displayed.

## Copyright of your own work

Current copyright legislation gives exclusive economic and moral rights to an individual who owns copyright, allowing that individual to:

- copy the work
- issue copies to the public
- rent or lend work to the public
- perform, show or play the work in public
- broadcast the work, or show it on a cable programme service
- adapt the work, or do any of the above in relation to an adaptation.

The four moral rights are the right to:

- be identified as the author or director of the work
- object to derogatory treatment of a work
- object to false attribution of a work
- privacy in certain photographs and films.

Copyright is owned by the author or creator of a work, although if that individual is an employee, copyright will belong to the employer unless there has been previous agreement to the contrary. For example, the copyright of articles written by reporters for a newspaper belongs to the owners of the newspaper, not the reporter. This can have important consequences for protection against allegedly libellous material published in the newspaper.

If there is more than one author (e.g. in a multi-author book such as this), agreement on copyright ownership for each contribution will have been reached between the overseeing editor and the publishers. That agreement will then have been incorporated into the individual contracts for each contributor. (For more information on book publishing, see Chapter 22.)

## Copyright Licensing Agency

In order to provide a simple method of obtaining authorisation to copy, and thereby preventing the need to contact the author or copyright holder on an individual basis on each occasion, in 1982 the UK Copyright Licensing Agency (CLA) was created. The CLA licenses users to copy extracts from books, journals, magazines and periodicals, and collects fees from them for doing so. It then distributes these fees to authors, publishers and artists, and institutes legal proceedings against those it believes to be in breach of copyright.

The CLA is owned by its 120 000 members, who are the authors and 1500 book, journal, magazine and periodical publishers that it represents: the Authors' Licensing and Collecting Society and the Publishers Licensing Society. The CLA recommends that any organisation carrying out photocopying and scanning of copyright works should have a licence. In addition, any organisation that makes multiple copies or distributes copies internally should have a licence.

Business licences are granted based on the type of business and the number of employees. In return for a licence, any organisation can copy prescribed amounts from over 3 million UK titles and from 16 million titles from a range of countries worldwide. Reciprocal agreements between the CLA and other countries permits access to a wide number of other countries' works.

Importantly for medical writing, in May 2004 the CLA and the Association of the British Pharmaceutical Industry (ABPI) introduced a new model licence for pharmaceutical companies. This permits the unlimited photocopying, scanning and email delivery of articles from books, magazines, journals and periodicals, removing the need for individual member companies to seek additional clearances through the CLA's Rapid Clearance Service.

The novel feature of this licence was the inclusion of permission for systematic electronic storage, allowing electronic copies of certain materials on an intranet within a company. Equally, international distribution to affiliated companies is allowed, plus the supply of copies to regulatory authorities when submitting marketing authorisation applications.

## Useful address

Copyright Licensing Agency Ltd
90 Tottenham Court Road
London W1T 4LP
Tel: 020 7631 5555
*www.cla.co.uk*

## Trademarks and patents

It may seem strange to consider trademarks and patents when undertaking medical writing, but the law covering these topics has always been relevant to the information industry. When you write for a particular publication, and if it has been established for many years, it is likely that its appearance will be very familiar and have stayed the same for a long time. This building of a recognisable image with positive connotations can be vitally important in maintaining customer loyalty to a publication. The publisher may then want to ensure that no other publisher attempts to 'cash in' on that image, by registering it under a trademark. However, as with many other aspects of the law affecting medical writing, the advent of the internet has significantly complicated the law governing trademarks. Advertising or images deemed to be protected in one jurisdiction may clash with a similar trademark used legally in another country.

In essence a trademark, as defined by the Concise Oxford Dictionary, is:

> *'The name or other symbol used by a manufacturer or dealer to distinguish his products from those of competitors'.*

The most important aspect of a trademark is that the term or symbol applied to a particular product is readily recognisable, simple in appearance and eye-catching. If you are involved in medical writing and the repeated use of a particular drug name, it will rapidly become apparent why an easy-to-spell and easy-to-use name is so important. It is far easier to remember, and remembering the name will enhance the likelihood that it will be prescribed by a GP or suggested for over-the-counter prescribing.

Readily recognised trademarks are so important for the success of pharmaceuticals because prescribing physicians must rapidly become familiar with the new names of the drug, both generic and proprietary. If they fail to do so this will lead to obscurity for the drug and potentially financial disaster for the company, and an inability to recoup the considerable investment that has gone into the new product.

Similarly, it is vital that the trademark name be distinctive. It has been recognised that protection of intellectual property, including safeguarding the trademarked name, is essential to the success of the research and development process.

## Legislative aspects

The first legal register of trademarks and Trade Marks Registry was opened in London in 1876. The register entry of a word or symbol (e.g. logo) determines that it is a trademark and who owns it. The owner has exclusive use of the trademark and can prevent unauthorised use by a legal action for infringement. Further major legislation on trademarks was enacted in 1883, 1905 and 1938. More recent legislation has included:

- The Trade Marks (Amendment) Act 1984
- The Patents, Designs, and Trade Marks Act 1986
- The Copyright, Designs, and Patents Act 1988 (which for the first time in the UK rendered it a criminal offence to forge a trademark).

The legislation currently applicable in the UK is the Trade Marks Act 1994, which ensures that British law corresponds with that of the EU and with international law, especially that of the USA. It also simplifies and accelerates the processing of trademark applications by the UK Patent Office.

The law relating to trademarks is also modified by various Statutory Instruments. A list of those that have been applied since the 1994 Act is given in Table 19.3.

## The UK Patent Office

The registration of UK trademarks is dealt with by the Patent Office, which has two main offices (see Useful addresses, below); a Central Enquiry Unit (CEU) is located at the Welsh office. The CEU can provide general information on all aspects of intellectual property.

**Table 19.3**  UK Statutory Instruments applicable to trademarks

| Year | SI No | Title |
|------|-------|-------|
| 2004 | 949 | The Community Trade Mark (Amendment) Regulations 2004 |
| 2004 | 948 | The Trade Marks (International Registration (Amendment) Order 2004 |
| 2004 | 947 | The Trade Marks (Amendment) Rules 2004 |
| 2004 | 946 | The Trade Marks (Proof of Use, etc.) Regulations 2004 |
| 2002 | 2749 | The Copyright etc. and Trade Marks (Offences and Enforcement) Act 1002 (Commencement) Order 2002 |
| 2002 | 692 | The Trade Marks (International Registration) (Amendment) Order 2002 |
| 2001 | 3832 | The Trade Marks (Amendment) Rules 2001 |
| 2000 | 138 | The Trade Marks (International Registration) (Amendment) Order 2000 |
| 2000 | 137 | The Trade Marks (Fees) Rules 2000 |
| 2000 | 136 | The Trade Marks Rules 2000 |
| 1999 | 1899 | The Patents and Trade Marks (World Trade Organisation) Regulations |
| 1999 | 983 | The Register of Patent Agents and the Register of Trade Mark Agents (Amendment) Rules 1999 |
| 1998 | 1776 | The Trade Marks (Fees) Rules 1998 (revoked by SI 2000/137) |
| 1998 | 925 | The Trade Marks (Amendment) Rules 1998 (revoked by SI 2000/136) |
| 1996 | 1942 | The Trade Marks (Fees) Rules 1996 (revoked by SI 1998/1776) |
| 1996 | 1908 | The Community Mark Regulations 1996 |
| 1996 | 715 | The Trade Marks (International Registration) (Fees) Rules (Amendment) 1996 (revoked by SI 1996/1942) |
| 1996 | 714 | The Trade Marks (International Registration) Order 1996 |
| 1995 | 3175 | The Community Trade Mark (Fees) Regulations 1995 |
| 1995 | 2997 | The Trade Marks (Claims to Priority from Relevant Countries) (Amendment) Order 1995 |
| 1995 | 1444 | The Trade Marks (EC Measures Relating to Counterfeit Goods) Regulations 1995 |
| 1994 | 2803 | The Trade Marks (Claims to Priority from Relevant Countries) Order 1994 |
| 1994 | 2625 | The Trade Marks (Customs) Regulations 1994 |
| 1994 | 2584 | The Trade Marks (Fees) Rules 1994 (revoked by SI 1968/1942) |
| 1994 | 2583 | The Trade Marks Rules 1994 (revoked by SI 2000/136) |

The CEU provides general information on the Patent Office and its operation, and issues free information packs and literature. It can provide specific information on the law and practice relating to patents, trademarks, design and copyright, and will give information on specific UK and European patents, designs or trademarks. Enquiries will usually be answered within 5 days.

Public trademark searches can also be arranged and supervised by the CEU. These can be undertaken by members of the public or by agents at the South Wales offices. The register can be scanned and copies taken of case details; a search can also be carried out. The CEU can assist in this by word-searching or searching for a device (logos, smells and sounds). However, CEU staff can neither advise on whether a proposed trademark is likely to be registered, nor give advice on infringement issues.

### Filing to register a UK trademark

The three criteria that the Patent Office must apply to an application for registration of a new trademark are that it must:

- be distinctive
- not be deceptive
- not conflict with other registered trademarks.

An application form (TM3) is available from the Patent Office or can be downloaded from the internet (www.patent.gov.uk/dtrademk/how toapp.html), and is accompanied by guidance notes to assist in its completion. The cost of submitting the form to register a trademark is £200 for one class of goods/services and £50 for each additional class. The fee is intended to cover the average cost of the examination of the application. If for any reason it is not possible to complete registration of the trademark, these fees are non-refundable.

### Registration of the trademark

A trademark is first advertised in the *Trade Marks Journal*, whereupon others can make 'observations' on the application or oppose it.

### 'Observations'
These can only be made if the application is made under the 1994 Act (see above).

### Opposing the application

Applications can be opposed using a Notice of Opposition form (TM7), stating why the application is being opposed and submitting a fee of £200. These items must be sent within the time limits specified by the Patent Office. The Registrar will send notice of the opposition to the applicant, who can submit a defence of their application. After an optional cooling-off period, hearings may be arranged (if requested by either party) after the evidence has been submitted. The Registrar will then issue a written decision, which usually includes an award of costs to be paid by the unsuccessful party to the successful one.

### Concluding the registration

If there is no opposition, and there are no remaining observations in its examination or proceedings in place against it, the trademark is formally recorded in the UK Register of Trade Marks 15 weeks later. The applicant becomes the 'proprietor' of the trademark (hence the term 'proprietary products' for pharmaceuticals).

Four weeks after recording in the Register, notice of registration is advertised in the *Trade Marks Journal* and the proprietor is issued with a Certificate of Registration. The date of registration is backdated to the date of application of the trademark.

All proprietors should recognise that the trademark is a valuable piece of intellectual property. To maintain it on the Register, it must be renewed every 10 years on the anniversary of the filing date. Changes that can be made to the trademark include:

- alterations in certain circumstances
- merging with other trademarks of which you are the proprietor
- licensing of its use by others with your permission
- surrendering the trademark partially or entirely.

If the owner of the trademark suspects that it is being counterfeited, the local Trading Standards Office, or Trading Standards Central, should be consulted.

### Useful addresses

The UK Patent Office
Cardiff Road
Newport
South Wales NP10 8QQ

Tel:          08459 500 505
Text phone: 08459 222 250
Fax:          01633 813 600
email:        *enquiries@patent.gov.uk*

or

The Patent Office
Harmsworth House
13–15 Bouverie Street
London EC4Y 8DP
Tel:   01633 813930
Fax:  01633 813 600

## Writing for the internet: legal aspects (see also Chapter 21)

In medical writing it may be necessary to assist in the preparation of websites that contain medical information. One of the objectives in making such information available on a website is to ensure that, when someone uses an internet search engine, that information is readily identified as a 'hit'.

### Meta-tags and trademark issues

Legally, one of the issues to be considered is the use of trademarks on the internet. One tool used in the preparation of websites to ensure that a 'hit' is as high as possible in the listings when a search is carried out is meta-tags. A meta-tag is hidden information that contains a summary of the information on the website. Basically, when a search engine is activated, the internet is scanned at very high speed and a database is created which consists of a list of words and information giving the location of the words being sought. If these 'hits' are also found in the meta-tags, the rating attached to the 'hit' will be higher than if they are not.

As the meta-tags may include one or more trademarks, following a test case the courts have determined that the Trade Marks Act 1994 (see above) does apply to them. As a consequence, registered trademarks belonging to others cannot be used within the meta-tags.

## Registering internet domain names

A domain name is an alphanumeric name that represents one or more IP (internet protocol) addresses and which is used in URLs (uniform resource locators) to point to specific websites. For example, the Royal Pharmaceutical Society's domain name is *www.rpsgb.org.uk*. This comprises rpsgb, which in this case is the registered trademark of the organisation that operates the website. The second portion of the domain name (in this case .org.uk, but other examples include .plc.uk and co.uk) is described as the top-level domain. There are many of these, some of which are listed below:

| | | |
|---|---|---|
| .com | .int | .pro |
| .net | .arpa | .info |
| .edu | .coop | .name |
| .gov | .aero | .museum |
| .mil | . biz | |

The third element is the country code top-level domain, of which there are about 240 worldwide. A registry maintains each element of the domain name: in the UK, applications to register the top-level domain .uk have to be made to Nominet (*www.nominet.org.uk*).

A mechanism for checking whether a domain name has previously been registered, called WHOIS, is available and can be found (among other places) at interNicUK (*www.internic.co.uk*). However, each of the other top-level domain names must be registered with separate organisations or through domain registration companies, which abound on the internet.

## Legal issues concerning domain names

When domain names first became available attempts were made by some individuals and organisations to register well-known names (so-called 'cyber squatting'). One intention was to seek payment — in some cases very high payments — from the organisations that might wish to use those names. Alternatively, the original purchaser of the domain name might be trying to take advantage of the fact that people would be drawn to their website (and to goods and services offered on it) because it appeared to be run by the well-known organisation.

Other problems have arisen in the registering of domain names where variants on a famous name have been registered but with some derogatory suffix — commonly 'sucks'.

In cases where legal disputes have arisen about the ownership and use of domain names, a number of different precedents have been set. The first relates to two organisations that want to use the same domain name because they have the same trading name, although the services they offer are different. In this case, the principle of 'first come, first served' has been upheld by the courts and that the Trade Marks Act 1994 has not been infringed.

In the case of cyber squatting, the courts have determined that, if the original purchaser of the domain name had been looking to act fraudulently, the domain name must be returned for the use of the company who would be recognised by most people as the owner of that particular trademark.

Disputes on the use and abuse of domain names are often referred for arbitration to a California-based global organisation, ICANN (the Internet Corporation for Assigned Names and Numbers), which was formed in 1998 (www.icann.org). As a result, there have been relatively few that have reached national or international courts. In most of the cases held under the auspices of ICANN the outcomes tended to reflect a balance between the rights of protection afforded to trademark owners and the right to free speech. In essence, a domain name will be allowed if it is not already being used, and if it is to be used honestly in the commercial field.

## Racist and religious language

Although it should never be a part of writing on medical topics, those writing for medical publications should be aware of the limitations that apply to the use of language that might incite racial or religious hatred. The UK law on racial hatred, the Public Order Act 1986, s.17, defines it as:

> '. . . hatred against a group of persons in Great Britain defined by reference to colour, race, nationality (including citizenship) or ethnic or national origins'.

There has been some confusion as to the meaning of some of the terms (e.g. 'ethnic') in this legislation. It has been determined in law that for a group of persons to be considered ethnic, the members of that group must consider themselves to be a distinct community defined by certain primary characteristics:

- a long shared history, of which the group is conscious as distinguishing it from other groups, and the memory of which is kept alive

- a cultural tradition of its own, including family and social customs and manners, often but not necessarily associated with religious observance.

These characteristics must also be recognized by others outside the group. Secondary features of an ethnic group include a common language, a common geographical origin, and a common religion different from that of neighbouring groups or of the general community surrounding it.

There are several offences relating to race hatred. In medical writing, the most important are those that concern non-broadcast material.

## Legal definitions for non-broadcast material

Under the 1986 Act it is an offence to use abusive, insulting or threatening behaviour or to display any written material which is threatening, abusive or insulting if that material is intended to stir up racial hatred. Equally, it is an offence to distribute or publish such material. It is important to recognise that, even if an article does not itself stir up or suggest racial hatred, the mere fact that its publication could lead to racial hatred being created makes it an offence for it to be published.

The seriousness of the offence is borne out by the maximum punishment being 7 years' imprisonment. Custodial sentences have also often been imposed by the courts.

There are also plans (November 2005) to introduce legislation to extend the existing criminal offence of incitement to racial hatred contained in the Public Order Act 1986 to create a new offence of incitement to religious hatred. The proposals will make it an offence to use words, behaviour or written material that is threatening, abusive or insulting with the intention or likely effect that hatred will be stirred up against a group of people targeted because of their religious beliefs or lack of them. It was felt that new legislation was needed to protect individuals from those who foment hatred against people because of their religious beliefs. The legislation prohibiting the incitement of racial hatred protects Sikhs and Jews, but not Muslims, Hindus, Rastafarians, Christians or others. This is because Sikhs and Jews are included in the definition of a racial group, but other religions are not. Some extremists have exploited this loophole, using religious terms to identify victims whom they would have previously identified using racial terms.

It is not intended that the new legislation will prevent people:

- telling jokes about, or making fun of, religions
- causing offence to followers of a religion
- debating or criticising the beliefs, teachings or practices of a religion or its followers, for example by claiming that they are false or harmful

- proselytising one's own religion, or urging followers of a different religion to cease practising theirs
- expressing antipathy or dislike of particular religions or their followers.

Rather, it is intended to protect the believer not the belief. There is a clear difference between criticism of a religion and the criminal act of inciting hatred against a person or persons on the basis of their religion (or lack thereof). Only if a person used threatening, abusive or insulting words, actions or material with the intent or likely effect that hatred would be stirred up by the actions listed above would they be at risk of prosecution.

At the time of going to press, the legislation had been debated in the UK House of Commons and passed to the House of Lords. However, the Lords had voted against the proposed legislation, and it has therefore not yet been passed into law.

## Patient consent issues

It is important not to breach confidentiality when undertaking medical writing, either of the patients whose clinical histories may form a part of that writing, or of the medical staff who have provided the information. The UK General Medical Council has issued guidance on giving information about patients to the press and in written information.

---

➤ Remember that information a doctor has acquired in their professional capacity should be regarded as confidential, whether or not that information is also in the public domain.

---

Whenever possible, obtain explicit consent from patients before discussing matters relating to their care, whether or not the patients' names or other identifying information is to be revealed. Explicit consent must be obtained if patients will be identifiable from the details disclosed.

---

➤ Remember that patients can be identified from information other than names and addresses. Details which in combination may reveal patients' identities include their condition or disease, their age, their occupation, the area in which they live, their medical history, and the size of their family.

---

Always consider and act in accordance with the best medical interests of patients when responding to invitations to speak to the media.

## Data Protection Act 1998

When considering patient consent issues, the Data Protection Act 1998 (which enforces EU Directive 95/46/EC) cannot be ignored. The government body that oversees its application is the Information Commissioner, and in May 2002 it published guidance on the application of the Act: *Use and Disclosure of Health Data*. In this, the personal data that are subject to a duty of confidence have the following characteristics:

- the information is not in the public domain, or readily available from another source.
- the information has a certain degree of sensitivity, such as medical data.
- the information has been provided with the expectation that it will only be used or disclosed for particular purposes.

The courts have recognised three exceptions to the duty of confidence:

- where there is a legal compulsion
- where there is an overriding duty to the public
- where the individual to whom the information relates has consented.

The EU Directive defines consent as:

> '... any freely given specific and informed indication of his wishes by which the data subject signifies his agreement to personal data relating to him being processed'.

Most importantly, any consent given by the individual must be informed: in other words, they must know what the information is likely to be used for. Secondly, there must be some degree of choice in giving that consent. Consent given under any form of coercion or duress is not consent at all. The consent given should be optional, and if it is withheld, without adverse consequences for the individual. Thirdly, there must be some sort of indication of the consent having been given. This may be implicit (without a formal record having been taken) or explicit (as is the case in drug trials, when all aspects of the course of treatment are laid before the individual).

## Ethical issues

One of the major difficulties faced in medical writing is being able to discern poor or potentially inappropriate material. Publishing medical information is big business. Equally important are the careers of those who seek to publish their results in leading medical journals: to add such journals to their CV can have significant consequences.

In light of real and perceived problems with the ethics and intellectual honesty of some of those undertaking research, in 1997 a Committee on Publication Ethics (COPE) was formed to try to bring respectability and uniformity of standards to medical publishing. A corresponding international organisation also exists (the World Association of Medical Editors — WAME).

## COPE

COPE (*www.publicationethics.org.uk*) is a forum where the editors of peer-reviewed journals can discuss issues related to the integrity of the scientific record. It supports and encourages editors to report, catalogue and instigate investigations into ethical problems in the publication process.

The major objective of COPE is to provide a sounding board for editors who were struggling with how best to deal with possible breaches in research and publication ethics. Its formation has been well received by an increasing number of publishers, practising physicians, authors, editors, and all those involved in the teaching of medicine and scientific research.

Individual cases are discussed at quarterly COPE meetings and via written submission to the committee; advice is offered through correspondence.

COPE's work was extended after preliminary discussions with the ethics committee of WAME (*www.wame.org*) to include:

- What happens when an editor suspects that data have been falsified or fabricated, but there is insufficient conclusive evidence?
- What should be done under these circumstances?
- What action should be taken?
- How soon should a response be made?
- Should a further investigation be conducted to obtain more evidence?
- What, if any, sanctions need to be applied?

Some of these issues are addressed in anonymous cases submitted to COPE. They illustrate particular aspects of the complexities of publication ethics, and also provide a framework for tackling this pervasive and pernicious form of research misconduct.

COPE produces guidelines on good publication practice and a code of conduct for editors of biomedical journals. The guidelines on good publication practice cover:

- study design and ethical approval
- data analysis
- authorship
- conflicts of interest
- the peer review process
- redundant publication
- plagiarism
- duties of editors
- media relations
- advertising
- how to deal with misconduct.

They also deal with some of the most pressing problems likely to be faced when involved in medical writing. For example, under 'Authorship', the guidance stresses that the number of authors stated should reflect only those who have had an active role in the work being submitted. Similarly, 'redundant publication' refers to the submission of two or more papers without full cross-reference that share the same hypothesis, data, discussion points or conclusions.

# 20

## Writing and editing books

*Paul J Weller*

Writing or editing a book can be a daunting, exhausting, but ultimately exhilarating experience. On rare occasions it may even be financially rewarding. This chapter aims to describe something about the book publishing industry, how to get published, and the mechanics of writing and editing books.

### The book publishing industry

Book publishing is very much a global industry and is dominated by a number of large multinational corporations that often have extensive commercial operations, of which publishing is only one. At the other end of the scale are smaller commercial businesses, family-run publishing houses, professional societies, and academic institutions that often concentrate on niche publishing for a specific audience.

Worldwide, it is estimated that approximately 1 million books are published annually. The UK leads the world in book publishing, with an estimated 160 000 titles produced in 2004, an increase of 35 000 over those published in 2002. For comparison, approximately 65 000 titles are published annually in the USA.

Broadly speaking, book publishing can be divided into two types: trade publishing, and academic or professional. Trade publishing includes fiction and non-fiction books that are aimed at the general reader. These titles have a potentially enormous market and sales can consequently be very large. Consider the 'Harry Potter' books by JK Rowling, for example, which have enthralled millions of children and adults worldwide and have made the author a multimillionaire.

In contrast, academic publishing caters for a smaller and more specialised audience, e.g. history, law, medicine, and accounts for about 40% of the books published in the UK. Academic publishing and publishers may be further divided into scientific, technical and medical (STM) publishers, and further still into individual subject specialties such as chemistry, engineering, medicine, nursing, pharmacy, etc. The distinction is important when considering a publisher for your book (see below). Out of the 160 000 or so titles currently published annually in the UK about 3500 are medical books.

## Where to start

The main difference between trade and academic publishing is the audience for the work. Trade publishing, as it is aimed at the general reader, requires particular publishers with the skills to market books to the public and bookstores and to compete against the best-selling titles. Trade publishing is extremely competitive and it is notoriously difficult for the novice to get published. Such publishing is outside the scope of this chapter, but there are many helpful publications and organisations that can provide advice for those tempted to try their hand at such writing.

With academic publishing, in contrast, it is relatively easier to have your book published. Indeed, if you reach a senior enough position in your chosen field, publish enough research papers, or speak regularly at conferences it is more than likely that you will be approached by a publisher inviting you to write or edit a book. In this instance, rather like being 'headhunted' for a job, the publisher will have identified you as a likely candidate to produce a book on a subject about which you have special knowledge and which they believe will have a ready audience. This is known as being commissioned. Although this is flattering, it is just the beginning of writing and publishing a book, and much the same processes have to be considered as if the idea for the book was your own.

## The idea

Although you're inspired to write a book, before doing anything more, and certainly before you rush off to start hitting your computer keyboard, think very carefully about your idea. Ask yourself:

- What is my book about?
- Who is it for?
- Why is my book needed?
- Am I qualified to write it — do I have the knowledge, ability, and most importantly the time?

You should think rationally about all of these questions and do some research to answer them. Even at this stage, the first rule of writing, or editing, a book is that planning and preparation are never wasted. Any publisher you approach will want detailed answers to these questions so that they can evaluate your book proposal.

## What is my book about?

Consider what has been the trigger to make you think of writing a book. Perhaps you are an academic who teaches undergraduates a specialist course, and are frustrated that there is no suitable textbook that you can recommend for them to read. Perhaps you are a researcher who wishes to bring together in a single volume a lifetime of research in a particular field. Whatever the topic of your book, think of a short descriptive title and then consider a brief description of what it is about — no more than a paragraph.

## Who are my readers?

Consider who you are writing the book for; think broadly, and consider both your main market and any secondary market. Perhaps it is a book for undergraduate medical students. Would it also be suitable for students of other healthcare disciplines, e.g. pharmacy? Would it be of interest in a number of countries, or just one? If you have an idea of the potential numbers of people who may be interested in your book then note this down; you should convey this information to any publisher you approach. For a publisher to even consider producing a book at a reasonable price it will probably need to sell at least 1000 copies. To do this, the potential market will need to be at least 10–20 times this number.

## Why is my book needed?

Consider why your book is needed. Perhaps your idea is a summary of a totally new field of research and is unique. Perhaps a previous book has been published on the subject but is now 20 years out of date. Perhaps there is a comprehensive and expensive book on the subject and you want to write a short, cheaper, introduction for a wider, non-specialist audience. Whatever your answer to this question, you should be diligent in your research of other similar titles that have been published. Look at bookshop and library holdings and web catalogues (such as Amazon) to consider similar titles. Note down their details, strengths, weaknesses, age, price, etc., and contrast them with your own proposed book. If you find a recently published book very similar to your own idea you may have a very hard time convincing any publisher to produce it. However, even if there are lots of books close to your own idea do not necessarily be disheartened. There is an old publishing saying: 'If there are 100 books on a subject then publish the 101st, because someone must be buying them'.

### Am I qualified to write the book?

Consider why you should be the one to write a book on a specific subject. Do you have particular knowledge or skills that make you an expert? Do you have the ability to write informatively for your chosen audience? Ideally, you should have some demonstrable previous writing experience, such as research papers, book chapters or a thesis. When approaching a publisher enclose a CV and a publications list to demonstrate your expertise or previous writing background. An experienced writer will probably be more highly valued than a novice. Likewise, a Nobel Prize-winner will be more highly sought-after than a PhD student.

Finally, consider the impact writing a book will have on your sanity, relationships and work. Writing a book, though rewarding in many ways, is enormously challenging and time-consuming and requires considerable determination. Most probably you will be writing as a 'hobby' in addition to all the other things that were previously happening in your life, and this will almost certainly mean you will have to give something up to make time for 'the book'. It is generally better to write little and often, and it is a good idea to think about your commitments. Could you devote every Sunday morning for the next 12 months to writing, for example? Writing a book should be enjoyable, so if you think it would become a chore it is probably better not to even start.

### Finding a publisher

The key to finding the right publisher is to do your homework. Again, look in bookstores, libraries and online book catalogues to identify publishers who publish work in your chosen subject. In addition, check the various publishing and writers' directories. Such directories list publishers and include the type of subject they publish; they also often indicate the number of titles published each year by them. This is obviously a useful guide to the scale of the publisher. The more titles published, the more infrastructure the publisher will have, for example it may have better global marketing capability than a smaller publisher. However, bigger doesn't always mean better, and size is no indicator of quality. Smaller publishers may have a niche market to themselves, or may have more prestige, e.g. be part of a professional body or society. Smaller publishers are generally also associated with a more personal relationship with authors, because they publish fewer works.

You should look for a publisher that has values that are similar to your own. If attention to quality is important to you then you should avoid publishers who have produced books you consider to be badly designed, copyedited or printed. If at all possible, ask friends and colleagues if they have worked with a particular publisher before, and consider their experience and recommendations.

## Approaching a publisher with a book proposal

Once you have identified a publisher for your book you should get in touch with them. Some authors will contact several publishers at the same time, although publishers dislike this. If you do so, you should inform the publisher that your proposal is also under consideration by others.

You should, if possible, look at a publisher's website for information on proposing book projects. Publishers will often have specific guidance on the type of information they require to consider your project. You should also try to identify a specific person to contact. This will usually be the Commissioning Editor (called the Acquisitions Editor in the US). Generally, publishers like to receive a formal written proposal for consideration. However, an informal email or phone call is appropriate if you are unsure whether you should submit the proposal to that publisher, i.e. you think your idea may not be in their specialist field.

Your proposal should ideally include the following (note the similarities to the information considered by you earlier):

- book title
- author details (enclose a CV and a publications list indicating previous writing experience)
- description of the book
- description of the market for the book (and potential market size if known)
- list of chapter titles, with a brief description of the content of each
- estimated length of the book in number of words
- estimated number of illustrations and photographs
- whether you think colour will be required

- proposed date for completing the book
- competing books — what features distinguishes your book from the competition?
- potential reviewers of your proposal
- sample chapter.

In many respects, submitting a book proposal is like applying for a job. A well-considered and presented proposal will convince a publisher that you are organised and capable of writing a book.

You should note that generally it is not a good idea to write an STM book without first approaching a publisher. To save a lot of wasted effort it is far better to prepare a detailed, well-written proposal and perhaps a sample chapter.

The publisher will review your proposal in-house with editorial, production, sales and marketing input, and often with external peer reviewers. A good publisher will provide constructive feedback on your proposal, often with detailed suggestions about the contents, style or proposed market. This may take several months. Even if the publisher rejects your idea you should consider their comments carefully, so that you can modify your proposal should you choose to submit it elsewhere.

If the publisher accepts your proposal they will then negotiate financial and other terms with you, which will be spelt out in a formal contract (see below). You should now start the writing process in earnest.

## Planning your book

Once you have established the broad scope and audience for your book it is vital to establish a detailed structure. Write down a table of contents, listing all of the chapter headings that should be included, and arrange them in a coherent order. This is the skeleton to which the flesh of your book — your words — will be attached. Consider what each chapter should contain, and write down appropriate subheadings showing the structure of individual chapters. You may want to establish a regular structure for every chapter, e.g. each one will begin with an introduction and end with a further reading section. You should also establish the tone and style of writing you intend to use: a professional reference work should read very differently from an undergraduate textbook. Consider whether you will include references: roughly how many per chapter, and what will the reference style be?

Ideally, ask some colleagues to peer-review your chapter outline. They may have some valuable suggestions about additional material that should be included, or how the contents should be structured. Remember when writing for a global audience that practice or methods elsewhere may be different from what you are familiar with. To make your book appeal to as wide a market as possible you should include examples from as wide a field as possible. This, of course, does not apply if you are writing for a clearly defined, narrower market, e.g. UK undergraduate pharmacology students.

Consider approximately how many illustrations, photographs, tables, bullet lists, etc. you think should be included with each chapter. It is particularly important to consider whether colour photographs or illustrations should be included, as this will add to the production expense incurred by the publisher. For a dermatology text, for example, colour photographs would probably be essential. It is increasingly common for textbooks to be lavishly illustrated in colour and imaginatively designed.

You should also carefully consider the size and length of the book. You should have in mind a vision of the book and its use. Do you see it as a substantial, expensive, hardback library reference book, or a short, cheaper, paperback textbook purchased by individual students? Look at similar published books to get an idea of the number of pages per chapter and per book. Typically, a published book will have 400 words per page. You should estimate the number of words per chapter, and stick to this guide when writing.

It is one of the bad writing sins to produce a book much bigger or smaller than originally proposed: be realistic at the outset about what is needed and how much you can write! Consider whether every chapter should be allocated the same number of words, or whether some should be longer or shorter. Typically you might want to write a book with 10 chapters, 100 000 words and 50 illustrations. Consider other pieces of writing you have done, such as magazine articles, research papers, etc. to get a feel for the number of words required to convey the information you want to impart in a book chapter.

Having considered all of the above, you should finally consider whether you are going to write the book entirely on your own. The options could be to do this, to work with another author or authors, or to edit the book, with the majority of the chapters being written by others. If you decide to write the book on your own you should carefully plan a writing schedule and set yourself a realistic deadline for completion. At least one year is a typical timescale. Your goal might then be to write every Sunday morning for 3 hours and to complete one chapter per month.

**Editing a book**

One of the key decisions in producing a book is to decide whether it is to be written by you alone or in collaboration with others. In STM publishing multicontributor edited works are very common. In theory, editing a book (such as this one) should be less work than writing it alone, as the majority of the text will be written by others. However, editing a book presents distinct challenges.

As editor, your first task is to plan the detailed structure of the book very clearly. You will then need to find authors willing to work on the project to a deadline that you specify. Individual authors should have relevant expertise that qualifies them to write the chapters, and should be given clear written and verbal guidance on what is required of them: the length of the chapter, the style of writing, number of references and figures etc. It is a good idea to inform chapter authors about the structure of the book as a whole, and for them to be aware of who is writing other chapters. Generally, it is a good idea to ask authors to produce a detailed chapter outline, with headings, which the editor then agrees is satisfactory.

The publisher will require from you contact details for each contributor and information about what they are writing and the writing schedule. The publisher will advise you about the financial and contractual arrangements for the individual contributors. Generally, it will be agreed that chapter authors will be clearly acknowledged in the published book and will receive a fee or a share of royalties for writing (see below). Chapter authors will usually also receive a copy of the book on publication.

In theory, edited books can be written more quickly, as many authors are working at the same time, but an edited book will proceed only at the pace of the slowest author. Typically, the editor should allow 3–6 months for an author to write a chapter. Any less and the author will probably decline to work on the project; any more and there is a risk that they will give the project a low priority and forget to complete the chapter (or even to begin writing). The editor should regularly keep in touch with chapter authors to monitor progress.

Although having many different authors involved in a book can be an advantage as they can bring their own specific experience to give a broad overview to a book, this can also be a disadvantage. Books with many contributors can be repetitive, and writing styles and extent of coverage can vary widely between chapters. A good editor will have prevented this by careful planning and briefing of chapter authors. Once all authors have submitted their chapters a good editor will also carefully move, delete, rewrite and generally improve the text to ensure a consistency of approach and emphasis throughout. To do this can take several months, and this should be allowed for in the schedule discussed with the publisher. Only once the work has been edited and all the material is complete is it ready to be submitted to the publisher.

Unfortunately, with an edited book, it is common for at least one chapter author to fail to complete their work to schedule. The editor then needs to decide whether the author's deadline should be extended, a replacement author found (sometimes the editor will have to write the chapter themselves), or to remove the chapter from the book. As an editor you will need to be ruthless on this point if you are to avoid your book being delayed excessively.

### Books with several authors

Instead of editing a book, with a different author or authors per chapter, you may decide to write a book with a handful of other authors. In such a case it is again important to plan the book's structure carefully and agree in advance the division of labour among your fellow authors. Individual authors may be assigned to write specific chapters, or may write parts of chapters. As with an edited work it is important that the final book is coherent and has a consistent style and 'voice'.

### Writing a book

Having thoroughly planned the outline of your book and found a publisher, it is now time to get down to the task of writing. It is a good idea to write a little and often: most authors will find things more manageable and satisfying if achievable goals are set, such as to complete one chapter every month. Once you have finished writing, it is a good idea to set the book aside and try to forget about it for a few weeks. Return to the text refreshed and read it through to edit and rewrite as necessary.

A good publisher will have provided some guidance on how to submit the completed book and will often provide detailed style or writing guides to assist authors. A publisher will appreciate your following their submission instructions. Generally these will specify such things as 'the author should submit a printed copy of the book along with an electronic copy as wordprocessed files on a disk'. Most publishers will ask that the electronic files are broken down into one per chapter. Publishers very rarely ask authors to use complex formatting, so long as the structure of the text layout, such as headings and subheadings, is clearly indicated.

You should always retain a secure electronic and printed copy of your work. It is not unknown for files or entire books to be lost in the post or corrupted via email, and it would be a tragedy to lose months — perhaps years — of work.

It may seem obvious, but the work submitted to the publisher should be the final version and should be complete. It should thus include all artwork, preliminary material (such as the contents list and preface) and index if you were required to produce one. At this stage you should also supply the publisher with any documentation giving permission from other copyright holders to reproduce work from other published sources that you have used in your book. Your publisher should have advised you about this. They should similarly have advised you about submitting photographs, diagrams or other artwork for inclusion in your book.

## Publishing contracts

Once you have verbally agreed to work with a publisher a formal written contract will be sent to you. This should be signed and dated by you, and by your co-authors if required. Someone representing the publisher will also sign the agreement; a signed copy will be returned to you for your records.

Publishing contracts vary in size and complexity but are generally fairly standard in the terms they specify. They are legal documents, and should you choose to do so you could ask a specialist to consider the contract on your behalf. Societies or organisations representing writers will often provide this service to members. The contract is important, as it formally commits both you and the publisher to work on a project. Books may take several years to produce, and the individuals who initially committed to publish your book may not be involved in the project once it becomes time to submit the manuscript. However, the contract remains as a written record of what was agreed between you and the publisher.

The following are selected important terms that a publishing contract will specify:

- author(s) or editor(s) of the project
- proposed title of the work
- completion date of the work (submission date to the publisher)

- format of the work (e.g. number of words, illustrations, photographs, etc.)
- rights assigned to the publisher
- financial terms (e.g. payments to the author and schedule)
- termination of the agreement and reversion of rights.

Of these, probably the one that causes most anxiety to authors is the completion date. Most publishers will be reasonably flexible to amend this date if necessary, although it is vital to keep them informed of your progress.

Probably the most important considerations are the financial aspects of the project, discussed below, and the rights (copyright) associated with the work.

Copyright is internationally recognised by law as a means to specify how the output of creative or intellectual endeavour may be distributed and used by others. The duration of copyright protection varies from country to country, but for written work is usually for the lifetime of the author plus either 50 or 70 years. Publishers will usually ask that authors assign copyright to them in its entirety, although this is generally not advisable as it could restrict your future options for using or exploiting your work. Today it is increasingly common for authors to retain the copyright in their work but to grant the publisher limited rights (a licence) to exploit it. For example, an author might grant the publisher the exclusive rights to publish their work in English only, or to sell the work only in North America rather than globally. It is also particularly important to consider what the contract says about future editions of the work: are you giving the publisher the rights to publish every edition, or only for a specific edition or number of editions? In addition, publishing contracts will specify rights relating to other formats of your work, not just the printed book, e.g. are you giving the publisher permission to publish your work electronically (i.e. online)? (For more information on copyright see page 369.)

In addition to the obligations you will have as an author, the publisher also has obligations to you and these should be clearly stated in the contract. Such obligations might include a commitment on how your name is represented in association with the published work, or a commitment to publish your work within a certain time after delivery of the manuscript.

Termination of the publishing agreement should also be stated clearly in any contract. You should consider, for example, what happens to your book, and your rights as an author, if the book goes out of print, or if the publisher is sold or ceases publishing activities.

Editors' publishing agreements are different from an author's publishing agreement, mainly in specifying the duties and role of the editor. With an edited work, the publisher will negotiate specific agreements with chapter contributors: these are often very simple documents compared to a sole author's or editor's contract.

You should remember that publishing contracts and the specific terms they contain are negotiable — up to a point. Ultimately, if you and the publisher wish to see your work published both parties must agree terms that they consider reasonable and practical.

## Finances

If financial gain is your sole motivation in writing books then you would probably be better advised to pursue other, more lucrative endeavours. Indeed, even other forms of writing, such as journalism, can be far more profitable than writing books. A Society of Authors survey in 2000 suggested that 61% of its members earned less than £10,000 per year from writing, and the situation is probably worse for STM authors. One doctor calculated that he earned the equivalent of less than 50p per hour of work from a textbook he wrote.[1]

However, writing books can occasionally be financially very rewarding, and there are many other non-financial motivations. Certainly having a book published will enhance your CV and advance your professional career. It will also mark you out as an expert in the field, and will probably lead to invitations to write other material and speak at conferences. For STM authors, knowing that they have completed a book and added to the body of work on a subject is also a source of considerable satisfaction.

## Royalties

Typically, an author will either receive a fee for writing a book or, more commonly, a royalty from the publisher. The royalty is usually a percentage of the revenue obtained from each copy sold, although sometimes it is calculated as a percentage of the list price of a book. On average, for each copy of a book sold a publisher will receive around 65% of the list price. The author royalty is usually 10%, although this can vary between 5% and 15%; a higher rate than this is exceptional. The income to the author is thus related to the number of copies of the book sold. Publishers usually pay royalties once or twice a year. In some cases a fee or an advance against the royalty may be paid. For example, the publisher might pay the author £500 on signing the contract, followed by a further £500 on delivery of the completed manuscript. If this fee is an advance against the royalty then the author will receive no further payments until sufficient copies have been sold equivalent to a royalty of £1000.

Financial terms can often be quite complicated with, for example, increased royalty rates being applied after a certain number of copies have been sold. Royalties may also be obtained from different rights granted to the publisher, e.g. if you grant the publisher electronic rights to your work you should receive a royalty from any revenues obtained from this delivery method.

For edited books, the editor will similarly usually receive a royalty based on the number of copies sold. Editors' royalty rates are generally lower than for authors: 5% is typical. Chapter contributors generally receive a one-off fee for their work (e.g. £50–£200), although they may receive a royalty from the publisher (e.g. 5% divided equally between all the contributors).

When more than one author or editor is involved in a project the publisher will divide the royalty or fee as advised by the authors or editors.

In addition to receiving a royalty or a fee for their work, authors and editors should clarify with the publisher (and have this written into the publishing agreement) any other benefits they will receive. This might include travelling expenses to attend meetings, or support to purchase equipment or materials.

The contract should also state the number of free copies of the published work that the authors or editors receive: typically this is around 10 copies each.

## What the publisher does

Authors often have a relatively vague idea of what publishers do and how long it will take to publish their work. The editorial goal of a good publisher is to help an author express themselves as clearly and accurately as possible. Typically, for an STM book the time taken from delivery of the manuscript to actual publication can be anything from 3 to 12 months. A publisher will usually indicate to an author who will be involved in the different stages of the publication process and when these will occur. Most people involved in the publication of your book will not actually work directly for the publisher but will be employed in a freelance capacity or on a contract basis to supply a service, such as typesetting.

On delivery of your manuscript, someone at the publisher, usually the Development or Desk Editor, will assess the work to make sure that it is complete and conforms to the specifications outlined in the publishing agreement. Often the work will be peer-reviewed and suggestions be made for changes or the inclusion of additional material before the manuscript is finally accepted.

## Copyediting

Unless you have been asked by the publisher to produce work designed as pages ready to print with no further intervention by the publisher (camera-ready copy) your work will be handed over to a copyeditor.

The copyeditor's role is to read through your work carefully to ensure accuracy and consistency in how the material is presented. This will mean checking the consistency of spellings, abbreviations and headings, ensuring that cited references are complete and accurate, etc. The copyeditor will usually be required also to improve the use of grammar and language to aid understanding of the text. Copyediting changes outside a publisher's standard 'style guide' will often involve discussion with the author. The copyeditor will also structure the text, tables, figures, etc. in such a way to facilitate typesetting of the book. They may also be required to check that all necessary permissions have been obtained from copyright holders where material from other published sources is reproduced.

Once the copyediting has been completed page proofs will be produced by the typesetters to a design specified by the publisher. Proofs will then be sent to the author for checking and correction. Before the widespread use of computers, making corrections to page proofs was very expensive. Although today the process is much easier and hence cheaper, changes to proofs can still be complicated, expensive, and cause delays in the production schedule. Any change also risks introducing errors in the text or page layout. Authors are therefore generally encouraged to confine themselves to essential changes only, either by correcting factual omissions or errors, or by improving the layout of the pages.

Publishers will usually employ a proofreader (a different person from the copyeditor), who will independently read through the proofs, the copyeditor's changes to the manuscript, and the author's corrections to the proofs to ensure that the typesetter can make final adjustments to the text ready for the pages to be printed.

If an index is to be included with the book it will be constructed at this time before also being typeset.

The book will then finally be printed and bound. This stage of the publishing process — essentially the physical manufacture of the book — can typically take 4–8 weeks. (For further information about the editing process, see page 451.)

### Publication and promotion

In addition to manufacturing a book, publishing is also about marketing and selling. Several months before publication the publisher will prepare a marketing plan to show how potential purchasers of your work will be alerted to its publication. Most publishers welcome marketing input from authors, although it should be remembered that they will be working to a finite budget. Advertising, direct mail, and increasingly electronic methods (websites and email) will all be used to alert bookstores, libraries and readers to your work. (For more information about marketing see page 459.)

## Indexing

If an index to a book is required the publisher will often arrange for it to be produced by a specialist indexer. However, sometimes the author or editor will be encouraged to supply one. This can be a daunting and time-consuming task for the inexperienced, but there are a number of tips that will help you to produce a useful, accurate index.

### Function of an index

The purpose of an index is to guide the reader rapidly to specific topics of interest in a book. It is therefore important to consider the readership and to produce an index with a sufficient level of detail to be comprehensive without being so detailed that it is unusable. As a general guide you should aim to have no more than three to five index entries from each page. These should be both concepts and proper names. Only pages where useful information about a topic is given should be included; passing references should be omitted. Generally, chapter headings and subheadings form the basis of index entries.

### Effective indexing methods

Work on the index may be started from your wordprocessor files, but ultimately you will need to incorporate final page numbers and so it is often easiest to work from numbered page proofs.

You should read through the proofs highlighting any text you think should be indexed — remember, this can be from headings, the main text or tables, and should include specific names, phrases or concepts. You should only include words or phrases that you believe a reader will look up. You should also include sub-entries, for example you may be indexing a chapter that discusses drugs used in heart disease — index the class of drug as well as the drug names:

Antihypertensives, 20
Atenolol, 24
Beta-blockers, atenolol, 24
Propranolol, 25
Beta-blockers, propranolol, 25
Antihypertensives, drug interactions, 30

Cross-references should also be included to navigate around the index and text:

Epinephrine see adrenaline
*and under adrenaline*:
Adrenaline, discovery and synthesis, 108
Adrenaline, sites of action, 110

Also include additional cross-references:

Malaria, 114 see also Antimalarials

It can be useful to include in the index words that are commonly used as synonyms for words or terms used in the text, especially if they appear separately in the index:

Renal failure see Kidney failure

Common abbreviations should also be indexed as cross-references:

EGF see Epidermal growth factor

Once you have created your list of index entries they should be keyed into a wordprocessor file and sorted. Index entries are generally best sorted on a letter-by-letter basis, i.e. ignoring spaces and hyphens. Once you have sorted the list, multiple entries can be organised into a single entry and sub-entries rationalised, e.g.:

Atenolol, 23,
Atenolol, 106
*to*
Atenolol, 23, 106

*and*
Adrenaline
discovery and synthesis, 108
sites of action, 110

The completed index should then be sent to the publisher for typesetting.

## Reference

1.   Jacobs A (2000) How true! Rapid responses to Tim Albert: How to become a book author. *Br Med J Career Focus*. Available on *http://careerfocus.bmjjournals. com/cgi/eletters/320/7237/S2-7237*. [accessed 16 May 2006]

## Further reading

Albert T (2000) How to become a book author. *Br Med J Career Focus* 320: S2–7237.
Banks M (1998) Get your book published. *BMJ* 317: 1715–1718.
*Directory of Publishing 2007*. London: Continuum International Publishing Group, 2006.
Turner B, ed (2005) *The Writer's Handbook 2005*. London: Macmillan.
*Writers' and Artists' Yearbook 2005*. London: A & C Black.

## Useful websites

Nielsen BookData
*www.whitaker.co.uk*

Publishers Association
*www.publishers.org.uk*

Society of Authors
*www.societyofauthors.net*

# 21

## Writing for the internet

*Sue Childs*

*Note: The web addresses of resources marked with * are given at the end of the chapter.*

## Introduction to internet-based media

### The internet

The internet is a global computer network comprising numerous smaller networks run by private or public sector organisations. These networks exchange packets of data according to standard protocols. From the users' point of view, the effect is almost instant transmission or receipt of data. The internet carries a number of services, such as:

- email
- the World Wide Web
- instant messaging or two-way chat.

### History

The internet evolved from ARPANET, developed by the US military in the late 1960s. ARPANET was a distributed computer network: if one computer facility was shut down messages could still be exchanged by using other routes within the network.

### Coordination

The Internet Society* is an international organisation providing for global coordination and cooperation on the internet. It houses the groups responsible for internet infrastructure standards. The Internet Corporation for Assigned Names and Numbers (ICANN*) is a not-for-profit organisation contracted by the US government to manage and coordinate the domain name system (DNS).

## Domain Name System

Every computer on the internet has a unique address — a string of numbers — called its Internet Protocol (IP) address, e.g. 62.128.130.76 (for The Royal Pharmaceutical Society of Great Britain — RPSGB). Via the DNS this IP address is translated into a more memorable set of letters, e.g. www.rpsgb.org.uk/. The DNS comprises a hierarchical directory of domain names and their corresponding computers and individuals or organisations registered to use them.

## The web

The World Wide Web (WWW, W3, the web) is one of the services that operates on the internet. Web pages are identified by their URL, e.g. http://www.rpsgb.org.uk/. The web was invented in the early 1990s by Tim Berners-Lee, then working at CERN (the European Organisation for Nuclear Research), as a method for physicists to exchange scientific information. The World Wide Web Consortium (W3C*) creates the web's standards and guidelines.

## Web browsers

A web browser is a software application that enables users to find and display web pages. Common browsers are Microsoft's Internet Explorer* and Mozilla Firefox*, a free, open source browser. To obtain a web page you either put the URL into the browser's search bar or you click on a hyperlink within a document or another web page. A hyperlink is a reference to a web page; it enables a piece of information on the web to be linked to any other piece of information. The browser finds the designated web page and displays it on the user's computer.

## Search engines

Search engines, e.g. Google*, help users find information on the web. Search engines continually search (crawl) the web for information and store links to web pages indexed by keywords. When a user types in a set of keywords into a search engine a list of the web pages indexed by those keywords is retrieved. There are medicine-specific search engines, e.g. MedHunt* and OmniMedicalSearch*. SearchEngineWatch* provides information about the search engine industry and tips on web searching.

## Electronic publishing

The web provides an excellent mechanism to make publications easily available via online databases, electronic journals (e-journals) and electronic books (e-books). Writing the content of e-journals and e-books is no different from writing for traditional print media. The difference lies in how they are submitted to the publisher (each individual journal has instructions for contributors) and how they are made available to the reader, e.g. via the web or on CD-ROM. (For more information on getting published see Chapter 22.)

### Access to subscription resources

Many of these resources require a paid subscription for access, either from individuals or from organisations on behalf of their staff. The National Core Content Project* makes a wide range of subscription databases, e-journals and e-books available, free to the end user, to NHS staff in England. Unfortunately, pharmacists not directly employed by an NHS Trust are excluded from this arrangement. The National electronic Library for Health (NeLH*)/National Library for Health (NLH*) provide free end-use access to additional subscription resources for NHS staff, patients and the public in England. Similar services are available in Scotland* and Northern Ireland*. Access to subscription resources in other countries will depend on national/local arrangements in the individual countries. Pharm-line*, the database for pharmacy practice and prescribing, requires a subscription, although 12 months of abstracts are available free of charge.

### Access to free resources

However, free databases and journals are available on the web, and for many subscription journals you can see contents pages and often abstracts for free.

Medline, the health and medicine database, is made available via the PubMed* interface. Other resources available via PubMed include TOXNET* (covering toxicology). The NHS Centre for Reviews and Dissemination* provides free access to databases of systematic reviews of effects, economic evaluations and technology assessments. Prodigy* is a source of evidence-based clinical knowledge.

Lists of e-journals can be found via FreeMedicalJournals* and The Directory of Open Access Journals*, for example, and e-books via e.g. FreeBooks4Doctors!*.

## Open access publishing

A current initiative is open access scholarly publishing: placing material on the web for free, full text access.[1] Resources for open access medical journals include PubMed Central*, from the US National Institutes of Health, BioMed Central*, a publishing company, and Public Library of Science (PLoS)*, a non-profit organisation.

### Funding

Some open access publishers, e.g. BioMed Central, obtain their funding via the 'author pays' model, i.e. the author of the article pays a processing charge. However, organisations can pay to join BioMed Central so that their staff do not have to pay the processing charge directly. The NHS in England is a member, as are many UK universities.

### Copyright

In traditional publishing, the author signs over their copyright to the publisher. In open access publishing the author retains the copyright but licenses others to copy, distribute and display their work as long as they are attributed and given the credit, e.g. via CreativeCommons* licenses. (For more information on copyright and legal aspects of writing for the internet, see page 381.)

### Institutional repositories

In 2003/4 the House of Commons Science and Technology Committee reviewed the scientific, technical and medical publishing industry.[2] They recommended that 'all UK higher education institutions establish institutional repositories on which their published output can be stored and from which it can be read, free of charge, online', e.g. e-Prints Soton*, at the University of Southampton. The Wellcome Trust, a major UK funder of medical research, now requires papers published from research they have supported to be placed in such repositories.

## Creating websites

To set up a website you need:

- a domain name
- a web hosting service
- a method of creating HTML.

## Website domain names

The URL (uniform resource locator) specifies the address of a web page. Note that in a URL characters before the first / are not case sensitive, but characters after the first / are case sensitive. The 'domain name' of a website is the first part of the web address, between http:// and the first /, e.g. in the URL http://www.rpsgb.org.uk/ the domain name is www.rpsgb.org.uk. This domain name uniquely identifies that organisation on the internet. Its different sections are as follows:

- http means 'hypertext transfer protocol'
- punctuation, which separates the various components of the URL
- www means World Wide web; usually present, but not always
- the specific part, e.g. rpsgb, which is the part of the domain name that the website owner can choose; it cannot be currently in use by anyone else
- codes representing the type of organisation and its country of origin (see Table 21.1).

For further information on legal issues concerning domain names, see page 382.

## Obtaining a domain name

You have to register your domain name with an organisation accredited by ICANN. A list of such organisations is available from the ICANN

**Table 21.1**  Domain name codes

Common organisational codes (top level domains, TLDs) include:
    .com (commercial organisations)
    .edu (educational organisations)
    .gov (governmental organisations)
    .org (organisations, usually non-commercial)
Country codes (country level domains) e.g.:
    no code (USA)
    .uk (UK)
Second level codes (second level domains, SLDs) e.g.:
    .ac.uk (UK educational organisations)
    .co.uk (UK commercial organisations)
    .gov.uk (UK governmental organisations)
    .nhs.uk (NHS organisations)
    .org.uk (UK organisations, usually non-commercial)

FAQs* web page. Nominet UK* is the Registry for .uk domain names and manages most UK second-level domains.

You have to pay to register but prices are not uniform. For a fee, companies will act as registration agents on your behalf. Consider buying your name with a range of organisational codes (e.g. .org, .org.uk, .com, .co.uk) as people often make errors when typing in a web address. These 'ghost' sites can be set to link automatically to your website.

You have exclusive right to your domain name for the registration period. However, it is important that you remember to renew your domain name before the end of this period — you don't want to lose your audience by losing your domain name.

If you are creating a section within an existing website, then follow the website's internal naming conventions.

## Web hosting services

For a fee, companies will provide web hosting services. The big internet service providers (ISPs) offer access to the internet as well as web hosting, domain name registration, etc. To find such a company, ask people for recommendations or look, for example, at the list of Nominet members*. ADSLguide* lists details of, and comments on, ISPs.

If you are creating a section within your organisation's website then contact the IT department for details of local procedures.

## HTML

Web pages are usually written in HyperText Markup Language (HTML). This gives instructions to the web browser so that your content on the page appears in your intended style and format. HTML is a plain text language, i.e. it is written in ASCII (American Standard Code for Information Interchange), the standard for coding computer characters. Anything written in ASCII can be understood by any system. Plain text is also easily transmitted. HTML is a markup language, i.e. instructions (tags) are embedded in the text.

### HTML code

See Table 21.2 for examples of HTML.

To see some real HTML open up any web page and click on the Menu options View / Source. A separate text window will open and you can then see the page's HTML coding.

**Table 21.2**   Examples of HTML

---

Defining structures or styles
<h2>Adverse effects</h2> — putting 'adverse effects' in the heading 2 style (large and bold)

Defining appearance
Drug — putting 'Drugs' in bold font

Defining a hypertext link
<a>href="http://www.rpsgb.org.uk/">RPSGB</a> — making 'RPSGB' a hyperlink to the RPSGB website

---

### Learning HTML

HTML is not complicated. There are tutorials on the web to give you a feel for it, e.g. Getting started with HTML*, HTML Source*. The current W3C HTML standard* is version 4.01.

### Writing HTML

You can write HTML with a text editor. Basic text editors come with your computer, e.g. Notepad and Wordpad in Windows (look in Programs / Accessories). A good, cheap text editor with more facilities is Textpad*. When you've created some text with HTML tags save the file as an HTML file. Then open the file with your web browser (menu option File / Open / specify file name or browse for file).

There are software applications you can purchase to help you produce web pages easily, e.g. Macromedia Dreamweaver*, Microsoft FrontPage*, Adobe GoLive*, but be careful that such applications do not introduce non-standard, proprietary extensions into your code.

If you are more experienced with writing HTML you may want to look at the W3C HTML standard*. W3C offers a range of information and support on its HTML pages*.

Animation and interactivity can be added to web pages using applications such as Adobe Flash*, Java applets* and JavaScript*. However, these applications need more knowledge from the website developer, may require users to have appropriate plug-ins installed on their machines, and may cause accessibility and usability problems.

### Content management systems

If you are producing pages for your organisation's website then you might have to use a content management system (CMS). This is a software application that enables collaborative creation and updating of a website. Usually the management sets the style and structure of the website, to ensure their corporate 'look and feel'. Individuals with permission to enter information will be supplied with an ID/password, and information will be input via electronic forms to preset templates: no knowledge of HTML is necessary. New content may need to be moderated before it becomes live.

### XML/XHTML

The next stage in the evolution of the web is the creation of the semantic web.[3] The aim here is to make the meaning (semantics) of web information understandable to computers as well as to humans. 'Agents' could then find information for you in much more useful ways, e.g. take your doctor's prescription, find the nearest chemist who would deliver your drugs, order them for you, and then remind you to take them at the specified time. Extensible Markup Language (XML) is being developed to describe the content (data) of web resources. XHTML, an application of XML, is the successor to HTML. However, HTML is still recommended for writing web pages.

## Quality issues for websites

There is concern that health information on the internet can be incomplete, inaccurate, even dangerous, particularly for drugs.[4,5] People could follow web advice to replace prescription drugs with crank therapies, or buy drugs or herbal products from websites without being prescribed the therapy or knowing what chemical they have actually been sent.

Many initiatives try to address this problem.[6] I have produced guidelines for judging the quality of health information websites (made available via the Judge* website) that would be useful to any beginner creating a website.

The most common quality initiative is the Health on the Net (HON) code of conduct, produced by the HON Foundation. The HONcode* comprises ethical principles that website producers should abide by (see Table 21.3) and reviews the website to check that it does so. If it does, the website can use a verifiable seal. This carries the HON logo, and when a user clicks on the seal they go to a HON page which confirms that the website has passed the HON review. However, the review process does not check that the content of a website is correct.

**Table 21.3**  HONcode principles

- Authority (medical advice should be given by medical staff)
- Complementary (information should support, not replace, a doctor's advice)
- Confidentiality
- Attribution (references should be given to source data)
- Justifiability (claims should be evidence-based)
- Transparency of authorship
- Transparency of sponsorship
- Honesty in advertising and editorial policy

## Producing good-quality websites

To produce a good-quality website you need to address the following issues:

- accessibility for people with disabilities
- accessibility by different software products
- usability
- writing style
- content.

### Accessibility for people with disabilities

The Disability Discrimination Act requires organisations to make their facilities and services accessible to disabled people. Aim to make your website easily accessible to all, and reduce barriers to its use by people with sight, hearing, physical or cognitive problems. W3C have set up a web Accessibility Initiative* and provide guidelines.

Careful use of fonts and graphics is very important, particularly to make your site accessible to people with visual problems, including those with colour blindness or dyslexia. The Royal National Institute for the Blind's Web Access Centre* provides advice:

- Use fonts (size and colour) that can be easily read, and/or changed by the user as required, e.g. through their browser settings.
- Avoid using graphics of text.
- Consider carefully your use of background colour and texture.
- Navigation around the website is vital, so don't use graphics or active content for navigation.
- Warn people if there are drop-down menus and pop-up windows.
- Be sparing in your use of graphics, and only use them if you have a good reason.

- If you use graphics to convey important content, always provide a text alternative.

You should also consider the needs of people with hearing problems if you include audio material on your website. Provide transcripts or captions.

There are resources that you can use to check the accessibility and usability of your website, e.g. Bobby*, webXACT*. W3C provides a list of accessibility tools*.

---

**Tips on use of fonts, colours and graphics**

- A sans serif font is easier to read on a screen.
- Underlined text means a hypertext link.
- Emphasise a piece of normal text by using bold font.
- Large sections of text completely in upper case or italics are difficult to read.
- Use alt-tags with all images or graphics: these briefly describes the image or icon.

---

## Accessibility by different software products

People use Apple MACs as well as PCs, and have different versions of software and web browsers, not just the most recent. Your website needs to be accessible to all these software products. This can be achieved by using the W3C open internet standards, rather than proprietary extensions.

Complex technical design and the use of additional software, such as plug-ins, can be irritating and are a barrier to people with older technology or inexperienced in using computers and the internet. They can also slow down page downloading.

Make sure that your website downloads quickly, especially the home page: as a general rule, some text must be readable within 10 seconds. Avoid large graphics as they can take a long time to download.

## Usability

Usability is a quality attribute — how easy, intuitive and pleasant it is for people to use your website.[7] If you think about what annoys you when you visit a website, avoid those things in your website and you won't go far wrong.

The top 10 web design mistakes of 2005 were:[8]

- legibility problems
- non-standard links
- unnecessary use of flash (animated graphics technology from macromedia)
- content not written specially for the web
- bad search
- browser incompatibility
- cumbersome forms
- no contact information or other company information
- frozen layouts with fixed page widths
- inadequate photo enlargement.

Users just want:[8]

- text they can read
- content that answers their questions
- navigation and search that help them find what they want
- short and simple forms
- no bugs, typos or corrupted data
- no linkrot [out of date links]
- no outdated content.

## Writing style for websites

Web pages are not as easy to read as printed pages. Therefore, aim to keep your text short and simple. Following the rules of Plain English* will help (see Chapter 2).

People tend to scan web pages quickly, so the use of headings and bulleted lists will make the text easier to read. On the whole, people do not like to scroll down a page, so if you can, restrict your content to one screen view.

If you want to convey a lot of information this is best done in the form of files (e.g. Word, PDF) which can be attached to the website for people to download, save, and view or print. Provide a text summary and specify the type and size of the files so that people can decide whether to download them. OASIS has developed a non-proprietary standard for an OpenDocument format* (ODF) for office applications.

### Copyright

The content on your website is copyrighted to you. Conversely, you must consider the copyright of other people's material that you may use. (For more information about copyright, see Chapter 19.)

One copyright issue particular to the web is the use of links to other sites. Links to the home page of another website are acceptable. However, there is some dispute as to whether or not 'deep linking', where you make a link directly to a page or resource inside a website and bypass the home page, could be interpreted as breaking that website's copyright.

- Check the terms and conditions of a website to see if they have given people permission to link to their website, particularly to deep link.
- If you are concerned, ask the organisation's permission to deep link to their website.

If your website uses frames and a user clicks on a link, the text from that other website is automatically 'included' in your website. This 'framing' is clearly breaking copyright. You must always ask an organisation's permission to do this.

It is good practice to indicate that the user is leaving your website when they click on an external link, or to make an external link open up in a new browser window. This makes it clear to a user that the linked website is nothing to do with your site.

## Data protection

The Data Protection Act covers the use of personal data, which is anything that could identify a living person. Anyone displaying or collecting personal data through their website must obey this law. This could apply if you have pictures or personal details of people on your website, or use cookies to automatically obtain data from your users, or provide an email address for feedback, as well as when you specifically request information from your users.

The Office of the Information Commissioner oversees the Data Protection Act and has published a website FAQs* document with guidance on this issue.

## Terms and conditions and disclaimers

Explain the terms and conditions under which you produce your website. Areas to cover could include:

- privacy: whether or not you ask for personal information, and what you do with such information
- copyright: any permissions that you give to use your copyright information, or to deep link to your site

- accuracy: your policy and procedures to ensure that your information is correct
- links to other websites: your policy for selecting and making links.

Include disclaimers so that people understand the limits to what your website can do. You might need to get legal advice on this. Areas to cover include:

- Medical information: This is not intended to replace consultation with a person's own doctor.
- Guarantees and responsibility for harm: You cannot guarantee the accuracy and currency of the information you provide. You cannot be held responsible for any problems users of your website might encounter or harm they might be caused.
- Availability: You cannot guarantee your website will always be available.
- Links to other websites: You do not endorse the organisation or its website; you do not guarantee the quality of their information; you do not guarantee that the website will be available.
- Virus protection: This disclaimer is only necessary if you provide information in non-HTML formats. People should always use antivirus software on any material downloaded from a website. You cannot accept responsibility if people are affected by a virus from using material available through your website.

Guidelines for UK government websites* gives examples.

### Writing content of web pages

The standard principle of writing good-quality content also applies to web pages. People want to know who has written the content, their authority and expertise to do so, when it was written, and what sources of information the author used. When the content comprises scientific information, then the evidence base for statements must be given.

On your website set up an 'About' page. Say who you are, your purpose in running the website, who funds, sponsors or supports you. Give contact details, including postal addresses and telephone numbers.

On every page give the date that the page was first written, when it was last updated, and the next revision date. Some material needs to be updated frequently. For material that changes little, it is still a good habit to check the content on a yearly basis. Many external links will have changed within a year. Even if the page does not have to be changed, still amend the updated and next revision dates. People expect websites to be current.

Where specific content has been written by other people, give their names and affiliations, plus the date the piece was written.

Documents attached to websites, e.g. Word, PDF or ODF files, still need full bibliographical details: author, affiliations, publisher, address of publisher, date.

### Metadata

Metadata are data about data, e.g. descriptive information about your website. This can be placed in the 'head' section of the HTML code. Using metadata increases the chances of your website being retrieved in response to someone's search query.

The types of information you can provide include:

> *<title>This is a context-rich title of my website</title>*
> *<meta name="Author" content="Fred Bloggs">*
> *<meta name="keywords" content="These are words and phrases, separated by commas, that define the subject content of my website">*

For an example of how to add metadata to a website look at the Nordic Metadata Project*.

## Email

Writing emails is such an everyday occurrence that it is easy to forget that careful thought must be given to their content and writing style.

Emails are not secure: your email and its contents are effectively in the public domain. It is easy for a recipient of your email to forward it to anyone, and messages in email discussion lists are crawled by search engines, so be very careful about including confidential, private or sensitive information in an email — particularly patient information, financial information, other people's contact information or personal details.

The formal structure of letters and the cues from verbal and face-to-face communication are missing in emails, and messages tend to be short and succinct. It is therefore easy to offend or upset someone with an email that might be perceived as brusque or even rude. Take care that your message cannot be misunderstood. Correct spelling and grammar are also important: readers will make judgements about you based on such things. Emails are 'official' documents, so keep copies of important messages.

Rules of appropriate behaviour are called net-etiquette or netiquette (see Table 21.4).

**Table 21.4** Email netiquette

- Use meaningful subject lines
- Use plain text format, not HTML
- Use a short, informative signature, e.g. postal address, phone and fax numbers, email address, website URL
- Think carefully about sending attachments: ask people if they would like you to email them the document individually, or post the document on a website and email the URL
- Don't include all the previous emails in a reply or thread — just include enough so the nature of the previous correspondence is clear

### Email discussion list netiquette, e.g.

Particular rules apply to email discussion lists: check the list service website for details, e.g. JISCmail*.

- Don't cross-post to a large number of lists — many people belong to more than one list
- Don't send attachments
- If you use 'out of office' messages, temporarily 'suspend' from the list before you go away, otherwise everyone on the list will receive your 'out of office' messages in response to every posting

Copyright also applies to emails: the writer of the message owns the copyright. When writing an email be careful not to break another person's copyright, e.g. when forwarding a message, or including published quotes.

## Discussion forums

Discussion forums include online chat or instant messaging, internet forums, newsgroups and bulletin/message boards, and email discussion lists. Online chat provides for real-time communication; the other methods are asynchronous.

Email discussion lists push the messages at subscribers; for other forums the user has to actively visit the site. Many such forums are for leisure activities, but they are increasingly being used in professional contexts, e.g. health topic forums for patients, carers and health professionals, and virtual classrooms and discussion lists in education.

Netiquette issues similar to those covered under email apply to discussion forums. As a member, you should stick to the subject coverage of the forum, be courteous and considerate, and respect other members' opinions, privacy and copyright.

Forums can be moderated, i.e. the manager of the forum checks that messages adhere to the forum's netiquette and acceptable use policies. Sanctions are to admonish unacceptable behaviour, terminate threads, or even cancel a person's membership. If you are managing a forum, then you need to establish the netiquette and acceptable use policies and moderation procedures. You can find lists of forums at, for example, Google Groups*.

## Blogging

A weblog or blog is an online publication that usually consists of short entries posted in reverse chronological order. Blogs can be:

- the diary of an individual
- a community of writers
- produced by organisations
- non-interactive sites
- interactive sites that encourage readers to leave comments.

Blogs can contain text, pictures, and links to sources of information. They are being produced by individual health professionals and by health organisations as a mechanism for disseminating information and engaging others. Services are available to create and run blogs for free, e.g. Blogger*, owned by Google. Alternatively, specialised software can be purchased for the task.

There are a number of key points to remember when writing a blog: the content is in the public domain, so:

- be careful of confidentiality and copyright issues.
- individual entries should be short.
- blogs should be added to on a regular basis — at least monthly if not weekly or daily.

To keep up with what's happening with blogs look at the Technorati* website.

## Wikis

Wikis are a type of website that allows collaborative authoring of content. Software applications to run wikis are available as open-source or paid-for products. For information about such applications see, for example, Choosing a wiki*. Wikis can be restricted to members only or be public sites. For a list of public wikis see WikiIndex*, for example.

The content of a wiki can be left completely up to the contributors, or there can be some form of moderation by the site's originators. However, by their very nature wikis are vulnerable to vandals. The best known wiki is Wikipedia*, the free, online encyclopaedia where anyone can create or edit entries.

## News

Writing news items for the internet is the same as writing any news (for more information on writing news see Chapter 151), although you should aim for short, succinct paragraphs. News can be provided as the whole or part content of your website.

You can advertise by email when your news has been updated. The email could be just an alert to say the website has been updated, with the URL given, or you can also include the new items as text within the email (do not send out news items as email attachments). You can either manage your list of email subscribers through your own software (which can be time consuming) or sign up to a free or fee-paid mailing list provider.

Another way to alert people to your new stories is via an RSS (Really Simple Syndication, or Rich Site Summary) feed (webfeed, news-feed). An RSS feed is a page of text coded with XML so that it can be read by an RSS reader and displayed in human-readable format. An RSS reader or aggregator keeps a list of the RSS feeds you have chosen to subscribe to, checks them regularly, and then displays their contents.

A range of RSS reader applications, free or on subscription, are available, e.g. at RSS Compendium*. There are also lists of feeds, e.g. Feedster* and NewsIsFree*. An NLH directory* lists good-quality health-related newsfeeds.

---

**In summary**

- Writing for the internet is mainly about using the technology to best effect.
- Facilities include electronic publishing, the web, email, discussion forums, blogs and wikis.
- Aim for easily accessible, usable outputs.
- Standard principles of good-quality writing also apply to writing for the internet.
- Aim for short, succinct, well laid-out, easily understood content.
- Copyright and data protection issues also apply to internet content.

**Examples of internet resources of interest to pharmacists**
A wide range of resources for the pharmacist can be found on the internet. The following examples give a flavour of what is available:

*Official bodies*

- Department of Health (http://www.dh.gov.uk/AboutUs/HeadsOf Profession/ChiefPharmaceuticalOfficer/fs/en)
- NHS Gateway (for the public) (http://www.nhs.uk/)
- Medicines and Healthcare Products Regulatory Agency (http:// www.mhra.gov.uk)
- Prescription Pricing Authority (http://www.ppa.org.uk/)

*Individual organisations*

- See RPSGB website links (http://www.rpsgb.org.uk/links.html)

*Individual pharmacists and pharmacies*

- NHS Gateway (http://www.nhs.uk/england/pharmacies/)
- PharmWeb database (http://www.pharmweb.net/pwmirror/uk/ chemistsuk.html)

*Information sources*

- British National Formulary (BNF) (http://bnf.org/bnf/)
- BNF for Children (http://www.bnfc.nhs.uk/bnfc/)
- electronic Medicines Compendium (http://emc.medicines.org.uk/)
- eMIMS (http://www.emims.net/)
- NHS dictionary of medicines and devices (http://www.dmd.nhs.uk/)
- UK Medicines Information (http://www.ukmi.nhs.uk/)
- International Federation of Pharmaceutical Manufacturers and Associations clinical trials portal (http://www.ifpma. org/clinicaltrials. html)

*Individual publications*

- Changing role of pharmacies (http://www.parliament.uk/documents/upload/POSTpn246.pdf)

*Gateways*

- SHOW (NHS Scotland) (http://www.show.scot.nhs.uk/)
- National electronic Library for Medicines (http://www.nelm.nhs. uk/home/default.aspx)
- PharmWeb ('online community of pharmacy, pharmaceutical and healthcare-related professionals') (http://www.pharmweb.net/)
- Intute: health and life sciences (catalogue of internet resources) (http://www.intute.ac.uk/healthandlifesciences/)

*Patient information*

- NHS Direct Online (http://www.nhsdirect.nhs.uk/)
- Patient UK (http://www.patient.co.uk/index.asp)
- MedlinePLUS (US information) (http://www.nlm.nih.gov/medline plus/)
- medicinechestonline (http://www.medicine-chest.co.uk/)

*Email discussion lists*

- Jiscmail lists (http://www.jiscmail.ac.uk)
- Pharmacy-related listservs, e.g. Pediatric-PRN and Pharma (http://www.pharmacy.org/lists.html)
- CataList (the official catalog of LISTSERV(r) lists) (http://www.lsoft.com/catalist.html)

*Internet forums*

- Mouth Cancer Foundation Online Support Group (http://rdoc.org.uk/eve/)
- Yahoo! Health Groups (http://health.dir.groups.yahoo.com/dir/Health_Wellness/Support)

*Blogs*

- DrugData Update (new acquisitions to DrugScope's library) (http://drugscope.blogspot.com/)
- Random Acts of Reality (by an emergency medical technician) (http://randomreality.blogware.com/)

*Other*

- Internet Pharmacist (online tutorial on internet information skills) (http://www.vts.rdn.ac.uk/tutorial/pharmacist)

## References

1. Bailey CW Jr (2006) The scholarly electronic publishing bibliography; The open access bibliography; The open access webliography. (http://info.lib.uh.edu/sepb/sepb.html)
2. House of Commons Science and Technology Committee (2004) *Scientific Publications: Free for All? Tenth Report of Session 2003–04*. London: The Stationery Office. (http://www.publications.parliament.uk/pa/cm200304/cmselect/cmsctech/399/399.pdf)
3. Berners-Lee T, Hendler J, Lassila O (2001) The semantic web. *Sci Am* (http://www.sciam.com/article.cfm?articleID=00048144–10D2–1C70–84A98 09EC588EF21&catID=2)

4. Anon (2002) Trust me, I'm a website. [issue on quality of health information on the internet]. *BMJ* 324. (http://bmj.bmjjournals.com/content/vol324/issue 7337/)
5. Eysenbach G, Powell J, Kuss O, Sa ER (2002) Empirical studies assessing the quality of health information for consumers on the world wide web: a systematic review. *JAMA* 287 2691–2700.
6. Childs S (2005) Judging the quality of internet-based health information. *Performance Measurement and Metrics* 6: 80–96.
7. Nielsen J (2003) Usability 101: Introduction to usability. Alertbox, August 25. (http://www.useit.com/alertbox/20030825.html)
8. Nielsen J (2005) Top ten web design mistakes of 2005. Alertbox, October 3. (http://www.useit.com/alertbox/designmistakes.html)

## Web addresses of resources covered in this chapter

(Listed alphabetically by name)

Adobe Flash (http://www.adobe.com/uk/products/)
Adobe GoLive (http://www.adobe.com/uk/products/)
ADSLguide (http://www.adslguide.org.uk/)
BioMed Central (http://www.biomedcentral.com/)
Blogger (http://www.blogger.com/start)
Bobby (http://www.mardiros.net/bobby-accessibility-tool.html)
Choosing a wiki (http://c2.com/cgi/wiki?ChoosingaWiki)
Creative Commons (http://creativecommons.org/)
Directory of Open Access Journals (http://www.doaj.org/)
e-Prints Soton (http://eprints.soton.ac.uk/)
Feedster (http://www.feedster.com/)
FreeBooks4Doctors! (http://www.freebooks4doctors.com/)
FreeMedicalJournals (http://www.freemedicaljournals.com/htm/index.htm)
Getting started with HTML (http://www.w3.org/MarkUp/Guide/)
Google (http://www.google.com or http://www.google.co.uk/)
Google Groups (http://groups.google.com/)
Guidelines for UK government websites (http://www.cabinetoffice.gov.uk/e-government/resources/handbook/html/1-10-9.asp)
HONcode (http://www.hon.ch/HONcode/Conduct.html)
HTML Source (http://www.yourhtmlsource.com/)
ICANN (http://www.icann.org/)
ICANN FAQs web page (http://www.icann.org/faq/)
Internet Society (http://www.isoc.org/index.shtml)
Java applets (http://java.sun.com/applets/)
JavaScript Tutorial (http://www.w3schools.com/js/default.asp)
JISCmail etiquette (http://www.jiscmail.ac.uk/help/policy/etiquette.htm)
Judge: websites for health (http://www.judgehealth.org.uk/)
Macromedia Dreamweaver (http://www.adobe.com/products/dreamweaver/)
MedHunt (http://www.hon.ch/MedHunt/)
Microsoft FrontPage (http://www.microsoft.com/frontpage/)

Microsoft Internet Explorer (http://www.microsoft.com/windows/ie/default.mspx)

Mozilla Firefox (http://www.mozilla.org/products/firefox/)

National Core Content (http://www.library.nhs.uk/corecontent)

NeLH (http://www.nelh.nhs.uk/)

NewsIsFree (http://www.newsisfree.com/)

NHS Centre for Reviews and Dissemination databases (http://www.york.ac.uk/inst/crd/crddatabases.htm)

NLH (http://www.library.nhs.uk/)

NLH newsfeeds directory (http://www.library.nhs.uk/rss/)

Nominet UK (http://www.nominet.org.uk)

Nominet members list (http://www.nominet.org.uk/governance/members/list/)

Nordic Metadata Project (http://www.lub.lu.se/cgi-bin/nmdc.pl?lang=en&save-info=on&simple=1)

Northern Ireland health gateway (http://www.honni.qub.ac.uk/OnlineResources/)

OpenDocument format (http://www.oasis-open.org/specs/index.php)

Office of the Information Commissioner, website FAQs (http://www.ico.gov.uk/documentUploads/Website%20FAQ.pdf)

OmniMedicalSearch (http://www.omnimedicalsearch.com/)

Pharm-line® (http://www.pharm-line.nhs.uk/home/default.aspx)

Plain English Campaign (http://www.plainenglish.co.uk/)

Prodigy (http://www.prodigy.nhs.uk/)

Public Library of Science (http://www.plos.org/)

PubMed (http://www.ncbi.nlm.nih.gov/entrez/query.fcgi)

PubMed Central (http://www.pubmedcentral.nih.gov/)

Royal National Institute for the Blind web access centre (http://www.rnib.org.uk/xpedio/groups/public/documents/code/public_rnib008789.hcsp)

RSS Compendium (http://allrss.com/rssreaders.html)

Scotland NHS e-library (http://www.elib.scot.nhs.uk/portal/elib/pages/index.aspx)

SearchEngineWatch (http://searchenginewatch.com/)

Technorati (http://www.technorati.com/)

Textpad (http://www.textpad.com/)

TOXNET (http://toxnet.nlm.nih.gov/)

W3C (http://www.w3.org/)

W3C HTML pages (http://www.w3.org/MarkUp/)

W3C HTML standard (http://www.w3.org/TR/html401/)

W3C list of accessibility tools (http://www.w3.org/WAI/ER/existingtools.html)

W3C web Accessibility Initiative (http://www.w3.org/WAI/)

webXACT (http://webxact.watchfire.com/)

WikiIndex (http://wikiindex.com/Wiki_Index)

Wikipedia (http://en.wikipedia.org/wiki/Main_Page)

# 22

## Getting published

*Mark C Stuart*

Having your work accepted for publication in a professional journal is highly regarded by the scientific and medical community and also with potential employers. On the other hand, publishing a lot of poor-quality work can be highly counterproductive. As well as the personal satisfaction involved, getting published can be an important step in becoming recognised as an expert or leader in your field.

This chapter is about how to get your work published. It covers the process of selecting a publisher and submitting your work to them, the editing process and the final production of the work. It covers the basic principles that apply to all types of publishing, with specific mention of best practice for scientific journals. For comprehensive and specific information about getting a book published see Chapter 20.

### Knowing your market and selecting a publisher

Knowing which publisher to approach is a key factor in getting your work published. There are many different health publications that cover the full spectrum of health topics, and knowing which to approach requires some homework. For scientific research, the choice of journal is somewhat easier than for more topical and publicly oriented articles, as the type of work published by specialist journals is usually quite obvious.

The best approach is to get a feel for the market before you start to write. If you choose the target publication first, you can tailor your article to its audience. The other approach is to search for a publisher after you have finished your manuscript — this can be much more difficult, and may mean that you need to edit your work somewhat to meet their requirements; this may require a substantive style overhaul or a reduction in the length of the work.

Most publishers issue guidelines for authors contributing to their publications. If you can get your hands on these you will be off to a flying start — knowledge of these issues could save you a lot of work. Things that publishers often specify are:

- length of work to be submitted
- style of writing suitable for the publication
- topics exclusively covered by the publication
- whether unsolicited material is accepted.

The most useful thing you can do is to read previously published work produced by the publisher you have in mind. If you are planning to write for a magazine, study some recent issues closely to get a feel for the way the writers address the reader and the general length of the articles. Structural features specific to the publication may also become evident. For example, a particular magazine may use a short introductory or 'taster' paragraph at the beginning of an article, or may consistently use summary boxes or highlighted quotes lifted from the regular text. You will be one step ahead if you work these specific features into your article before submitting it to the editor or publisher.

If you are considering writing a book your local library is probably the best place to start. University libraries or libraries attached to medical societies will be the best place to find a good range of specialist textbooks and journals. For pharmacy-related issues, the Royal Pharmaceutical Society has an extensive library.

The same goes for any piece of writing you do: if you are writing a letter to the editor of a journal, check the style, length and tone of previously published ones. If writing text for a website, study the angle taken by other text on the site.

> Remember: Editorial policy may change frequently. Don't base your research on last year's guidelines, or old editions of the publication.

One of the best ways to get an overall picture of the publishing market is through the *Writer's & Artists' Yearbook* (see further reading at the end of this chapter). This comes out once a year and has a comprehensive list of UK and global publishers (including health titles and journals). It also gives an outline of the type of work they publish, often with details about fees, length of articles to be submitted, and sometimes whether or not the publisher accepts unsolicited work.

## Choosing a publisher

The choice of publisher is most often governed by the specific interest the publisher has in certain topics.

If your work is about a particular medical specialty, you could start by contacting the related medical or academic institution. Many of these have a publishing division that may be keen to accept your work. For example, Pharmaceutical Press is the publishing division of the Royal Pharmaceutical Society. Consider researching the types of publications put out by your own governing institution.

Another useful start would be to consult either the *Writers' & Artists' Yearbook* or *The Writer's Handbook* for lists of the major publishers and their areas of interest. You could also look for similar publications at a bookshop or local specialist medical library and note the publishers.

When choosing a scientific journal to submit your work to, take time to research the types of articles they publish. Some journals devote different proportions of each issue to particular types of article. These usually include a combination of research articles, editorials, commentary, scientific review articles, letters to the editor, articles on historical issues, book and website reviews, conference proceedings, medical case studies, and continuing education self-assessment articles. Always take a look through some recent issues to get a feel for the type of information included, the style of the information, and the audience it is aimed at.

---

➤ Visit the library of a university with a medical or pharmacy department, or the library of a large medical organisation. They are likely to subscribe to a good range of medical journals that you can compare and assess for suitability for your work.

---

Key questions to ask yourself when selecting a publication are:

*   Does it publish the kind of topic I have written about?
*   Is my work in the general writing style of the publication?
*   Is my article suitable for the audience the publication is aimed at?

## Types of publisher

### Consumer (or trade) publishers

These publishers produce books for the general consumer and sell them through specific channels that have been set up for books, such as bookshops and wholesalers. This is the most high-profile type of publishing and the most commercially focused. Publications can include both fiction and non-fiction for both adults and children.

### Scientific, technical and medical (STM) publishers

These publishers produce books and journals specifically written for and marketed to professionals in a wide variety of industries, such as medicine, law, business, technology, science and the humanities. They are more likely to be involved in commissioning books and journals than are trade publishers.

### Educational publishers

These publishers produce textbooks, workbooks, tests, software, CD-ROMs and maps.

### University presses

These publish material aimed at the academic and specialist markets. They may be non-profit departments of universities, colleges and museums. They may also market their products to the general consumer.

### Independent publishers

These are usually privately owned and publish all types of books and other products.

### Vanity publishers

These companies offer publication services for a fee paid by the author. They will usually own the copyright to the book, but do not usually help to promote or sell it. Some bookshops will refuse to purchase books published this way, and such books are rarely reviewed.

### Contract publishers

These publishers provide editing, design, marketing and distribution services to authors for a fee paid by the author.

### Regional publishers

These publishers specialise in publications relevant to a geographical region, the products being sold almost entirely in that area. They may be particularly interested in books of historical interest to the region, or which address health issues prevalent in the area.

*Self-publishing*

Do-it-yourself publishing has been made possible with the easy availability of desktop publishing methods. With this type of publishing, you do everything a publisher would do, including editing, designing, proofreading, finding and negotiating with a printer, and promoting and distributing the final product. You also incur all the costs and business risks.

## Approaching the publisher

Be business-like when approaching the publisher: after all, you are selling them a product — your written work. Keep enquiry letters to the point. When putting your idea across, be clear and direct and support the proposal with examples of what you intend to write. If there is evidence to support your proposal, use it. For example, if you are proposing a new edited textbook, inform the publisher about similar books on the market, the gap that you see needs to be filled, and how you expect your text to be received by your intended audience.

Do not plead with the publisher to take your work — this will not be successful. Publishers are looking for products that will make a profit for the company: they are not in the business to publish out of sympathy for an over-zealous author.

Many large publishing companies have editors dedicated to commissioning work in particular fields. Always direct your enquiry to the commissioning editor responsible for the topic you are presenting.

Most often the publisher's website will contain all the contact details you require. Do not hesitate to telephone the editorial office if you have any queries. I find that I get better results talking to someone in person when making first contact with a publisher — you can often get a good initial idea about whether it is worth presenting that publisher with a detailed submission.

If you are writing regularly for a particular publication, a personal rapport with the editor concerned is always an advantage and can often lead to additional work. However, as with enquiry letters, keep the initial telephone contact polite, directed, professional and to the point.

When you contact the publisher, have a clear outline of the proposed work ready. This may include sample pictures, excerpts from a section, examples of overall layout, notes on your target audience, or even the first couple of chapters. Be prepared to expand on the concepts you present if asked.

In your initial outline, make it clear what your intention is for the project and include enough information to sell the project effectively, but be cautious about giving too much information away. An effective taster of your work will evoke either a positive or a negative response from the publisher. If they are serious about taking the project on, they will probably ask for a much more detailed submission. This may require actual word estimates for particular sections, or suggestions for authors for an edited work.

Be prepared to accept advice and criticism: in fact, if your manuscript or idea is rejected the first time you submit it and you are not given a reason, ask for one, and whether they can offer you any practical suggestions. This is invaluable and may give you a better understanding of the market from the experts.

Be persistent. There are many publishers to approach if you do not get an offer the first time around.

## Using an agent

Agents act as mediators and negotiators between authors and publishers. If your work is of a particularly commercial nature, such as a consumer health title, or relates to television or radio, an agent may easily facilitate your entry into the market.

You will need to convince an agent to take you on — you may have to submit your CV and attend an interview. Agents will also usually have submission requirements for all manuscripts, similar to those of publishers. The *Writer's & Artist's Yearbook* is an excellent place to start if you are considering exploring this route.

### Using a public relations agency

Public relations (PR) companies can be a great way to build a writing portfolio and can lead to great publishing opportunities. If you are a specialist in a particular field and keen to talk to journalists, or even write articles on the topic for various publications, it may be worth registering your expertise with one or more of the medical PR companies.

PR agencies get a range of requests from different media, including newspapers, magazines, television and radio. They may be asked by their clients to provide an expert on a particular topic that is in the public spotlight. If this topic relates to your particular expertise, you may be contacted and asked to either discuss the topic with a journalist or even provide your own article to a magazine or newspaper. It can be a good way to get some good public recognition and quickly establish your own portfolio.

The downside to this approach is that sometimes you can spend considerable time providing information for other journalists without much more recognition than a mention of your name in their article.

The other more active (and more costly) approach is to pay the agency to search for experts and sources of information you can base your own work on.

## The publishing process

Table 22.1 is an overview of the publishing process.

## Preparing the manuscript for submission

The way your manuscript is presented can be the deciding factor in getting your work published — getting this right is crucial. Editors will not spend hours trying to understand the content of a manuscript that is poorly written, does not contain the information requested, or worst of all, is not in the style and format required by the publication.

### The basics

*Manuscript format*

All editors appreciate work that is clear and easy to read and that has enough space for them to make editorial marks on the page. One of the most effective ways of doing this is to provide a double-spaced document (i.e. with the equivalent of one whole line of space between lines of text) with sufficient space in the margin for annotations (see Appendix 4) when the document is printed. In Microsoft Word it is easy to set up double spacing in the paragraph format, and page margins can be set in the 'page set-up' section of the program. A good margin for submission is around 3.5 cm.

Publishers will usually specify the size of font to be used: 11 or 12 point is commonly preferred.

**Table 22.1**   Overview of the publishing process

### Step 1 — Submit your manuscript
You submit your manuscript to the editor.

### Step 2 — Senior editor requests author revisions
The usual process starts with the senior editor requesting any changes from the author. This may include cutting the document size, or revising the content.

### Step 3 — Senior editor does a substantive edit
After the revised document has come back from the author, the senior editor may then either do a substantive edit themselves, or pass it on to another senior editor. At this stage broad issues would be addressed and the document be reduced to the desired size.

### Step 4 — Technical editor edits the document
The document is then usually passed to a 'technical' or 'copy' editor. This person will apply the house style to the document, which could include preferred spellings, terminology, reference styles, and check the representation of figures, statistical information, and dosing information. This editor will also add specific instructions to the typesetter about how the document should look, for example specifying heading levels, table layout, or emphasised text.

### Step 5 — Typesetter
The document is sent to the typesetter, who lays it out electronically as it will appear in print. The document may be sent back to the editor in an electronic format to ensure that the information has been presented correctly.

### Step 6 — Document sent to printer
The typesetter will then send the document in electronic format to the printer.

### Step 7 — Printer's proofs sent to editors
The printer will prepare a set of proofs. This is an exact paper copy of how the finished document will look. The technical editor or proofreader will then read the text against the original edited document to check that nothing has been left out and that the layout is appropriate. Changes can still be made at this stage (although it can be more awkward than making changes in-house in the previous stages).

### Step 8 — Final sign-off from most senior editor
At this point there is no going back — the proofs are despatched to the printers for the final production stage.

### Step 9 — Printing and distribution
The document is printed and despatched to a distribution centre or the warehouse of the publishing company.

## Paper

If the publisher requests a printed submission, use good-quality white A4 paper (not coloured or continuous-feed computer paper) and print only on one side. Start new chapters or major sections on a new page.

## Spelling

If you are working on a PC, always run a spell check on your document. Use this tool as a guide only and consider each prompt for a spelling change carefully — its suggestions may not always be the best. Set your program to the language you intend to publish in, and be aware of the spelling differences between the USA and the UK. The standard spell-checking programs often have a limited scientific vocabulary, so always check technical terms manually, particularly the spelling of long chemical or drug names.

## Capitalisation

Maintain consistency with capitalisation. If there is no house style available from the publisher with regard to capitalisation, decide on your own style and use it throughout. For example, you may decide to capitalise specific events or job titles, such as 'the Garlic Festival' (compared with 'the garlic festival') or 'Director of Operations, Ms Renmark' (compared to 'director of operations, Ms Renmark').

## Punctuation and meaning

Always re-read you work and scrutinise for punctuation and meaning — make sure the message you want to convey is clear and that the language cannot be misinterpreted. Get someone else to read the work and address any problems they had understanding it.

## Facts and figures

Check all facts and figures used in the manuscript against the original source. Pay particular attention to any symbols used, such as greater than ($>$) or less than ($<$), and that statistical information follows the standard conventions. Also check the spelling of people's names (including their correct title) and any organisations mentioned.

If your information contains drug doses that will be used in a clinical setting, it is good practice to get a second and even third check before they are printed. If these are wrong, there is the potential for harm to the patient.

### Headings within text

Check that your headings and subheadings are clearly recognisable as such, and ensure that the headings clearly indicate the various sections and subsections. For example, the title could be in bold upper case, the first-level heading could be bold upper and lower case, the second level bold italic, and the third level plain italic; the main text should be in 12-point roman for clarity.

### References

Once again, check the referencing requirements of the journal you are submitting to. Some will require the Vancouver system and some the Harvard or another convention (see Chapter 3). There may also be specifications for the layout of reference lists at the end of a document.

### Footnotes

Whether the document is on screen or on paper, check that any footnotes appear on the correct page and that the numbering or symbol system is consistent with the publisher's requirements. Footnotes are a common cause of error when it comes to formatting and typesetting a document. In many cases publishers prefer that footnotes be taken into the text itself (in parentheses if necessary), as embedded footnotes can cause problems for the copyeditor and typesetter (see later).

### Typeface

The following points apply:

- Use a plain typeface (or font) for the document to be submitted. Times New Roman or Arial are standard typefaces and are clear and easy to read.
- Keep the same typeface throughout the document, including headings for images.
- Use either bold or italic font only for specific words needing emphasis, or to follow scientific conventions (for example in the formal naming of bacteria).

- Decide on a font size for different heading levels (for example headings and subheadings) and keep these consistent throughout the document.
- Avoid decorative or unusual fonts — they often look unprofessional and can be more difficult for the editor to read.
- Eleven- or 12-point is the usual standard font size requested for the body text of a submitted manuscript.

## Graphs and tables

- Use a cross-hatching pattern to shade graphs and technical diagrams — they will appear consistent whether the document is printed in colour or black and white. They will also appear consistent on computer screens set at different display settings.
- Label your tables or graphs using alphabetical references (such as 'Table A' or 'Figure B') and be sure to include the appropriate cross-references from the text.

## Units of measurement

It is a good idea to spell out in words unusual units of measurement to ensure that they are not misinterpreted.

## Abbreviations

Remember to check that you have spelt out all abbreviations at first mention of the term. Remember that the editor may not be an expert in the topic you are presenting and so may not be familiar with standard terms used in your particular field.

## Terminology

Always check if a publication specifies that work submitted should comply with specific nomenclature standards. This may include receptor terminology preferred. Terminology and scientific conventions may also vary between countries. If you are submitting to an overseas journal, ensure that the terminology is that used locally — be aware that there are many spelling differences between UK and USA medical terminology.

### Get your colleagues and friends to read it

Before submitting your work to a publisher, always get your colleagues or peers to read through it and give you some feedback: chances are that if they do not understand any aspect of it, neither will the editor reading it or the readers of the publication. Often journals have very wide audiences and may be read by people of little or no prior knowledge of the topic. To check that the information is accessible to a variety of readers, it is also a good idea to get someone with little knowledge of the topic to read it.

## Electronic submission of manuscripts

Most publishers now prefer electronic submission of manuscripts and often have provision for uploading electronic documents through their websites. With effective tools for tracking editorial changes and marking up electronic documents, most editorial departments, whether for journals or other publications, now edit onscreen and have streamlined electronic editorial processes. This certainly speeds up the submission, review and publishing process, particularly when the manuscript is circulated to external reviewers.

Online submission processes, particularly for journals, may include a number of different online forms and prompts to indicate the location of your manuscripts on your personal computer. The documents will be uploaded to the publisher from these locations. At the end of the online submission process you will usually be given a specific identification number for your manuscript that you should record, and quote in any further correspondence.[1]

Some journal publishers offer an online tracking system for manuscript submissions. This is usually accessed online with your specific manuscript identification number and shows the stage of the process your manuscript is at.

### File types

Publishers will often give specifications about the type of file they will accept, e.g. Word, WordPerfect, EPS, LaTeX, text, PostScript or RTF. Images may be requested in TIFF, GIF, JPG, PostScript or EPS format and should be prepared at the same size as you would expect them to appear. (JPG files are often preferred because they are quite small compared to other formats.) The publishers may even go to the extent of specifying how many dots per inch should make up the graphic (150 dpi is a standard request). It is best to present figures and tables separately in the correct format: embedded figures cause no end of problems for the copyeditor and the first thing the publisher asks for is that they strip them out and present them as separate files for the typesetter, whose software will be different from Word and often unable to deal with embedded material.

If you are not very computer literate, it is a good idea to get someone who is to check that the technical formatting of your work matches the publisher's specifications. This may avoid unnecessary delays caused by your work being returned because the editor could not open your file, or because the images you have provided are not suitable for printing.

Always follow the specific directions for submitting electronic documents for publication. Such directions are usually given on the publication's website.

### Submitting a manuscript as an electronic file on a disk

Some publishers require authors to submit a disk (floppy or compact disk) containing an electronic copy of the manuscript. When doing so, always do the following:

- Provide a covering letter stating the file format used.
- Provide a printout of the manuscript.
- Name the file in a way that briefly describes the content of the manuscript.
- Only provide the latest version.
- Label the disk with the name of the file and the format used.
- Keep a copy for yourself.

### Paper submission

Publishers will also have specific requirements for the submission of paper documents, so check these carefully. They will often include size and format specifications for printed text, and the number of printed copies to be submitted for distribution to peer reviewers and editors. The instructions for contributors may specify that the text should be double spaced and printed on one side of the paper only. Always choose a guaranteed and secure method of postage for printed matter.

After you have submitted your manuscript to a scientific publication, you should be sent notification that your work has been received.

### Submitting your article to a journal

See Table 22.2.

**Table 22.2**   Types of journal articles

**Research papers**
These are written after a study has been conducted to answer a specific question (see Chapter 4)
**Case reports**
These are reports about medical conditions and treatment in individual patients. They are used to highlight the care provided in specific situations to illustrate medical technique (see Chapter 6)
**Review article**
These consist of a literature search of a number of studies, to bring together findings about a particular topic (see Chapter 5)
**Letter to the editor**
This is a letter to a medical or scientific journal, expressing your opinions with reasonable supporting evidence (see Chapter 9)

*Usual format of scientific manuscripts*

Although each journal usually will have slightly different format requirements, generally the publisher will ask that your manuscript contain the following subsections:

- Title page — Check the journal specifications for length of title and specific content of this page
  - Author names in the format of: first name, initials, surname
  - The organisation or institution you represent
  - Name and contact details of a contact author(s)
  - Name and contact details of a contact author to receive reprint requests
  - Funding details (such as grants used for the project)
  - A short title
  - Any disclaimers
- Conflict of interest notification page
- Summary — Check journal specifications for length and if keywords or standard abbreviations are to be included
- Abstract — Keep the abstract to the length specified for the journal you are submitting your work to. This is usually between 150 and 250 words.
- Body of text
  - Introduction — The aim of the paper
  - Methods — Outline of the procedures undertaken
  - Results — Results of the investigation
  - Discussion — Findings of the investigation and conclusion

- **Acknowledgements** — Sources of support, including individuals or organisations
- **References** — Check the specific format requirements of the journal
- **Tables** — Check the specific requirements of the journal
- **Illustrations** — Check the specific requirements of the journal

For detailed information about the format of scientific manuscripts see Chapter 4.

### Usual steps in manuscript submission and peer review for medical journals

1. You submit the manuscript.
2. Quality checks are carried out by the editorial office.
3. A specific staff editor is assigned to the manuscript.
4. The staff editor assigns referees.
5. The referees review the manuscript.
6. The staff editor makes a recommendation to the executive editor.
7. The executive editor decides whether the manuscript is to be published.
8. You are contacted with the result of the decision.

The following information will explain each of these steps.

---

➤ Important: Always check the specific guidelines of publishers before submitting work.

---

### The covering letter

Convince the editor

This is your chance to convince the editor that your work should be published in their journal. It is a good idea to explain why your work is suitable for that journal rather than any other: for example, if you are approaching a general international medical journal, you could explain why you think it is more appropriate than a more specialised local journal. You may wish to explain that because of the topic, your work may appeal to a wider audience than a more specialist publication attracts. Keep your explanations and reasons clear and concise.

Offer suggestions for alternative formats

Often scientific research papers are very lengthy and will not be suitable for printing in their entirety. After accepting the paper, the editor of the journal may choose to shorten it to a review. It is very useful to the editor or reviewers if, in the covering letter, you pre-empt this by suggesting ways of shortening the paper. You may suggest tables or graphs that could be removed, appendices that could be omitted, or references that could be prioritised. Some journals will publish some sections of the paper online and provide a reference to it in the printed journal.

### Provide contact details

In the covering letter, provide contact details of the author(s) and the nominated author or contact who can deal with editorial issues before publication. Email is usually the preferred route for correspondence.

Most journals provide readers with a route by which they can comment on or question published work, and will usually offer the authors of the paper the opportunity to respond. It is useful to specify a nominated author who will coordinate these public responses.

### Author statement

Include a statement to say that the authors listed meet the criteria for authorship and that they have read and endorse the information in the manuscript.

### Redundant papers

State in your letter if you know of any other manuscripts submitted previously, either by you or by another author (which may have already been published) that may be regarded as redundant in light of your manuscript. Copies of these papers should also be submitted with your work for the consideration of the editor.

### Author details

Some journals ask for the specific details of individual authors who participated in the study at the time of submission of the paper. The International Committee of Medical Journal Editors recommends that credit should be given to authors who:

- have made substantial contributions to conception and design, or acquisition of data, or analysis and interpretation of data;
- and have drafted the article or revised it critically for important intellectual content;
- and who have approved the final version to be published.[2]

These details can usually be added at the end of the text. Many journals will require an additional individual signed statement from each contributing author. *The Lancet* suggests that the following format is used for papers submitted to the journal:

*'I declare that I participated in the [list contributions made to the study] and that I have seen and approved the final version. I have the following conflicts of interest [list conflicts of interest here]'*[3]

Some journals may request for an author to be nominated as guarantor for the work. This person would be responsible for the integrity of the work throughout all the stages leading up to publication.

Contributors who do not meet the requirements for authorship should be listed, along with their individual contribution, in an acknowledgement section at the end of the paper. This section could be broken into sections such as 'clinical investigators' or 'participating investigators'.[4]

### Conflicts of interest

A conflict of interest is defined as a situation where someone may stand to profit from decisions made in an official capacity. For example, if an author of a scientific study inappropriately influences the outcome of a study in favour of a drug from a company they own shares in. Financial relationships such as employment, consultancies, share ownership and honoraria are the most likely to undermine the credibility of both the paper and the journal that publishes it. These interests may be declared with the paper, particularly if the editor believes it is necessary for a fair judgement to be made by the reader.

Most medical publications require authors to submit the details of any financial or personal relationships that may be seen as a potential conflict of interest. Journals will often not publish work if any of the authors have recently owned any shares, have been employed by a company with a financial interest, or have been asked by an organisation to write the paper being submitted.

### Sources of funding

The source of funding for a scientific study may also be considered a potential conflict of interest. When submitting your manuscript to a journal these sources must be listed, either in the Methods section or as an acknowledgement at the end of the paper. Describe the role of the sponsor (if any) in designing the study, collection and interpretation of the data, writing the report, or submitting the work for publication. If the sponsor had no input it is also important to make this clear. Journals may reject a manuscript if an organisation or sponsor with a financial interest in the project has asserted any control over the author's right to publish.

## Patient confidentiality

Before submitting your work, remove all personal information about people who participated in the study, e.g. names, addresses, initials, hospital numbers or photographs. If you consider it necessary to include specific patient details, this must be done with the informed and written consent of the person after they have been given the opportunity to read the manuscript. This is usually a mandatory prerequisite for medical journals, and the consent obtained is often stated in the published article. Informed consent is particularly important for clinical case studies.

## Ethical standards

If your study involved an experiment on humans, when you submit your work to a journal you should declare whether the experiment complied with the ethical standards of the responsible committee on human experimentation and the 1975 Helsinki Declaration. If your study involved animal experiments, you should state whether the national guidelines for the care of laboratory animals were followed.[5]

## Search terms

The editor of the journal may ask that authors provide a number of key words or phrases that will be used to assist electronic searching of the document and in the indexing process (for information about indexing, see page 403).

## Submitting to more than one journal

It is best to submit your work to one journal at a time. Most journals will not consider papers that are also currently being considered by another journal. This is partly because they want to avoid any conflict regarding copyright, and also to avoid wasting resources on an unnecessary peer-review process. Rarely, two journals may simultaneously publish the same article if it is in the best interest of public health (see Table 22.3).

**Table 22.3**  Things to avoid when submitting journal articles

- Submitting two or more papers based on a single piece of research
- Submitting a series of articles based on the same piece of research (this is sometimes done to allow each member of a group of authors to be the leading author at least once)
- Coming to conclusions or extrapolations that suggest more impressive results than were actually found (this may be used to generate media attention)
- Submitting the same article to more than one journal at the same time
- Criticising the work of others in an unconstructive way within the article (a fair comparison within a trial is acceptable)
- Resubmitting the same article to the same journal after it has been rejected once

## Retracting a journal article

If after submission of an article you discover that the content is incorrect or fraudulent (such as flawed evidence used during your research) you must notify the editor immediately. Withdrawal of the article is usually (and probably encouraged by the editor) possible before it has been accepted for publication or during the review period. If the article has already been published, you should prepare a letter on behalf of all contributing authors, outlining the reasons for your retraction. This will normally be published by the journal.

## Submitting work to a professional medical organisation

This is often quite a different process from submitting to commercial publications or journals, as the information will often be published as 'official' information issued by the organisation. It is commonplace for medical institutions to commission research or data gathering from external authors for their own use. In larger organisations this information may pass through the editorial department prior to publication. If you are preparing a manuscript for submission to a professional body, bear in mind the following:

- Obtain the style guide for the organisation (if one exists) and become familiar with it before starting to write. The closer you can get your document to the house style requirements, the less it will need amending later.
- Check the preferred format for submitted documents.
- Ask if there are any electronic templates you should use as the basis of your document. For example, if an organisation regularly publishes a

particular type of document, there may be a pre-formatted template that already contains standard wording about the organisation.

- Check the organisation's style for what content usually goes in the headings.
- Check the policy for using images (for example, in the UK the NHS has guidelines for the use of images in their documents).
- Check requirements for referencing before you start. It can be very time-consuming to convert to a different style later.
- Check the preferred method of correspondence (emails may not be favoured for confidential patient information or commercial-in-confidence information).

▶ In the UK the NHS has formatting specifications for documents issued under the NHS identity. This includes specifications for font size, logo placement, colour and presentation of patient information. This information can be found at www.nhsidentity.nhs.uk.

## Peer review

Peer review is the process by which other experts critically review your work. The editor may not be an expert in your particular field and will have to do some research to locate people with suitable knowledge and expertise to do this. Some editors appreciate suggestions for suitable reviewers. This may be particularly important when you have written a textbook or contributed a chapter to a book. It is in your best interests that your work has been professionally scrutinised and considered an accurate representation of the subject by other experts. This can also be an added safety precaution when presenting guidance for clinicians about treatment methods, particularly when specific drug doses and dosing frequencies are discussed.

### Peer review for a journal article

A journal article will only move to the peer-review stage if the editor believes that the work is suitable, in terms of both subject matter and quality. After the first screening, the manuscript is sent to a number of referees, each of whom evaluates the work and prepares a report on it. Most often, this will have a section for the editor only as well as a section for the author(s). After all the reviews have been submitted by the referees, the editor decides whether or not to go ahead and publish the work. At this stage, you should receive notification about the decision.

The peer review panel for a medical or scientific journal is usually made up of experts from a range of academic and research backgrounds. Not all of them will be given your work to review: the editor will normally select a number of reviewers who have specific expertise or an interest in the topic of your work, and who collectively would have the expertise to comment on a broad range of aspects related to it.

Peer reviewers usually work on a voluntary basis. They must be considered by the editor to be knowledgeable on the topic, be able to pass fair judgement, to maintain confidentiality, be unbiased (the reviewer's conflicts of interests may have to be declared), have knowledge of research procedures and statistical analysis, and be able to review the manuscript within the required time (see Table 22.4).

## Rejection

For a scientific journal, peer-review reports are most often the cause of rejection. If this is the case with your paper you can ask to see the reports, which can be extremely useful with regard to both your research procedure and your write-up and presentation style. Given this expert opinion, you may consider that your work can be improved to a standard more suitable for publication. If the feedback related to the presentation only, you might wish to revamp the piece and resubmit it, either to the same journal or to a different one, but if the review process highlighted considerable flaws in your research method or review procedure, or that your conclusion was not supported by the data, you might need to rethink the actual content of your work.

If you choose to resubmit your work to the same publication, make sure that you have formatted it to their exact requirements and provide a letter outlining clearly and rationally why the editor should reconsider your work.

**Table 22.4**  The types of questions peer reviewers are asked

- Do they think the work is original?
- What are the importance and implications of the information?
- Are the scientific methods valid and reproducible?
- Is the design of the study appropriate?
- Is the discussion relevant?
- Does the conclusion accurately reflect the findings?

## Copyright

Always clarify the terms of copyright when you hand over your work to any publication. Most medical journals specify that authors must transfer copyright to the publisher: always clarify the terms of this process with the editor. The publishing contract may offer you the chance to request that you be consulted if your work is to be published subsequently in another publication or in another format (such as online, on CD-ROM, or in a different language). In some circumstances this transfer of copyright can be waived, for example if the information cannot be copyrighted, such as if it comes from a government source.

Many journals now just require that authors give the journal the exclusive rights to publish the article in print and electronically, but the author retains copyright. This arrangement can also be requested for chapters contributed to edited books. If you are a contributing author this type of arrangement is probably the best, because it means you are free to use your work elsewhere without having to obtain permission.

### The right to use your own work again

In addition to getting your work published in print, you may want to use it for personal projects that you are involved with. For example, you may regularly speak on a particular topic and want to reproduce your work to hand out at such events. You may also have your own website relating to your specialty, where you may wish to post your work.

Some publishers do not require that you grant them copyright, so that you are free to reuse the information in the future. You may be able to agree on the terms of this personal use beforehand.

Also consider whether you want to also publish your article on your personal website. Some publishers will only allow you to link from your website to an article that has been published online by them. Others allow you to use the work on your own website, with written permission, but may specify that you reference the original published source of the document. For more information on copyright see Chapter 19.

## Permissions

If you are reproducing any material in your manuscript, such as photographs or copyrighted extracts from other documents, always supply documentation when you submit the work that shows you have obtained the necessary permissions to reproduce the items in the context of your article.

If you are submitting a chapter to a book, always read the terms of your contract carefully, especially with regard to permissions. Often it is the individual author's responsibility to obtain permissions for material (such as photographs) to be reproduced, rather than the editor's. The editor of the book, or the publisher, may require written proof that this process has been carried out. They can usually offer assistance with regard to the best approach to requesting permission from an original source.

## Using images

Sometimes the editor will assign images to accompany your article, or will ask you for suitable suggestions. However, if you require a specialised diagram or photograph to enable the reader to understand your work, you should offer suggestions or locate a suitable image at the time of presentation. It is also common for the author to provide their own images as necessary.

Almost all medical publications contain images of some sort. Publishers will usually have preferred formats for the submission of artwork. Always check with them before submitting any work containing pictures.

Artwork needs to be planned sooner rather than later. If you are contributing to an edited book, the editor will have to take any space required for images into consideration in the early planning stages. If you are using images from other sources, allow plenty of time to request permission to use them, as well as to source new images if permission is denied.

For photographs of patients, for example in a case report or an article on a particular disease, patient confidentiality should always be taken into account. If such photographs are necessary, written permission should be obtained from the patient after they have been informed of your intended use of the image.

Ways to acquire a suitable image:

* create your own
* commission an artist to draw the picture
* purchase from an image supplier
* request permission to reproduce an image already published.

Medical texts frequently require highly specialised diagrams, which can often be purchased. There are some good image libraries online where you can purchase images. The organisations in Table 22.5 are also good sources.

The cost of purchasing an image can depend on where and how you intend to use it, and can vary considerably, so always shop around. The following factors can influence the cost:

- the size of the image (quarter-page size may be cheaper than half-page)
- whether you are using it on the cover of a publication
- the distribution of the publication (generally, the higher the distribution, the more costly the image)
- the purpose of its use (such as advertisement, logo, billboard).

If your image has to be hand drawn or is an original photograph, allow time to find an artist to draw it or to source the photograph. You will need to give the artist a clear brief stating your requirements and the purpose of the image. Artists specialising in medical illustration usually charge per picture at a pre-agreed rate. It is also common for the publisher to commission an artist from their many contacts in the profession.

➤ When searching for a suitable artist, ask to see their folio of previous illustrations. This will give you an idea of the style they specialise in.

**Table 22.5**   Resources for medical images

**The Wellcome Trust Medical Photo Library**
http://medphoto.wellcome.ac.uk

**Getty Images**
www.gettyimages.co.uk

**Science Photo Library**
www.sciencephoto.com

**Corbis**
www.corbis.com

**Alamy Images**
www.alamy.com

➤ For more consumer-type publications an in-house picture editor may decide on a suitable image to accompany your article and will often be responsible for sourcing one. The space available and commercial advertising may be factors in deciding what picture best fits with your article.

➤ Regardless of the publication you are submitting your work to, give the editor suggestions for possibly suitable (or unsuitable) images to accompany it.

## The editing process

Rarely will an editor decide to publish your work exactly as you submitted it. After official acceptance of the work it is usual practice for an editor to ask the author(s) to revise it, perhaps in response to suggestions from the peer reviewers (such as to provide additional evidence on a particular section, for example). The editor may also offer to publish the work in a different format. For example, you may be asked to cut the article considerably, or to reconstruct it in the form of a letter to the editor (see Chapter 9) or a brief report.

### The role of the editor

Editors have different roles depending on the type of publication they work on. The editor of a scientific journal is responsible for the overall management of the production process of the journal. They must maintain the objectives of the journal through the use of appropriate content, maintain quality and credibility, and manage all the other staff, including the other editors. Some publications have more than one executive editor, with shared management responsibilities.

The editor is going to be your contact during the publication process and so it is important that you establish a good working relationship in the early stages.

The editor makes the final decision about the acceptance or rejection of an article, based on the recommendations of the peer reviewers or any editorial board that may also exist.

After the editor has decided to accept your work, the document may be returned to you for changes or to reconsider various aspects of it. It is important to understand the motivation behind the actions of an editor when reviewing the alterations to your work. Suggestions for change should not necessarily be taken as criticism, but more the need to make your work fit with the overall mission and style of the publication. Respond to these requests after careful consideration. If a suggested change, addition or deletion is inappropriate, make it clear why (rather than becoming defensive). After all, the editor's aim is to produce a high-quality publication, which is in the best interests of all concerned.

An editor's responsibilities can vary greatly and their role depends on the specific nature of the publication. They are also often the public representative of the publication and will attend press conferences and be the point of contact for the media.

## Communicating with the editor

▶ An effective way to audit changes and exchange comments on electronic manuscripts is to use the tracking and electronic note functions of wordprocessing software.

Most correspondence is now carried out electronically. A common method for editors to make comments and annotate changes is to use electronic tracking within a document. This feature is available within Microsoft Word. By switching the function on before you change the document, every change you make can be viewed by someone else. The reviewer can accept or reject changes electronically and leave an audit trail of changes made. Attaching an electronic comment to a specific section of text is also an effective way to communicate between author and editor. Editors sometimes assume that authors are familiar with electronic reviewing tools such as 'track changes', but if you are not, ask the editor how to use them.

The other common method of annotating electronic text is to use square brackets, whereby comments can be slotted in at the relevant points in the text. To make these comments even clearer, consider using bold type or coloured highlights. As each issue is addressed, these comments can be easily located and stripped out of the document.

## Editorial teams

Whether it is a scientific journal, a glossy consumer magazine or a large government or medical organisation, editorial departments generally have a similar structure and the process leading to final publication is often very similar. However, depending on the size of the team, not all functions of the process may be undertaken in house. It is not unusual for publishers to make use of freelance editors, proofreaders, designers, artists and typesetters, as and when required.

It is important to understand the roles of the different people who may work on your manuscript before publication. Table 22.6 illustrates how different editors and desktop publishers with varying responsibilities may be involved in getting your work to press.

**Table 22.6**  Varying responsibilities of different editors and desktop publishers

**Consultant editor/Executive editor/Editor-in-chief**
These titles are usually used for the most senior editor of a publication. This person will usually be responsible for the overall content of the publication and will usually have final sign-off before it goes to press. They will usually be the public face of the publication and will oversee the full production process, have budgeting responsibilities, and manage the other editors.

**Assistant editor/Deputy editor/Associate editor**
These editors will usually work closely with the managing editor and, depending on the size of the organisation, have management responsibilities for other members of the editorial team.

**Development editor/Acquisitions editor/Commissioning editor/Managing editor**
These titles are generally used for people who commission new titles for publishing houses. This is the person you would approach if you had a proposal for a new book. These editors would also be responsible for maintaining the range of journal titles that a publishing house owns. They would oversee the financial aspects, sales, marketing, and manage any administrative staff, including editorial assistants. The managing editor may take the lead on publishing issues and overseeing the management of any associated electronic or online products.

**Editorial board members**
These people make up the editorial board of a journal, and as a team will govern the editorial direction of the journal. The editorial board often comprises experts in the field covered by the journal.

**Web editor**
This person may be responsible for managing the specific content of a website. Their role may involve uploading information to the site in an appropriate format, updating news sections, links, monitoring web-based notice boards and emails from viewers.                                                   (continued)

**Table 22.6** *Continued*

### Technical editor/Copyeditor/Subeditor

These editors are usually responsible for the technical aspects of the document. They may:

- apply house style to a document
- check facts and figures
- add page cross-references
- compile the index
- format references
- format images
- correct punctuation
- check spelling
- check a document for sense and clarity
- raise queries for the author to address.

Copyeditors usually enter the process after the managing or more senior editors have done a more substantive edit. They may also re-check the documents after they have been typeset (this stage is known as proofreading).

### Desktop publisher/Typesetter

These people are responsible for the layout of a publication. Often this is done using software such as QuarkXPress or Adobe InDesign. They may format text and images to comply with the specific design standards of the publication.

### Designer

This person may be responsible for designing the overall look of a publication, including logos, colour schemes, and the look of associated products such as websites and stationery.

### Picture editor/Photo editor

This person is responsible for acquiring suitable images for use alongside an article.

### Book editor

For a book containing contributions from a number of authors, they may also be responsible for inviting specialist authors to contribute to relevant sections. They will set schedules for submission of contributor's work in line with the dates agreed with the publisher. The book editor may also be responsible for initiating and coordinating a peer review process for specific sections of the book, or reviews for the book in its entirety.

### Editor for an organisation

Many large medical organisations employ editors to work on documents that they issue. Many of the royal medical colleges, NHS organisations, medical charities and medical research organisations will have an in-house editorial department.

## The copy (or technical) edit

Copyediting by a copyeditor or technical editor is usually one of the last stages in the editorial process. Depending on the publisher's policy, this editor may send you a marked-up version of your document, showing any inserted or deleted text and any changes made to conform with house style, together with any queries or requests for clarification. Some of the text may have been rewritten to make your work clearer — you will need to review these changes carefully to ensure that the correct message has been retained. The copyeditor may have added subheadings, broken up long paragraphs and sentences, and made amendments to make the document conform to house style. In making these changes, the original meaning and emphasis should have been retained.

This may be done on a marked-up paper version and annotated using standard editorial marks to indicate alterations. It is a good idea to become familiar with the basic editorial marks before you begin to review the edited work. A list of these can be found on pages 474–475 (Appendix 4). However, it is far more common nowadays for files to be submitted electronically and the editing to take place on screen, so the use of 'track changes' can be very helpful.

### Responding to queries

In responding to the queries raised by the copyeditor, answer each question directly and aim to resolve the issue with your answer. If you disagree with any changes, state your reasons clearly and provide suitable replacement text for the particular section. Just disagreeing with a change is not enough and will probably lead to the work being returned to you for further review, after the editor has tried to address the issue for you — this may lead to delays in publication.

**This is the last chance you have to make any major changes to the document prior to publication!**

## Proofreading

In the final stages of production you may be sent a printer's proof, but this is not necessarily standard practice for all journals. The proof is a copy of how exactly the final document will look in print. It is crucial that you check this proof thoroughly, because there is no going back once it is approved for printing. Small changes can be made at this stage, but it can be more difficult and can be expensive, as the document has already been typeset and will usually be in a fixed format document (such as a PDF file). This is not the time to make major changes to the content.

---

➤  Always find out when the proofs will be sent to you and set aside time to proofread them carefully. Often at this stage the printing schedule will be tight and proofreading will need to be done within a period of hours or days.

---

**Proofreading checklist**

☑  Compare the original edited manuscript with the proof — check that every insertion, change and deletion of text has carried though to the final document.
☑  Do a paragraph-by-paragraph check against the original to see that all blocks of text have been retained.
☑  Read the whole manuscript from start to finish, checking for sense and to see that nothing has been inadvertently left out.
☑  Check spelling, especially specialist scientific terminology.
☑  Check the spelling of names and places.
☑  Check the end of each line to see that words and figures have been split appropriately.
☑  Check all drug doses and frequency of administration very carefully — ensure that doses have not been split over two lines. A common example is when the number and the units are separated by a line break — this could potentially lead to dosing errors.
☑  Check that tables are complete and that rows and columns correspond correctly.
☑  Check that cross-references to other pages and sections are correct.
☑  Check the numbering and content of footnotes.
☑  Check scale, position, colour and content of all images.
☑  Check page numbering is correct.
☑  Check page headers and footers.
☑  Recheck any calculations represented.
☑  Check any mention of dates.

## How errors are introduced

Mistakes can be introduced in a number of ways. Be aware and particularly vigilant at these points in the publishing process where errors are commonly introduced (see Table 22.7).

**Table 22.7**   Common sources of error

- Author's original submitted writing
- Copyediting stage
- Typesetting stage
- Converting the original document into a different format for use with desktop publishing software
- Spell-checking software (don't assume the suggested change to spelling or grammar is always correct)
- Automatic text changes by computer software
- The use of a global find and replace process, without checking that individual changes made by the software are appropriate
- Having more than one working version (changes may be made to one but not the other)
- Last-minute changes that are not subject to such rigorous review as the other information at the various production stages

➤ Warning: If your manuscript contains drug doses, always check them against the original source at proof stage. It is good practice to get an independent checker to confirm their accuracy against authoritative texts (such as the *British National Formulary* or *MIMS*). Keep in mind that even if your information is not intended for use as a prescribing resource, it may be.

## Production and distribution

After the document has been edited and typeset, the printing process is begun. This involves:

- selection of a printing company (this may involve a tender for the job)
- determining the size of the print run
- assignment of an ISBN (International Standard Book Number) — this is a unique number assigned to a book title by its publisher for tracking and ordering purposes
- arranging for printers' proofs to be reviewed by the editorial team
- setting printing schedules
- uploading the information on any associated website
- distribution to subscribers and other buyers, either directly from the printers or from the publisher's own warehouse.

## Offprints

Offprints of articles or complete journal issues are usually more expensive after the initial print run has been completed. If you require a substantial number of copies of your work, it is best to ask for them before the printing stage. Publishers will often supply authors with a number of free copies, and will usually offer subsequent copies either at cost price or at a discounted rate for professional use (such as to distribute to colleagues).

If you are a contributing author to a book you will usually receive at least one free copy. As a sole author or editor you will probably receive around 10 copies. As a courtesy, most journals will also supply a dozen or so copies of the journal or article to contributing authors.

The cost of purchasing offprints has reduced considerably in recent years thanks to digital printing techniques, most printers being able to supply small numbers of offprints on a supply-and-demand basis.

Supplying drug companies with offprints of particular articles that favour their drug can also provide additional revenue for publishers. These are often bound as individual booklets and are used by drug companies as promotional material for conferences and marketing.

## Pre-production copies

You may want to obtain copies of the printer's proofs to distribute to colleagues prior to publication. This will depend on the individual policy of the publication. If the article contains sensitive or controversial information, the publisher may require a strict embargo. As the copyright to the article often belongs to the publisher after initial submission, always check before you circulate the article to anyone prior to official release.

## Selling the final product

The marketing department of a publishing house is responsible for promoting and selling the final work and making a profit for the publisher. Marketing may involve the following:

*   selling advertising space within a journal
*   promotional point-of-sale material
*   promotional launches
*   advertising the publication in related publications

- producing catalogues of the titles produced by the publisher
- advertising on related websites
- writing a press release to coincide with the launch of a book
- arranging a review to be written about the book in another publication
- targeted email campaigns
- promoting licences for online viewing of journals published electronically.

## Advertising

Advertising is often a main source of revenue for journals, but most will have strict criteria for the use of printed advertisements. This may include the amount of space an advertisement may take up, and restrictions on the type of advertisement used. The placement of advertisements in any publication can be difficult: finding a balance between a suitable place for the advertisement next to an article without conflicting messages can be an ongoing battle between the editorial and advertising teams.

Ethical considerations are also taken into account when placing advertisements. Many journals will not publish an advertisement for a product near a research article that either supports or condemns its use.

The majority of advertisements in medical publications come from drug companies, or from other medical publications promoting journals or websites. For more information on advertising, see Chapter 12.

## Marketing

Unless you are publishing your own work, marketing is usually undertaken by the publisher. Publishing companies usually have their own marketing teams who are specialists in selling the final products. If you are the editor of a book, you will probably be asked for suggestions about how the publisher should direct their marketing and advertising. This will involve looking at your target audience, competitor texts and avenues for promotion. For example, you may offer the names of leading websites or journals that have a similar audience to your book, where the publisher could consider placing advertisements.

## Press releases

These are a good way for publishers to notify a wide audience about recent or imminent publications of interest. Obviously, they can be a great source of publicity and will help to generate sales. On the other hand, if the work is in any way controversial, a press release can draw attention to it and generate public and media debate on the issue.

### Embargoes

Sometimes, copies of a work may be issued ahead of general release of the book or journal. An embargo is usually placed on such releases, meaning that those given prior access to the article must agree not to publish anything about the topic before the official publication date. This gives journalists and news organisations time to read the work and prepare any stories or reviews, so they are ready for press on the official launch day.

Publishers should usually inform you about the press release and may ask you to review the document or contribute to the information it contains.

## Dealing with the media

You may also be approached by the media for further information about your work.

---

➤ Before your work is published, ask the editor or publisher how to best handle media enquiries.

---

Publication of your work may affect a range of sensitive areas. If your work is a research article with an outcome favouring a particular drug, news of its publication may considerably affect the price of shares in the company or its competitors. Likewise, news of a new side effect can lead to alarmist reports in the popular press, which could have serious implications for public health. An example of this is the publicity the MMR vaccine received when reports were published that linked it to autism. This affected the numbers of children receiving the vaccine.

Remember that as soon as your work was accepted for publication, ownership of the copyright may have passed to the publisher, who may therefore have the right to decide whether any information is disclosed prior to the official publication date. If in doubt, always refer media or professional enquiries to the editor, who will be experienced in dealing with such interest.

## Professional organisations

European Medical Writers Association
*www.emwa.org*

European Association of Science Editors
*www.ease.org.uk*

Medical Journalists' Association
*www.mja-uk.org/*

The Society of Authors
*www.societyofauthors.net*

The Publishers Association
*www.publishers.org.uk*

Australasian Medical Writers Association
*http://www.medicalwriters.org/pub.asp?page=news&pubid=1&issid=1*

American Medical Writers Association
*www.amwa.org*

International Committee of Medical Journal Editors
*www.icmje.org*

The World Association of Medical Editors
*www.wame.org*

Council of Science Editors
*www.councilscienceeditors.org*

## References

1. Uniform Requirements for Manuscripts Submitted to Biomedical Journals: Writing and Editing for Biomedical Publication (Updated October 2004) International Committee of Medical Journal Editors *http://www.icmje.org/* accessed October 6 2005.
2. Uniform Requirements for Manuscripts Submitted to Biomedical Journals: Writing and Editing for Biomedical Publication (Updated October 2004) International Committee of Medical Journal Editors *http://www.icmje.org/* accessed October 6 2005.
3. *http://www.thelancet.com/authors/lancet/authorinfo* accessed October 6 2005 — Information for Authors *www.thelancet.com*.
4. Uniform Requirements for Manuscripts Submitted to Biomedical Journals: Writing and Editing for Biomedical Publication (Updated October 2004) International Committee of Medical Journal Editors *http://www.icmje.org/* accessed October 6 2005.

5.  Uniform Requirements for Manuscripts Submitted to Biomedical Journals: Writing and Editing for Biomedical Publication (Updated October 2004) International Committee of Medical Journal Editors *http://www.icmje.org/* accessed October 6 2005.

## Further reading

Hall GM (2003) *How to Write a Paper.* London: BMJ Books.

Huth EJ (1999) *Writing and Publishing in Medicine.* Baltimore, MD: Williams & Wilkins.

McCallum C (2003) *The Writers' Guide to Getting Published.* Oxford, UK: How-to Books.

Richardson P (2002) *A Guide to Medical Publishing and Writing.* Wiltshire, UK: Mark Allen Publishing.

Taylor RB (2005) *The Clinician's Guide to Medical Writing.* Oregon: Springer.

*Writers' & Artists' Yearbook* (2005) London: A & C Black.

# Appendix 1

## Common medical abbreviations

*Melissa McClean*

Medical abbreviations are commonly used in hospital, medical and dental records, product information leaflets and literature (see Table A1.1).

**Table A1.1** Common medical abbreviations

| Abbreviation | Definition | Abbreviation | Definition |
|---|---|---|---|
| aa | equal part of each | ALT | alanine aminotransferase |
| AA | affected area | AMA | against medical advice |
| AAA | abdominal aortic aneurysm | AMI | acute myocardial infarction |
| AAS | acute abdominal series | AML | acute myelogenous leukaemia |
| Ab | antibody | | |
| abd. | abdomen | ANA | antinuclear antibody |
| ABG | arterial blood gases | ANF | antinuclear factor |
| ACE | angiotensin-converting enzyme | AODM | adult-onset diabetes mellitus |
| acid phos. | acid phosphate | app. | application |
| ACTH | adrenocortocotrophic hormone | approx. | approximately |
| | | ARC | AIDS-related complex |
| ADH | antidiuretic hormone | ARDS | acute respiratory distress syndrome |
| ADHD | attention deficit hyperactivity disorder | ASAP | as soon as possible |
| AER | aerosol | ASD | atrial septal defect |
| AF | atrial fibrillation | ASHD | atherosclerotic heart disease |
| AIDS | acquired immunodeficiency syndrome | ASO | antistreptolysin O |
| | | AST | aspartate aminotransferase |
| alb. | albumin | | |
| alc. | alcohol | ATN | acute tubular necrosis |
| alk. phos. | alkaline phosphate | AV | atrioventricular |
| ALL | acute lymphocytic leukaemia | BBB | bundle branch block |
| | | BCAA | branched chain amino acids |

*(continued)*

**Table A1.1** *Continued*

| Abbreviation | Definition | Abbreviation | Definition |
|---|---|---|---|
| BMI | body mass index | COPD | chronic obstructive pulmonary disease |
| BMR | basal metabolic rate | | |
| BMT | bone marrow transplant | CPAP | continuous positive airway pressure |
| BP | blood pressure | | |
| bpm | beats per minute | CPK | creatinine phosphokinase |
| BS | blood sugar or bowel sound | | |
| | | CPR | cardiopulmonary resuscitation |
| BUN | blood–urea–nitrogen | | |
| BW | body weight | CrCl | creatinine clearance |
| c. | with | CRF | chronic renal failure |
| Ca | calcium | crm | cream |
| CAA | crystalline amino acids | CSF | cerebrospinal fluid |
| CABG | coronary artery bypass graft | CT | computerised tomography |
| CAD | coronary artery disease | CV | cardiovascular |
| cap(s). | capsule(s) | CVP | central venous pressure |
| CAPD | chronic ambulatory peritoneal dialysis | CXR | chest X-ray |
| | | DAP | distal airway pressure |
| CAT | computerised axial tomography | DAW | dispense as written |
| | | d/c | discontinue |
| cath. | catheterise | D5W | 5% dextrose in water |
| CBC | complete blood count | D50W | 50% dextrose in water |
| CBG | capillary blood gas | DI | diabetes insipidus |
| CCF | congestive heart failure | DKA | diabetes ketoacidosis |
| CEA | carcinoembryonic antigen | DM | diabetes mellitus |
| | | DNA | deoxyribonucleic acid |
| CF | cystic fibrosis | DU | duodenal ulcer |
| CGL | chronic granulocytic leukaemia | DVT | deep vein thrombosis |
| | | EAA | essential amino acids |
| CHF | congestive heart failure | EBV | Epstein–Barr virus |
| CHO | carbohydrate | e/c | enteric-coated |
| CI | cardiac index or colour index | ECG | electrocardiogram |
| | | ECT | electroconvulsive therapy |
| Cl | chloride | EEG | electroencephalogram |
| CLL | chronic lymphoblastic leukemia | EFAD | essential fatty acid deficiency |
| CML | chronic myelogenous leukaemia | EKG | electrocardiogram |
| | | ELISA | enzyme-linked immunosorbent assay |
| CMV | cytomegalovirus | | |
| CNS | central nervous system | EMG | electromyogram |
| CO | cardiac output | ENT | ear/nose/throat |

Common medical abbreviations 465

**Table A1.1**  *Continued*

| Abbreviation | Definition | Abbreviation | Definition |
|---|---|---|---|
| ESR | erythrocyte sedimentation rate | HR | heart rate |
| | | HSV | herpes simplex virus |
| ET | endotracheal | IBD | inflammatory bowel disease |
| ETOH | ethanol | | |
| FBS | fasting blood sugar | ICP | intracranial pressure |
| f/c | film-coated | ICU | intensive care unit |
| FEV | forced expiratory volume | IDL | intermediate-density lipoprotein |
| FFP | fresh frozen plasma | | |
| FRC | functional residual capacity | IDDM | insulin-dependent diabetes mellitus |
| FSH | follicle-stimulating hormone | Ig | immunoglobulin |
| | | IHD | ischaemic heart disease |
| FTA | fluorescent treponemal antibody test | IM | intramuscular |
| | | inj. | injection |
| FVC | forced vital capacity | INR | international normalised ratio |
| G6PD | glucose 6-phosphate dehydrogenase | | |
| | | IRDM | insulin-resistant diabetes mellitus |
| GABA | gamma-aminobutyric acid | ITP | idiopathic thrombocytic purpura |
| GFR | glomerular filtration rate | | |
| GI | gastrointestinal | IV | intravenous(ly) |
| gr | grain | IVC | inferior vena cava |
| GTT | glucose tolerance test | IVF | in vitro fertilisation |
| HAART | highly active antiretroviral therapy | JVP | jugular venous pressure |
| | | K | potassium |
| HAV | hepatitis A virus | KCl | potassium chloride |
| Hb | haemoglobin | LA | left atrium |
| HBP | high blood pressure | LBBB | left bundle branch block |
| HBV | hepatitis B virus | LDH | lactate dehydrogenase |
| HCG | human chorionic gonadotrophin | LDL | low-density lipoprotein |
| | | LFT | liver function test |
| Hct | haematocrit | LH | luteinising hormone |
| HDL | high-density lipoprotein | liq. | liquid |
| HIV | human immunodeficiency virus | LV | left ventricle |
| | | LVF | left ventricular failure |
| HLA | human lymphocyte antigens | MAOI | monoamine-oxidase inhibitor |
| HLB | hydrophilic–lipophilic balance | MAP | mean arterial pressure |
| | | max. | maximum |
| HOCM | hypertrophic obstruction cardiomyopathy | MBC | mimimum bacterial concentration |

(*continued*)

**Table A1.1** *Continued*

| Abbreviation | Definition | Abbreviation | Definition |
|---|---|---|---|
| MCH | mean corpuscular haemoglobin | $paO_2$ | plasma partial pressure (concentration) of oxygen |
| MCV | mean corpuscular volume | PAS | para-amino salicylic acid |
| MD | muscular dystrophy | Pb | lead |
| MDI | metered dose inhaler | $pCO_2$ | plasma partial pressure (concentration) of carbon dioxide |
| Mg | magnesium | | |
| MI | myocardial infarction | | |
| m/r | modified release | PCV | packed cell volume |
| MRI | magnetic resonance imaging | PDA | patent ductus arteriosus |
| | | PEEP | positive end-expiratory pressure |
| MSU | midstream specimen of urine | | |
| | | PEF | peak expiratory flow |
| MTP | metatarsophalangeal | $pO_2$ | plasma partial pressure (concentration) of oxygen |
| n. | nerve | | |
| $N_2$ | nitrogen | | |
| $N_2O$ | nitrous oxide | PPD | purified protein derivative |
| Na | sodium | | |
| NaCl | sodium chloride | p.r. | per rectum |
| NB | note well | PTH | parathyroid hormone |
| NM | neuromuscular | PT | prothrombin time |
| NMR | nuclear magnetic resonance | PTT | partial prothrombin time |
| | | pulv. | powder |
| NSAID | non-steroidal anti-inflammatory drug | PUO | pyrexia of unknown origin |
| O | oral | p.v. | per vaginam |
| $O_2$ | oxygen | q.n.s. | quantity not sufficient |
| $O_2$ cap. | oxygen capacity | q.s. | quantity sufficient |
| $O_2$ sat. | oxygen saturation | RA | rheumatoid arthritis |
| OCP | oral contraceptive pill | RAD | right axis deviation |
| OGTT | oral glucose tolerance test | RAG | R antigen |
| | | RAST | radioallergosorbency test |
| oint. | ointment | RBC | red blood cell |
| o/w | oil-in-water | RD | respiratory distress |
| PA | pulmonary artery | RD | rheumatic heart disease |
| PABA | para-amino benzoic acid | resp. | respiratory |
| $paCO_2$ | arterial plasma partial pressure (concentration) of carbon dioxide | RF | rheumatic fever |
| | | Rh. | rhesus blood factor |
| | | RNA | ribonucleic acid |

**Table A1.1**  *Continued*

| Abbreviation | Definition | Abbreviation | Definition |
|---|---|---|---|
| RSV | respiratory syncytial virus | SVT | supraventricular tachycardia |
| RV | residual volume | $T_3$ | tri-iodothyronine |
| RVF | right ventricular failure | $T_4$ | total serum thyroxine |
| SaO$_2$ | arterial oxygen saturation | tab. | tablet |
|  |  | TLC | total lung capacity |
| SBE | subacute bacterial endocarditis | UA | urine analysis |
| s.c. | subcutaneous | ung. | ointment |
| s/c | sugar-coated | URI | upper respiratory infection |
| SIDS | sudden infant death syndrome | UV | ultraviolet light |
| sig. | directions | VLDL | very low-density lipoprotein |
| SLE | systemic lupus erythematosus | VSD | ventricular septal defect |
|  |  | VS | vital signs |
| ss | one half | VT | ventricular tachycardia |
| stat. | now/immediately | WBC | white blood cell count |
| supp. | suppository | w/o | water-in-oil |

Latin abbreviations are also common in medical literature. It is useful to know the English meaning of them, and so although the Latin meaning is not required knowledge it is included in Table A1.2 for interest.

**Table A1.2**  Latin abbreviations and their English meanings

| Latin abbreviation | English meaning | Latin |
|---|---|---|
| a.c. | before food | *ante cibum* |
| A.D. | right ear | *auris dexter* |
| a.h. | every other hour | *alternis horis* |
| ad. lib. | as desired | *ad libitum* |
| a.m. | before noon | *ante meridiem* |
| aq. | water/aqueous | *aqua* |
| A.S. | left ear | *auris sinister* |
| A.U. | each ear | *auris utro* |
| b.d. | twice daily | *bis die* |
| b.i.d. | twice daily | *Bis in die* |
| gtt. | a drop | *gutta* |
| h.s. | at bedtime | *hora somni* |
| o.d. | every day | *omni die* |

(continued)

**Table A1.2** *Continued*

| Latin abbreviation | English meaning | Latin |
| --- | --- | --- |
| O.D. | right eye | *oculus dexter* |
| o.m. | every morning | *omni mane* |
| o.n. | every night | *omni nocte* |
| O.S. | left eye | *oculus sinister* |
| O.U. | each eye | *oculus utro* |
| p.c. | after food | *post cibum* |
| p.m. | after noon | *post meridiem* |
| p.o. | by mouth | *per os* |
| p.r.n. | as needed | *pro re nata* |
| q | every | *quater* |
| q.a.m. | every morning | *quater ante meridiem* |
| q.d. | every day | *quater die* |
| q.d.s. | to be taken four times a day | *quater die sumendus* |
| q.h. | every hour | *quater hora* |
| q.i.d. | four times a day | *quater in die* |
| q.i.w. | four times a week | |
| q.l. | as much as desired | *quantum libet* |
| q.n. | every night | *quater nocte* |
| q.o.d. | every other day | *quaque altera die* |
| q.o.n. | every other night | |
| q.p. | as much as you please | *quantum placet* |
| q.p.m. | every evening | *quarter post meridiem* |
| q.q.h. | every 4 hours | *quarta quaque hora* |
| q.s. | as much as is required | *quantum sufficit* |
| q.w. | every week | |
| q2h | every 2 hours | *quaque 2 hora* |
| q4h | every 4 hours | *quaque 4 hora* |
| q6h | every 6 hours | *quaque 6 hora* |
| s.i.d. | once a day | *semel in die* |
| S.L. | under the tongue | *sub linguam* |
| t.d.s. | to be taken three times a day | *ter die sumendus* |
| t.i.d. | three times daily | *ter in die* |
| u.d. | as directed | *ut dictum* |

# Appendix 2

## Measurements

*Melissa McClean*

Various symbols for weights and measures are used in medical writing. The International System of Units (SI) is a modernised version of the metric system that has been established by international agreement. It is the most widely used system of units in science, industry and commerce. The system has seven basic units: length, time, mass, temperature, electric current, luminous intensity and amount of substance. All other units are derived from them.

A number of non-SI or conventional units are accepted for use with SI units. These have been included because of their practical importance, their continuous everyday use and their technical importance.

The rules for using SI units include:

- All unit names are either written in full or represented by their correct symbol.
- All units names are written in lower case except for Celsius.
- All symbols are lower case except for symbols derived from a person's name, e.g. the symbol for pressure is Pa after Blaise Pascal. The one exception to this rule is litre, which is written L as the lower case l looks too similar to the number 1.
- Symbols are written in upright (Roman) type.
- Symbols are not altered to indicate plurals.
- Symbols are not an abbreviation, so do not place a full stop after them unless it is the end of a sentence.
- Number and symbol are separated by a space, e.g. 2 kg.
- Multiplication of one unit by another results in the symbol being separated by a space or a centre dot, e.g. N m or N·m.
- Division of one unit by another results in the symbol being separated by a forward slash (/) or given a negative exponent, e.g. metres per second = m/s or $ms^{-1}$.
- Do not mix unit names and unit symbols, e.g. square cm.
- Spelling and pronunciation vary from language to language, but the symbols are international.

**Table A2.1.**   SI and conventional units of weights and measures commonly used in medical writing

| Name of SI unit | Symbol | Name of SI unit | Symbol |
|---|---|---|---|
| ampere | A | millimole | mmol |
| arbitrary units | a.u. | millisecond | ms |
| calorie | cal | millivolt | mV |
| centimetre | cm | minute | min |
| coulomb | C | molar | M |
| cubic centimeter | cc or cm³ | mole | mol |
| day | d | molecular weight | MW or mol.wt |
| decibel | dB | nanogram | ng |
| decilitre | dL | nanometre | nm |
| decimetre | dm | newton | N |
| degrees Celsius | °C | ohm | Ω |
| degrees Fahrenheit | °F | parts per million | ppm |
| farad | F | parts per billion | ppb |
| fluid ounce | fl oz | pascal | Pa |
| gram | g | picogram | pg |
| hertz | Hz | pint | pt |
| hour | h | pound | lb |
| joule | J | quart | qrt |
| kelvin | K | second | s |
| kilocalorie | kcal | seimens | S |
| kilogram | kg | square centimetre | cm² |
| kilohertz | kHz | tablespoon | tbsp |
| kilojoule | kJ | teaspoon | tsp |
| litre | L | unit | U |
| litres per minute | L/min | volt | V |
| metre | m | volume | vol |
| microgram | μg | volume in volume | v/v |
| microlitre | μL or μl | volume in weight | v/w |
| micrometre | μm | weight | wt |
| micromolar | μM | weight in volume | w/v |
| micromole | μmol | weight in weight | w/w |
| milliampere | mA | | |
| milligram | mg | | |
| milligrams per decilitre | mg/dL | | |
| milligrams per 100 mL | mg.% | | |
| millilitre | mL or ml | | |
| millimetre | mm | | |
| millimetres of mercury | mmHg | | |
| millimolar | mM | | |

# Appendix 3

## Normal values for common laboratory tests

*Melissa McClean*

Normal laboratory values are used to provide reference ranges for apparently healthy individuals. Every laboratory is independent and should have developed its own normal values for all tests it performs. These values may be affected by gender, age, diet, drugs taken, time of day and the position of the patient when the specimen is taken.

Normal laboratory values are calculated by performing the test on 'healthy' people in the age range or of the gender that is of interest. The test results are then averaged (mean) and a standard deviation (SD) is calculated. The normal range includes values in the range defined by mean $\pm$ 1.96 SD, which should include 95% of all normal results.

Table A3.1 contains the most common laboratory tests performed and their normal laboratory values. Remember that each laboratory has its own values, which could differ from those given below.

**Table A3.1**  Normal values for a range of common laboratory tests (Note: SI units are used)

| Test | Specimen | Normal laboratory values |
| --- | --- | --- |
| Activated partial thromboplastin time (APTT) | Whole blood | 25–35 s |
| Alanine aminotransferase (ALT) | Serum | ≤0.80 μkat/L |
| Albumin | Serum | 35–50 g/L |
| Alkaline phosphate (ALP) – total | Serum | 0.33–2.08 μkat/L |
| Amylase | Serum | 0.50–2.83 μkat/L |
| Aspartate transferase (AST) | Serum | <0.7 μkat/L |
| Bicarbonate | Serum | 18–23 mmol/L |
| Bilirubin – direct | Serum | ≤7 μmol/L |
| Bilirubin – indirect | Serum | ≤22 μmol/L |

(*continued*)

**Table A3.1** *Continued*

| Test | Specimen | Normal laboratory values |
| --- | --- | --- |
| Bleeding time – Ivy's method | Blood from skin | 2.5–9.5 min |
| Calcium – total | Serum | 2.12–2.57 mmol/L |
| Chloride | Serum | 95–108 mmol/L |
| Cholesterol – total | Serum | Desirable: < 5.17 mmol/L<br>Borderline high:<br>5.17–6.18 mmol/L<br>High: ≥6.21 mmol/L |
| Creatinine | Serum | ≤106 µmol/L |
| Creatinine kinase (CK) | Serum | Male: ≤3.92 µkat/L<br>Female: ≤3.17 µkat/L |
| Erythrocyte sedimentation rate (ESR) | Whole blood | Male: 0–15 mm/h<br>Female: 0–20 mm/h |
| Gamma-glutamyl transferase (GGT) | Serum | Male: 9–50 U/L<br>Female: 8–40 U/L |
| Glucose fasting | Plasma | <6.1 mmol/L |
| Glucose random | Serum | 3.9–6.9 mmol/L |
| Haemoglobin (Hb) | Whole blood | Male: 138–172 g/L<br>Female: 120–156 g/L |
| Haematocrit (Hct) | Whole blood | Male: 0.41–0.50<br>Female: 0.35–0.46 |
| Insulin | Serum | 36–179 pmol/L |
| Iron | Serum | 4–30 µmol/L |
| Lactate dehydrogenase (LD) | Serum | ≤4.5 µkat/L |
| Leukocyte count | Whole blood | 4.5–11 × $10^9$ cells/L |
| Lipase | Serum | 0.12–1.00 µkat/L |
| Magnesium | Serum | 0.6–1.0 mmol/L |
| Mean corpuscular haemoglobin (MCH) | Whole blood | 27–33 pg |
| Mean corpuscular volume (MCV) | Whole blood | 78–102 fL |
| pH | Whole blood – arterial | 7.35–7.45 |
| $pO_2$ | Whole blood – arterial | 11–14.4 kPa |
| $pCO_2$ | Whole blood – arterial | 4.66–5.99 kPa |

**Table A3.1**  *Continued*

| Test | Specimen | Normal laboratory values |
|---|---|---|
| Phosphorus | Serum | 0.81–1.45 mmol/L |
| Platelet count | Whole blood | 130–400 × 10⁹/L |
| Potassium | Serum/plasma | 3.5–5.3 mmol/L |
| Protein–total | Serum/urine | 60–85 g/L <150 mg/day |
| Prothrombin time (PT) – one stage | Whole blood | 10.0–12.5 s |
| Red blood count (RBC) | Whole blood | Male: 4.4–5.8 × 10¹²/L<br>Female: 3.9–5.2 × 10¹²/L |
| Reticulocyte count | Whole blood | 0.005–0.023 of RBCs |
| Sodium | Serum | 136–146 mmol/L |
| Urea nitrogen | Serum | 2.5–10.7 mmol urea/L |
| Uric acid 1.2–4.5 mmol/L | Serum/urine | Male: 238–506 µmol/L<br>Female: 149–446 µmol/L |
| White blood cell (WBC) count | Whole blood | 3.8–10.8 × 10⁹/L |
| WBC differential – absolute neutrophils | Whole blood | 1.5–7.8 × 10⁹/L |
| WBC differential – absolute eosinophils | Whole blood | 0.05–0.55 × 10⁹/L |
| WBC differential – absolute basophils | Whole blood | 0–0.2 × 10⁹/L |
| WBC differential – absolute lumphocytes | Whole blood | 0.85–4.10 × 10⁹/L |
| WBC differential – absolute monocytes | Whole blood | 0.2–1.1 × 10⁹/L |

kat, katal.

Source: Adapted from: The Merck Manual [Online], Chapter 296, Normal Laboratory Values. Available at: URL: http://www.merck.com/mrkshared/mmanual/tables/296tb2a.jsp. 8th May 2006.

# Appendix 4

## Proof correction marks

(based on BS 5261 part 2 and ISO 5776)

| Instruction | Textual mark | Margin mark | Comment |
|---|---|---|---|
| No corrections on this page | [ None ] | / | Mark indicates that the page has been looked at. |
| Leave unchanged ('stet') | InterColor consortium | ✓ (circled) | Often added to cancel an instruction wrongly requested. |
| Remove unwanted marks | under no circumstances | ✗ | May be applied to blemishes in reprographics |
| Refer to appropriate authority | (InterColor) consortium | ? | For use when the proofreader is unsure, or where a style guide can be referred to |
| Insert new matter | The red hen | little / | |
| Insert additional matter | required. However, as | ⟨A⟩ | Additional matter is supplied on a separate sheet marked with reference letter. |
| Delete | See the table on page 5. | ∂ | (In practice, these are usually the same in modern type-setting: 'close up' can be inferred from context.) |
| Delete & close up | See the table on page 5. | ∂ | |
| Substitute character | The little red hyn | e | |
| Substitute string of characters e.g. word | The little red hen | black | Vertical marks at end of line help to indicate boundaries. |
| Wrong type font used; replace with correct font | Too (many) cooks | ⊗ | (May also need to refer to style guide or give type specifications.) |
| Insert a full point | This sentence must end / | ⊙ | (The encircling ring helps to identify the character, which might otherwise be mistaken for a spot on the proof.) |
| Insert a colon | This clause has a point / | ⊙ | |
| Insert a semi-colon | This is wrong, I should | ; | (In this example, a semi-colon is being substituted rather than inserted.) |
| Insert a comma | Fish chips and peas | , or ⊙ | (As a comma is so small, to circle it might be wise.) |
| Insert single quotes | The liberated territory | ⸲ ⸲ | The additional mark under the punctuation helps to indicate the superscript positioning |
| Insert double quotes | The liberated territory | ⸲⸲ ⸲⸲ | |
| Insert apostrophe | The child pajamas | ⸲ | |
| Substitute character in superscript or subscript position | 23,500 m$^2$ of lumber | $^3$ | |
| | An escape of $CO_2$ gas | $_2$ | |

This card was prepared by Conrad Taylor of PopComm — Tel. [+44] (0) 1746 765605 — see http://www.popcomm.co.uk

| Instruction | Textual mark | Margin mark | Comment |
|---|---|---|---|
| Set in or change to italics | An incredible fortune | ⊔⊔ | |
| Set in or change to bold | An incredible fortune | ∿ | |
| Set in or change to bold italics | An incredible fortune | ⊔⊔ | |
| Set in or change to capitals | When in Rome, do as… | ▦ | |
| Set in or change to small capitals | When in Rome, do as… | = | (Some typefaces have a complementary 'expert set' containing true small capitals.) |
| Capitals for initials; rest in small capitals | When in Rome, do as… | ≡ | |
| Change capitals to lower case | FAILURE is seen… | ≠ | |
| Change small capitals to lower case | FAILURE is seen… | ≠ | |
| Change italic to roman | An incredible fortune | ⁴⁄ | |
| Start new paragraph | are confirmed. The new name for the company is | ⌐ | |
| No new paragraph; run on | are confirmed. The new name for the | ⌒ | |
| Insert space between characters/words | This typeface is called | Y or Y# | # is typographer's shorthand for 'space'. |
| Close space between characters/words | This type face is called or This type face is called | ⌒ or ↑ | The first method implies 'close up' – the second 'remove space' |
| Indent text by amount indicated | are confirmed. The new name for the company | ⌐ 1em | (An em is a space equal to the body size of the type; other units of measure could also be used e.g. millimetres.) |
| Cancel indent | are confirmed. ⊢The new name for the company | ⊐ | |
| Transpose characters | Accidents ha ppen | ⊓ | (Also for words, phrases) |
| Take over to new line | Cider apples have been a major source of income | ⊏ | |
| Take back to preceding line | Cider apples have been a major source of income | ⊐ | |

Reproduced with permission.

# Appendix 5

## A to Z of medical terms in plain English

### The Plain English Campaign

Medical terms or phrases can often baffle your patients or customers.
Try to watch out for this, and use ordinary language where possible. Be
prepared to explain technical terms if you need to use them. What follows in this A to Z is a selection of words that people may find troublesome. These terms are meant as explanations, not definitions. This is
not a 'correct' medical dictionary, and it is by no means complete — but
it's a start!

### A

| | |
|---|---|
| A and E | accident and emergency |
| AID | artificial insemination by a donor |
| AIDS | acquired immune deficiency syndrome |
| amnesia | loss of memory |
| analgesic | something that reduces pain |
| anastomosing | joining together |
| aneurysm | a swelling in an artery |
| antibiotic | a chemical used to treat infections caused by bacteria |
| antipyretic | a substance that reduces temperature |
| arthroplasty | repairing a joint (such as a hip replacement) |
| astigmatism | uneven curvature of the eye that can lead to blurring or lack of focus |
| atrium | a chamber in the heart |
| atrophy | a wasting away (of tissues, such as muscles) |

### B

| | |
|---|---|
| biopsy | removing a small amount of tissue to be examined in the laboratory |
| booked admissions | allowing patients to arrange with the hospital a date to come in for an operation |
| bronchoscopy | examining the airways with a small flexible camera tube (an endoscope) |

### C

| | |
|---|---|
| cardiology | study and treatment of the heart |
| cardiothoracic | to do with the heart and lungs |

| | |
|---|---|
| chemotherapy | in terms of treatment for cancer, using drugs to destroy cancer cells or prevent their growth |
| chronic | a long-lasting disease that changes slowly |
| cirrhosis | long-term damage to the liver (often associated with alcohol abuse) |
| coeliac | to do with the abdomen (usually the small intestine) |
| colonoscopy | examining the colon (bowel) with an endoscope |
| colorectal | to do with the colon and rectum |
| colposcopy | examining the vagina or cervix with an endoscope |
| CPM | continuous passive motion — a machine with a motor to help flex limbs |
| CT scan | 'computerised tomography' — a type of three-dimensional X-ray. It provides far more information than a standard X-ray |
| cystoscopy | examining the bladder with an endoscope |

## D

| | |
|---|---|
| D & C | dilation and curettage — widening the cervix and taking a sample of the lining of the womb |
| dialysis | filtering the blood, cleaning it |
| discharge | leaving hospital |
| diuretics | a drug that helps to remove excess water from the body |
| dysfunction | not working properly |
| dyspepsia | indigestion; upset stomach |

## E

| | |
|---|---|
| ECG | electrocardiogram — a graph showing the electrical activity of the heart, including the heartbeat |
| ECT | electroconvulsive (electroshock) treatment |
| ectopic | outside — so an ectopic pregnancy is a baby developing outside the womb |
| electrocardiogram | a graph showing the electrical activity of the heart, including the heartbeat |
| electrocardiograph | a machine used to produce an electrocardiogram |
| embolism | blocking of an artery (by a blood clot or air bubble) |
| encephalitis | inflammation of the brain |
| endometriosis | the presence of tissue similar to the lining of the womb at other sites in the pelvis |
| endoscope | various types of flexible tube with a fibreoptic camera for seeing inside organs |
| endoscopy | process of examining the inside of the body using an endoscope |
| enuresis | bed-wetting |
| epidural | a form of pain relief given by an injection in the lower spine, often given during childbirth |

# F

faeces                  solid waste from the bowel; poo
femur                   thigh bone

# G

gastroenterology        study and treatment of the stomach and intestines
GU                      genitourinary (as in 'GU' department) — the branch of
                        medicine concerned with reproduction and urination,
                        usually involving sexually transmitted infections
gynaecology             study and treatment of the female reproductive system

# H

haematology             study of the blood
haemophilia             a bleeding disorder where there is severe bleeding
                        without clotting
haemorrhoids            piles
hepatic                 to do with the liver
HIV                     human immunodeficiency virus — the cause of AIDS

# I

ICU                     intensive care unit
image intensifier       instant X-ray images on a TV monitor

# J

jaundice                a yellowing of the skin or the whites of the eyes due to
                        liver disease
jugular                 of the neck or throat

# K

keratic                 horny; hardening of the skin
keratitis               inflammation of the cornea of the eye
kidney                  an organ that filters blood and produces urine
kymograph               an instrument that measures blood pressure and flow

# L

labial                  relating to lips
labyrinthitis           inflammation of the inner ear, causing dizziness
lachrymal duct          the channel near the eye that produces tears; tear duct
lactation               producing breast milk
laparoscopy             examining the abdomen with an endoscope
laryngitis              inflammation of the vocal chords (larynx)
laxative                treatment for constipation
ligature                a tight bandage or tie, especially to stop bleeding
lithotripsy             breaking up kidney stones or gallstones using ultra-
                        sound

# M

| | |
|---|---|
| mammography | examining the breasts by X-ray |
| maxillofacial | to do with the face or jaw |
| metastasis | a secondary cancerous tumour (one that has spread from a primary cancer to another part of the body); the process of cancer cells spreading to other parts of the body |
| miscible | able to be mixed with another liquid |
| MMR | measles, mumps, rubella — the three-in-one vaccination for children |
| motor neuron disease | a progressive wasting disease of the nerves that control the muscles |
| myocardial infarction | basically, a heart attack — sudden death of part of the heart muscle |

# N

| | |
|---|---|
| nasal | to do with the nose |
| nauseous | feeling sick |
| necrotic | used to describe dead cells or tissue |
| neoplasm | a tumour |
| neurology | study of the nervous system |
| neurophysiology | study of the changes associated with the activity of the nervous system |

# O

| | |
|---|---|
| obstetrics | care and control of pregnancy and childbirth |
| oedema | swelling caused by fluid |
| oncology | study and treatment of tumours, cancers |
| ophthalmic | to do with the eye |
| orthodontics | dentistry specialising in correcting tooth problems |
| orthopaedics | treatment of bones and muscles (originally in children) |
| osteopathy | treatment of muscles and bones by manipulation and massage |
| osteoporosis | brittle bones; weakening of the bones |
| otolaryngology | treatment of diseases of the ear and throat |

# P

| | |
|---|---|
| paediatrics | the study and treatment of children and their diseases |
| palliative care | reducing symptoms of a disorder without curing it |
| paraplegia | paralysis of the legs |
| patella | the kneecap |
| pathology | study of the causes of disease; testing samples of tissue to check for disease |
| pertussis | whooping cough |
| phenylketonuria | inherited difficulty in processing an amino acid — can lead to learning disabilities |

| | |
|---|---|
| physiotherapy | use of physical methods, such as massage, manipulation and exercise, to promote healing |
| podiatry | a branch of chiropody (medical care of feet) |
| postop, postoperative | after the operation |
| pre-assessment | a hospital appointment before the operation date to check details |
| premed, premedication | drug given before an anaesthetic to calm the nerves before an operation |
| prophylactic | a drug procedure or piece of equipment used to prevent something, such as disease or pregnancy |

## Q

| | |
|---|---|
| quadriplegia | paralysis of all four limbs |
| quarantine | isolation of someone with an infectious or contagious disease (originally for 40 days) |
| quinsy | abscess on or near the tonsils |

## R

| | |
|---|---|
| radiography | taking X-rays; the X-ray department |
| radiotherapy | using radiation for treatment (especially of cancer) |
| renal | to do with the kidneys |
| rhinitis | inflammation in the nose |

## S

| | |
|---|---|
| sigmoidoscopy | examining the inside of the colon (bowel) |
| sinusitis | inflammation of the sinuses — air-filled 'tubes' around the nose |
| sutures | stitches |
| syndrome | the set of symptoms associated with a particular disease |

## T

| | |
|---|---|
| thrombolysis | dissolving a blood clot |
| tomogram | the image produced by tomography (a three-dimensional X-ray) |
| trachea | the windpipe |
| trauma | a wound or injury; emotional shock |
| triage | prioritising patients according to how urgently they need treatment |

## U

| | |
|---|---|
| urethra | the 'tube' that carries urine from the bladder |
| urology | the study and treatment of the urinary system |

## V

| | |
|---|---|
| venereal disease | 'VD'; sexually transmitted infection |
| ventricle | a cavity or chamber in the heart or brain |

# X

**xanthoma**  a yellowish deposit of fatty material in the skin

# Y

**yellow fever**  a disease carried by mosquitoes, causing jaundice and possibly death

# Z

**zygote**  fertilised egg at conception — it becomes the fetus

# Index